Essentials of
Nutrition

FOR THE HEALTH PROFESSIONS

SUSAN R. HOLMAN, MS, RD

Nutrition Educator, Joslin Diabetes Center
Boston, Massachusetts

J. B. Lippincott Company   Philadelphia
London   Mexico City   New York
St. Louis   São Paulo   Sydney

Sponsoring Editor: Paul Hill
Manuscript Editor: Lorraine D. Smith
Indexer: Alberta Morrison
Design Director: Tracy Baldwin
Design Coordinator: Anne O'Donnell
Designer: Quarasan
Production Manager: Kathleen P. Dunn
Production Coordinator: Caren Erlichman
Compositor: Progressive Typographers
Printer/Binder: R. R. Donnelley & Sons
                          Company

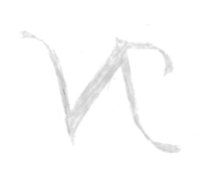

6   5   4

Library of Congress Cataloging in Publication Data
Holman, Susan R.
    Essentials of nutrition for the health professions

    Includes bibliographies and index.
    1. Diet therapy.   2. Nutrition.   I. Title.
[DNLM: 1. Diet Therapy. 2. Nutrition. 3. Nutrition
Disorders. QU 145 H7474e]
RM216.H74 1987   615.8'54   86-10437
ISBN 0-397-54504-5

The author and publisher have exerted every effort to ensure that drug selection and dosage set forth in this text are in accord with current recommendations and practice at the time of publication. However, in view of ongoing research, changes in government regulations, and the constant flow of information relating to drug therapy and drug reactions, the reader is urged to check the package insert for each drug for any change in indications and dosage and for added warnings and precautions. This is particularly important when the recommended agent is a new or infrequently employed drug.

*"And the Lord said to Moses,
'Who made man's mouth?'"*

Exodus 4:11

PREFACE

"Students find nutrition boring." That's what one nutrition teacher told me when I first began research to determine just what educators want most in a short, basic clinical nutrition text. She didn't explain her statement, but I could understand why it might be true. I, too, once scorned my home economics teachers in favor of the more personally appealing fad diet and health books. Nutrition is an art as well as a science, but often white lab coats, precise calculations, hours of chemistry and physiology, and sterile, premeasured food do bore. Yes, as a science, nutrition must be precise and accurate. But, as an art, it must appeal. This book is an attempt to reach both goals.

The text is divided into two sections: nutrition for the healthy person (Chapters 1–20) and a discussion of nutrition-related problems or diseases (Chapters 21–41). While they progress generally from basic concepts to more complex problems, each chapter is designed to stand alone if it must. Many contemporary nutrition issues and questions are covered briefly, with a list of references at the end of each chapter for the reader who wants to pursue the subject to a greater degree. Each chapter and section considers one or more of the many roles food plays in our lives.

First, food is an essential component in our general health. The more accurately we understand the physiology and biochemistry of nutrition, the more predictably and effectively we may use food to help ourselves—and others—remain healthy. The first eleven chapters of the book explain these systems and requirements as clearly and simply as possible. Illness and effective treatment mean little unless we understand health.

Second, food is part of "growing up." Toddlers have "food jags." Amidst all the crises of puberty, teens have growth spurts. Pregnant women have cravings and morning sickness. Adult needs change periodically. Everyone must eat—even if nutrition is boring. Chapters 12–17 serve as guidelines to help determine what comprises an adequate diet—and how to maintain it throughout the shifting patterns of life.

Third, food is part of our culture, our relationships, our belief systems. In this area it is most easily an art and a tool to help us express who we are. And it is in this area that it easily may be used and abused. This, too, we must understand. Chapters 18–20, 32 and 37 address these issues more specifically.

Fourth, food is part of compassionate medical treatment. The modified hospital diet should also be the chicken soup and cinnamon toast of ongoing medical care at home. We use and modify food to compensate for our weaknesses, illnesses, and handicaps. Food is not a panacea drug or a cure-all. Together with good medical care, though, it can be an attractive and creative means to help us achieve the greatest possible independence—for ourselves, those we love, and those we help to treat. The latter areas are addressed in the last 20 chapters of the book, where the most common types of diet therapy in disease are discussed in detail, with specific, practical guidelines for application.

This text will not meet all the needs of all its readers. However, I hope it will at least be a useful measure by which to evaluate the world of nutrition in health and disease, both locally and cross-culturally. I hope it will be a springboard for more reading and discussion. And perhaps it will not be boring.

Thanks are due to many persons for their help and support with this project. Carol Jean Suitor, MS, RD, Dr. Johanna T. Dwyer, and the structure of the dietetic internship at New England Medical Center first encouraged me to dream, while Bernice Heller and Paul Hill, editors at J. B. Lippincott, brought the dream to reality. Rhonda Dickson of the South End Health Center made it possible for me both to write and to work, while Joanna Douglas, Ann Hemenway, Marilyn Rodriguez, and Lela Silverstein provided staff relief, help with photos, and endless encouragement. Thanks also to Mary Kay Ebzery, MS, RD, nutritionist at Frances Stern Nutrition Center, for her invaluable comments, and to Linda Jo Stern, MS, RD, former acting director of the Massachusetts WIC program, for being there. Any errors that have slipped by are, of course, my own.

Susan R. Holman, MS, RD

CONTENTS

SECTION 2

Therapeutic Nutrition

UNIT 3

Nutrient-Controlled Diets

Normal Nutrition

UNIT 1

Basic Principles of Nutrition

CHAPTER 1

The Digestive System

OBJECTIVES

1. To help the student obtain a clear and complete picture of the digestive tract and its functions
2. To teach the role of each component part of the tract in digestion and absorption
3. To prepare the student to understand the rationale for pathology of the system and its consequent effects on nutritional status
4. To help dispel potential myths about dieting and food fads by helping the student understand what aspects of the digestive tract functions can and cannot be altered or modified by diet.

The process of nourishing the body with food and drink begins in the *digestive tract*.* A person must have a healthy, functioning digestive or *alimentary tract* in order to best use the nutrients provided in food, drink, and food supplements. Here all foods, liquids, and many or most oral medications must be digested before they can be absorbed into the bloodstream to be used by the body.

The alimentary tract is similar to a tubular canal; it begins in the mouth, or *oral cavity,* and

extends about 18 feet to 20 feet (in the average adult) to its end at the anus. In humans, this system is established (but still immature) by 3½ weeks following conception, when a cavity, lined with tissue and connected to a major blood vessel, is formed within the embryo.

As the alimentary tract develops, this primitive canal becomes differentiated into either (a) distinct parts of the digestive tract itself or into (b) the organs that connect to it. These organs include the pancreas, the liver, the bile ducts, and the gallbladder.

An understanding of the digestive system is essential to an understanding of nutrition. Any defect, problem, or change that occurs in the long, moist tube of the alimentary canal could alter the body's ability to digest what passes through it. Food, beverages, and some drugs that are not digested cannot be used by the body, and this may lead to problems. Other drugs are designed to affect digestion; this is part of their pharmacologic (drug) function. This will be discussed in more detail in Section II of this text.

The normal digestive tract resembles an actual canal in several ways. It is a contained space that is constantly being lubricated. Saliva, mucus, and site-specific digestive juices are always being produced by glands in the underlying tissue, just as water is constantly being supplied to a canal. The digestive tract has selective access to and from the organs and tissues outside of itself. For example, the fluid called *bile* flows into the digestive tract through a channel that connects the gallbladder and pancreas to the tract. This channel is called the *common bile*

---

* Throughout the text, key words are italicized and defined in the Glossary.

duct. Later on, in the intestines, nutrients and water can leave the canal through its semipermeable lining to enter adjacent blood vessels.

The alimentary tract is *unlike* a canal in that it is self-propelling. Normal walls of the tract include two layers of smooth muscle. The movement of these muscles propels foods, fluids, nutrients, and oral medications through the tract. This muscle movement *(motility)* is called *peristalsis.* It is controlled by autonomic nerve fibers, which also lie in the tissue walls. Normal motility is vital in transporting whatever is in one area of the alimentary tract into the next area.

COMPONENT PARTS OF THE ALIMENTARY CANAL

The distinct areas of the alimentary tract are

1. Oral cavity (the mouth)
2. Pharynx
3. Esophagus (about 10 inches long)
4. Stomach (about 5 inches long)
5. Small intestine (10 feet to 12 feet long), consisting of
   a. Duodenum
   b. Jejunum
   c. Ileum
6. Large intestine (about 5 feet long), consisting of
   a. Cecum
   b. Appendix
   c. Ascending *colon*
   d. Transverse colon
   e. Descending colon
   f. Rectum
   g. Anal canal

Figure 1-1 shows the location of major components of the digestive system; each is discussed below.

Oral Cavity

In the oral cavity, nutritional status is influenced by two things: the condition of the teeth and gums and the adequacy of saliva. Normal, healthy teeth, firmly rooted in healthy gum allow for good nutrition because of their ability to chew (or masticate) a large variety of foods. When foods are extremely limited, either by choice, financial restrictions, or availability, deficiencies in certain nutrients may occur. This in turn may affect the health of the gums and the teeth. Healthy, functioning teeth and gums help masticate or break down food into tiny pieces and thus expose it more completely to the saliva in the mouth.

The saliva contains *enzymes,* primarily salivary amylase. Salivary amylase further breaks down the food particles. This partly digested food then passes into the pharynx.

Pharynx

The pharynx extends from the nose to the esophagus and is used for the passage of nasal secretions, for the passage of food, and for breathing. The upper half of the pharynx has no role in digestion. The lower half has only a passive role. It receives food and helps it to pass on into the esophagus. At the lower end of the pharynx, two tubes, the esophagus and the larynx, are positioned like a fork in a road. Food particles are meant to go into the esophagus. Only air should travel down the other passageway, which leads to the lungs, although sometimes excited talking or laughing at a meal directs food "down the wrong way." The act of swallowing should close off the entrance into the lungs and permit food to pass only into the esophagus, which is closer to the back of the human body. Thus a person should not be able to breathe during the act of swallowing (try it).

Esophagus

The esophagus, which is about 25 centimeters long, carries food from the pharynx to the stomach. Like the pharynx, it does not digest food further. Also like the pharynx it is lined with epithelial tissue that resists abrasion.

The esophagus ends in a circular band of muscle called the *esophageal sphincter.* This muscle opens to let food into the stomach; normally it is closed to prevent the contents of the stomach from being regurgitated. Frequent exposure to highly acid juices in the stomach could

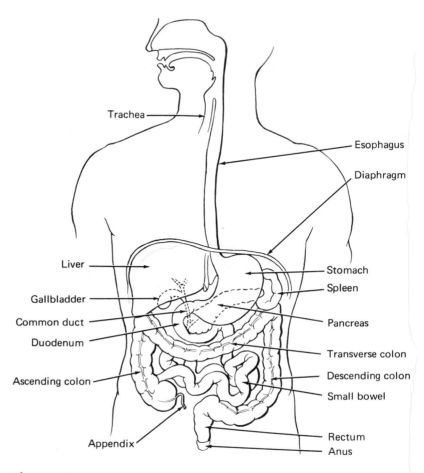

Figure 1-1
The digestive system. (Scherer JC: Introductory Medical-Surgical Nursing, 4th ed, p 399. Philadelphia, JB Lippincott, 1986)

eat away and damage the esophageal tissue wall. Gastric reflux and vomiting are two instances in which the esophageal sphincter is forced open from the stomach, causing unpleasant side-effects owing to acid reflux. The esophageal sphincter also helps the digestive tract pump and keep its contents flowing in the right direction.

Stomach

The stomach functions as a "storage bag" for food, which is gradually pumped from it into the small intestine. The most agressive breakdown of foods occurs in the stomach.

The normal gastric or digestive juices are more *acidic* (i.e., they have a lower "*p*H") in the stomach than in any other part of the alimentary tract. Thus they are generally more destructive to whatever they encounter than are the other digestive fluids throughout the tract. With a *p*H of 0.9 to 2.0, they are even more acidic than lemon juice or cranberry juice (which have a *p*H of 2.6 to 2.8) or vinegar (with a *p*H of 2.3 to 3.2). The continuous mucus lining around the inside of the stomach is the only protective element that keeps these acids from the stomach wall and keeps the stomach contents from destroying the stomach itself. Problems with the mucus wall can lead to damage of the stomach.

The body stimulates the stomach to begin producing its secretion in two ways. First, the sensations and the presence of food stimulate secretion. The smell, sight, or taste of food stimulates production of 50 ml to 150 ml of gastric juices. When food actually enters the stomach and comes in contact with its parts, these actions stimulate an additional secretion of 600 ml to 750 ml of gastric juice.

Together, the acidity of the gastric juice and the muscle movement of the stomach digest food into a mass called *chyme.* Almost everything that goes into the stomach is digested in this way. Only (a) medications that have been *enteric-coated* and (b) fiber (or indigestible components of food) can pass whole into the small intestine. Ethyl alcohol, on the other hand, never reaches the small intestine but is absorbed directly from the stomach into the blood stream.

The stomach also has a valvelike muscle called the *pyloric sphincter.* The sphincter is located at the point of entry from the stomach into the small intestine. The main role of this sphincter is to regulate the passage of chyme.

Small Intestine

In the intestines, the digestive process continues, chiefly in the small intestine. Chyme is broken down still further into its nutrients—not by more acid, but now by *enzymes.*

The three parts of the small intestine—the duodenum, the jejunum, and the ileum—are differentiated chiefly by the nutrients each absorbs. That is, different vitamins, minerals, and other nutrients are able to leave the digestive tract individually at points specific for them. Once completely digested, they flow or are absorbed through the walls of the alimentary canal and into the blood. Then the blood carries them to the organs of the body where they are used. These sites are outlined schematically in Figure 1-2.

The first section of the small intestine, the duodenum, is where much of the action occurs. Bile, produced by the gallbladder enters the duodenum. Bile is essential for fat digestion. Active proteins called *enzymes* also enter the duode-

num from the pancreas through the same channel (the *common bile duct*) and these enzymes are used to digest fats, fat-soluble vitamins, complex carbohydrates and proteins. Other enzymes are present in the intestinal fluid. Enzymes are very sensitive proteins and are easily destroyed by acids. Enzymes are highly specific about the substance on which they act (called the *substrate*). By their chemical makeup, acids destroy more indiscriminately than enzymes. Enzymes activate selectively. Enzymes are present in digestive juices, in the cells of the body (where they are protected from acidic destruction), and in the lining of the small intestine, where they are used to digest carbohydrate. Amylase, sucrase, lactase, and maltase are, for example, the specific enzymes that must be present in the lining of the small intestine to break down the carbohydrates amylose, sucrose, lactose, and maltose, respectively.

The bile and pancreatic enzymes entering the duodenum mix with the chyme, dilute it, and make it less acidic. As the mixture becomes less acidic and more *alkaline* the enzymes are able to begin their work digesting the nutrients.

The small intestine has an internal appearance totally different from that of the large intestine. The walls of the normal small intestine are made up of many folds and covered with hairlike projections called *villi* (the singular of the word is *villus*). Figure 1-3 graphically illustrates the folds as well as the villi of the small intestine. The chief advantage of these folds is that they create an extremely large surface area available for nutrient *absorption.* Although the large intestine is also folded slightly upon itself, it completely lacks villi.

Large Intestine

By the time the fluid mixture reaches the cecum, or entryway into the large intestine, the major portion of the digestive process is complete. However, *electrolytes* such as sodium, chloride, and potassium pass through the intestinal wall in the large intestine, along with water. Gaseous by-products of fiber (such as the gas produced after eating a large quantity of dry, cooked beans) may also be produced and partly absorbed here.

Most of the water we drink is absorbed

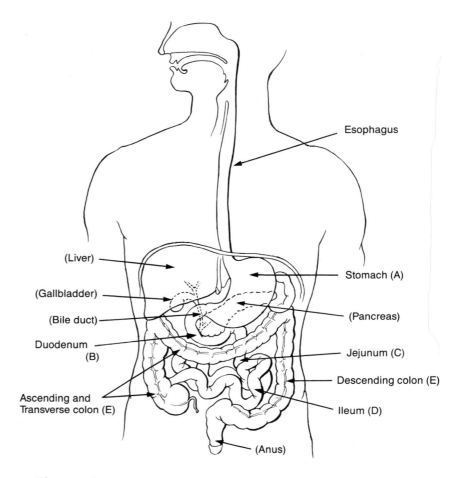

Figure 1-2
Where nutrient absorption occurs: (A) Water and ethyl alcohol. (B) Monosaccharides glucose and galactose, minerals, especially calcium (Ca*), magnesium (Mg), iron (Fe) and zinc (Zn), and some vitamins. (C) Most fat- and water-soluble vitamins and most energy-producing nutrients: glucose, galactose, sucrose, maltose, lactose, short- and long-chain fatty acids, protein, and amino acids; also chloride (Cl^-) and some water. (D) Vitamins K and B_{12}, sodium (Na^+), potassium (K^+), Chloride (Cl), water (H_2O), bile salts, and remaining vitamins and energy nutrients not already absorbed. (E) Vitamin K, short-chain fatty acids, H_2O, Na^+, Cl^-, K^+, biotin (?), and possibly gases and nutrients from soluble fiber. (Suitor CJW, Crowley MF: Nutrition, 2nd ed, p 220. Philadelphia, JB Lippincott, 1984)

through the large intestine. It then enters the tissues and blood before it is filtered through the kidneys into the bladder for urination. The only water that will be directly excreted at the end of the digestive tract is the water contained in the stool. The water content of the stool depends on what substances remain that have not been digested and how much water they can hold. This

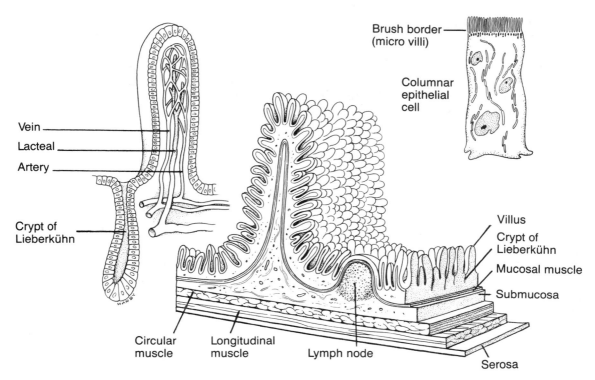

Vein

Lacteal

Artery

Crypt of
Lieberkühn

Brush border
(micro villi)

Columnar
epithelial
cell

Villus

Crypt of
Lieberkühn

Mucosal muscle

Submucosa

Circular
muscle

Longitudinal
muscle

Lymph node

Serosa

Figure 1-3
Diagram of the intestinal villi and columnar epithelial cells. (Adapted from
Chaffee E, Lytle I: Basic Physiology and Anatomy, 4th ed. In Suitor CJW, Crowley
MF [eds]: Nutrition, 2nd ed, p 218. Philadelphia, JB Lippincott, 1984)

mass gradually forms in the three parts of the colon and then moves into the rectum and anal canal for excretion. Two muscles at the anal sphincter help control excretion. One is an involuntary muscle and the other can be voluntarily controlled. So, although the alimentary tract is largely controlled by muscle, it is only at the beginning and the end that any voluntary muscle control is possible.

The digestive system involves not only the alimentary tract itself but also the absorption, *metabolism,* utilization, and excretion of nutrients. These four processes are discussed as they relate to individual nutrients in the following chapters. Body functions and how they may be affected by the digestive tract are discussed further in Section II.

STUDY QUESTIONS

1. By what point in human development is the digestive tract established?
2. Gravity has a small role in moving food through the digestive tract. What has the greatest role in this process? What is this movement called?
3. List the six parts of the digestive tract or alimentary canal.
4. What enzyme breaks down foods in the mouth?
5. What is the function of the pharynx?
6. Name the two muscles at the entrance and exit of the stomach. Describe the function of each.

7. If lemon juice, cranberry juice, and vinegar were consumed by a person in separate doses, which of the three, if any, would make the stomach more acid? Explain your answer.

8. If a person were taking enzyme pills that were not enteric-coated, would the pills be effective in the small intestine? Why or why not?

9. How does the small intestine differ from the large intestine in appearance and function?

10. What is the function of pancreatic enzymes? Of bile? Of amylase, lactase, and sucrase?

CHAPTER 2

Energy

OBJECTIVES

1. To emphasize the importance of food energy

2. To identify factors that affect energy requirements, and to explain each factor

3. To explain and illustrate the concept of energy balance and its relationship to weight gain, weight loss, and weight maintenance

4. To identify the principal sources of food energy: protein, carbohydrate, and fat

5. To introduce the concept that each of the three nutrient sources plays a distinct role in providing energy for the body

6. To introduce briefly the types and characteristics of energy-deficient malnutrition

7. To define the units by which energy is measured

While the body needs food for many reasons, the most important reason is energy. Food in the body is like fuel in a furnace: the food breaks down to make energy or power that is used by all the parts of the body in order to keep functioning. This energy made by food is used

1. To keep the heart, lungs, and other body systems working well

2. To stabilize the temperature of the body

3. To allow for growth and activity

4. To ensure that the other nutrients in food (proteins, vitamins, minerals, water, and electrolytes) are used properly

The lowest rate at which the body uses fuel or energy is called the *basal metabolic rate*, or *BMR*. Basal metabolism is defined as "the amount of energy needed for maintenance of life when the subject is at digestive, physical, and emotional rest." [1] As soon as a person begins to move, to eat, or to become physically stressed, his need for energy increases. The only way that energy can be provided, directly or indirectly, is through food.

The amount of food a person needs to provide energy depends upon many factors. These factors do not affect energy needs alone. They also influence a person's needs for many other nutrients as well.

FACTORS THAT AFFECT ENERGY REQUIREMENTS

Age. Basal metabolism varies throughout the lifespan. In infancy, the BMR is high and growth needs are great. In the prepubertal years when growth is fast once again, the energy needs are high; they lower slightly in the late teen years but still are high. In adulthood, the BMR begins to slow down at a rate of about 2% per decade. [2]

Activity. All body movements require energy. The more strenuous the moves, the more energy is needed. This is why exercise is one of the most effective ways to lose weight.

Body Size. A large body needs more energy than does a small body. An overweight person might compensate for this, though, by avoiding sports and moving as little as possible. As a person loses weight, the energy he needs to move his body will decrease.

Body Composition. The percentage of fat versus muscle in a body affects its energy needs. Muscles and organs require more energy than fat (adipose tissue) requires to stay healthy.

Climate. Whenever the difference between body temperature and external temperature increases, BMR increases. As a general rule, people in a cold climate need more energy than do those in a warm climate.

Eating. The BMR increases *slightly* for up to 12 hours after a meal. Digestion, absorption, and metabolism of food require energy.

Pregnancy and Lactation. The pregnant woman is providing nourishment, energy, and warmth for her unborn child, thus placing high demands on her body. Lactation (breast-feeding) uses energy by giving that energy directly to the child. Nutrient and energy needs in pregnancy and lactation will be discussed in more detail in Chapters 13 and 14.

Disease. Almost every disease state increases the BMR. The body needs extra energy to repair any damage done to it. The need depends upon the disease, the extent of damage, and the loss of heat by fever. This is discussed in more detail in Chapter 39.

Sex. Men have higher BMRs than women. This is probably due to the difference in body composition (men have proportionately more muscle mass than fat tissue). Women, even athletic women whose weight is normal, will have a higher percentage of fat stores than do their male counterparts.

Stress. Emotional or physical stress may increase the BMR. The increase is probably quite small and is not well defined. It depends upon the individual and the degree of stress.

Each person must take in enough food daily to meet his energy needs. If a person does not get the energy needed from the food he eats in one day, energy is drawn from the body's reserves. The person may lose weight, depending on how much of the body's reserves are used. If too much food is eaten, the extra food energy is stored. When the energy (fat) stores increase, the person gains weight. This concept of energy balance is illustrated in Figure 2-1. There is no other way (short of surgery) to gain or lose body tissue. The amount of water stored in the body can be changed slightly (i.e., with diet pills or diuretics), but this change is always temporary. An individual who wants to gain weight must take in more food energy than his body burns. Someone who wants to lose weight must burn up more energy than he acquires through food and beverages.

HOW THE BODY MAKES ENERGY

All foods are made of carbohydrate, protein, or fat or some combination of these three, plus vitamins, minerals, and water. When food is eaten and broken down in the small intestine into nutrients, these nutrients are actually drawn through the intestinal walls. The three nutrients that produce energy are *carbohydrate, protein,* and *fat.* (Note: alcohol also provides food energy but is discussed separately in Chapter 11.) These three nutrients will be discussed individually in the following chapters. When broken down, all of them are carried into the blood and are then carried by the blood (the circulatory system) to each cell in the body. It is in the cells that metabolism occurs and where the nutrients are converted into energy.

There is a common pathway in the cells through which all three nutrients must pass in order to be utilized by the body. This is called the *common metabolic pathway.* By passing through this pathway, as illustrated in Figure 2-2, nutrients manufacture energy. This chemical cycle could be called the "furnace" of energy production. The products of this chemical cycle, nicotinamide-adenine dinucleotide (NADH) and flavin adenine dinucleotide ($FADH_2$) produce energy as they are converted to water in the cell. This energy is in the form of adenosine triphosphate *(ATP)* and it is ATP that the cell needs and uses in order to function.

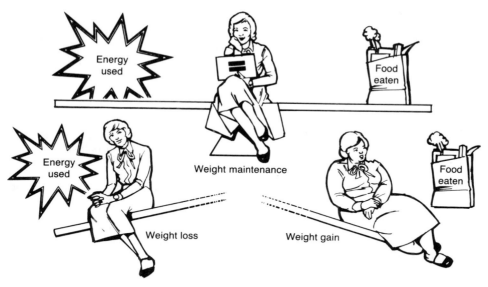

Figure 2-1
Energy balance

WHEN THERE IS NOT SUFFICIENT ENERGY

A day or two without enough food will not cause problems in the healthy body, but when a person is not able to acquire the energy he needs over a longer period of time many changes occur.

Carbohydrate is the most efficient source of energy. One hundred percent can be readily converted to energy. In the absence of sufficient carbohydrate, however, protein and fat can be utilized for energy. The process might be compared to a house heated by woodburning fireplaces. To run out of carbohydrate is to run out of ordinary firewood; the need for body heat does not stop. When this occurs, the body may suffer. Stored fat is burned. While the body uses fat for energy because there is not sufficient carbohydrate, it also uses protein. The protein comes from muscle stores, from any protein in food, and from blood. Over a long period of time, protein loss in starvation or severe dieting may cause problems.

The body protects itself by using the "cheapest" energy fuel (carbohydrate) first, then fat

and protein. Just as in the case of the house, it is when nothing is left that the fire goes out or the house begins to consume itself. Only after a long period of starvation does the body begin to break itself down (and damage major organs) for energy. Measurable malnutrition may be categorized as *protein-calorie malnutrition, kwashiorkor, marasmus,* or *stunting.*

Protein-calorie malnutrition (PCM) is the term for starvation that results from a protracted diet that does not provide sufficient energy or protein. It appears in children more often than in adults and it is most common in underdeveloped nations and in very poor areas of developed nations. Table 2-1 lists the characteristics of PCM. It may also be called *PEM* or protein-energy malnutrition.

Kwashiorkor is another type of malnutrition. In kwashiorkor, a child may receive enough energy through his food, but not sufficient protein. This condition was first noticed in African children whose mothers stopped nursing them because additional children were born. The child may not look skinny; rather he may look fat because of *edema* (excess water). When treat-

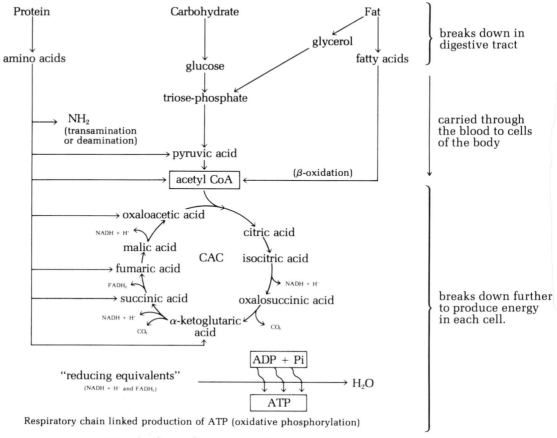

Respiratory chain linked production of ATP (oxidative phosphorylation)

(ATP is the form of energy used by the body)

Figure 2-2

The common pathway of human metabolism, called the common metabolic pathway, the Krebs Cycle, or the Citric Acid Cycle. (Adapted from Anderson L, Dibble MV, Turkki PR, Mitchell HS et al: Nutrition in Health and Disease, 17th ed, p 176. Philadelphia, JB Lippincott, 1983)

ment starts, edema disappears and starvation is more apparent.

A child with marasmus is severely malnourished. This child has not been receiving enough energy, protein, or fat for a long period of time. Many children with marasmus die of minor colds or infections. Their bodies are too weak to fight any bacteria. Refeeding must be done under very careful medical supervision.

Dwarfing, or stunting, is the result of pro-tracted mild malnutrition. A child who is stunted does not appear skinny, but he is short for his age. In many cultures where food is scarce, the people may all be small. It may be hard to distinguish between a child who is short because of genetics and one who is short because he has not eaten enough food throughout his life. Some studies seem to show that stunting occurs more frequently among poor children than among children of the same culture and

Table 2-1

Simplified Classification of Protein-Calorie Malnutrition

Categories	Body Weight, % Standard	Body Height	Edema	Weight/Height Deficit
Kwashiorkor	80%–60%	Affected	Yes	Marked
Marasmus	Under 60%	Affected	No	Marked
Mixed form	Under 60%	Affected	Yes	Marked
Moderate PCM (underweight)	80%–60%	Affected	No	Minimal
Stunted growth (nutritional dwarfing)	Under 60%	Markedly short for age	No	Minimal

Berg A, Scrimshaw NS, Call DL (eds): Nutrition, National Development and Planning. Cambridge, MIT Press, 1973

race who are not poor, since the more well-to-do members of the same ethnic group often seem to be taller and heavier.*

MEASURES OF ENERGY

In the United States, food energy is measured in *kilocalories,* or Kcal, popularly called *calories.* The kilocalorie, a unit of heat, is defined as the amount of heat needed to raise the temperature of one kilogram of water one degree centigrade (from 15°C to 16°C). Another unit of measure, the *joule,* is less commonly used but may become more prevalent in the future. One kilocalorie is approximately equal to 4.2 kilojoules. Throughout this text the term "calorie" refers to kilocalories.

When a person wants to gain weight, he must eat about 3500 *more* calories than the body uses in order to gain 1 pound. To lose 1 pound, an individual must eat 3500 calories *less* than the body needs for energy. If a person eats 500 calories less than he needs each day, it will take 7 days to lose 1 pound (7 days × 500 cal).

Although these unit measures and numbers are not precise, using them helps to ensure that a person acquires the food energy needed to maintain life and normal activity. The energy needs of individuals will be discussed further in Chapter 5.

REFERENCES

1. Taber's Cyclopedic Medical Dictionary, 15th ed, p B-16. Philadelphia, FA Davis, 1985
2. Food and Nutrition Board, National Academy of Sciences: Recommended Dietary Allowances, 9th ed, p 22. Washington, National Research Council, 1980

STUDY QUESTIONS

1. Why does the body need energy?
2. What are the three major components in food that provide energy? Which of the three is the most efficient for energy production?
3. What happens if this component is not available?
4. Where in the body is energy actually manufactured? Where is it used? In what form does it come?

---

* A study done (1983) by the Massachusetts Department of Public Health showed that 9.8% of children under the age of 6 from poor families suffered from stunted growth, as compared to a rate of 5% among all children.

5. List the factors that determine individual energy needs. Explain three of them. Do they increase or decrease energy needs, and how do they do so?

6. A hospitalized patient is assigned to you. She is a 60-year-old woman who recently lost her husband. She had an infection for several weeks and was admitted when her fever was so high she could not ignore it. She is losing weight because she says she doesn't want to eat.

   a. What factors contribute to her special energy needs? Why?

   b. What factors do you think can be changed? Why?

   c. How could she gain weight?

CHAPTER 3

Protein

While all foods contain energy, only certain foods have protein.

It is the protein portion of food that makes it possible for the body to

- Replace damaged tissues and constantly dying cells
- Maintain muscle tissue
- Form enzymes
- Make essential hormones, antibodies, and other glandular secretions

The body, therefore, must have enough usable protein or it cannot maintain itself. When a person's diet, or daily eating pattern, contains sufficient carbohydrate to produce energy, the protein can then be "spared." This means that the protein portion of the food is spared *from* being used simply as fuel for energy and spared *for* the functions that only protein can perform. If protein must be used for energy over a long period of time, there may not be enough of it left for these other essential functions. Disease may develop. The normal, healthy adult body needs at least 0.8 grams of protein per kilogram of body weight per day to maintain itself.

PROTEIN AND NITROGEN

What differentiates protein from carbohydrates and fats is that protein contains nitrogen. The proteins in the body, such as muscles, the enzymes, *antibodies*, and *hormones*, all need nitrogen. When protein breaks down, the nitrogen cannot be completely utilized so it must somehow be excreted from the body. It is usually lost in the urine via the kidneys. Nitrogen is also excreted in feces, sweat, and sloughed off nails, hair, and skin.

Just as "energy balance" is measured by weight gain or weight loss, protein "balance" is most accurately measured by nitrogen. The same factors that affect energy needs also affect protein needs. Some conditions, such as disease, may increase protein needs proportionately more than the need for energy. If the person who is sick is not eating enough protein foods to meet these increased needs, his body will lose protein tissue. The person may not lose weight, though, since energy needs may be met. A body in this state is in *negative nitrogen balance*. It is difficult to measure nitrogen balance precisely, but negative balance, over a long period of time, may become apparent in certain laboratory tests. Abnormal levels of creatinine, blood urea nitrogen (BUN), red blood cell count, and albumin may all signal a problem in protein balance and/or metabolism.

PROTEIN AND ENERGY NEEDS

It takes 6.25 grams of protein to provide 1 gram of nitrogen. In order to ensure that this nitrogen will be well used by the body, and not for energy, a person's diet should contain about 150 calories for ever gram of nitrogen. This allows the protein to be "spared" for its essential functions.

The easiest way for a person to determine how much protein he needs each day is to use the *Recommended Dietary Allowances* (reproduced in Table 3-1). The Recommended Dietary Allowances (RDAs) are designed to meet the needs of almost all healthy persons. The RDAs are divided by age groups and sex, and there is an RDA for every vitamin and mineral for which there is a proven need, as well as for energy, for fat, and for protein. Although the RDA of a nutrient may be more than an individual requires, protein is so important to the body that a diet slightly higher than the RDA for protein will not be harmful to the normal, healthy individual. The American diet tends to provide far more protein than most persons actually need. This usually is not true in underdeveloped nations. The RDAs will be discussed in more detail in Chapter 12.

AMINO ACIDS

"Protein" is actually a general term for a combination of about 22 small, building-blocklike compounds called *amino acids*. Like members of the same family, each amino acid has the same basic structure but different individual features and functions. Each amino acid contains nitrogen. Some amino acids can be made in the body from other amino acids. Eight or nine of them however, cannot be made and must be provided in foods. Those that the body

Table 3-1

Recommended Dietary Allowances for Protein

Age	Protein (grams)
Infants	
0–6 mo	kg body weight $\times$ 2.2
7–12 mo	kg body weight $\times$ 2.0
Children	
1–3	23
4–6	30
7–10	34
Males	
11–14	45
15–18	56
19–22	56
23–50	56
n 51+	56
Females	
11–14	46
15–18	46
19–22	44
23–50	44
51+	44
Pregnant	+30
Lactating	+20

Adapted from information from the Food and Nutrition Board, National Academy of Sciences: Recommended Dietary Allowances, 9th ed. Washington, National Research Council, 1980

cannot make are called the *essential amino acids* because they *must* be provided in the diet, in the right amount and in the right proportions. If they are not, the protein consumed cannot be well used. The essential and nonessential amino acids are listed on the opposite page.

Protein is broken down into the amino acids in the small intestine. The acids then travel through the blood to the cells. Once it arrives at the cell, each amino acid has a different function. They have many different roles in metabolism and enter into the common metabolic pathway at several different points. This is why the body needs different amounts of each essential amino acid. And since these acids work together, they must all be present in the right combinations before any one acid can be completely utilized. To arrive at the cell in the right combi-

ESSENTIAL AND NONESSENTIAL AMINO ACIDS

Essential	Nonessential
Histidine˙	Alanine
Isoleucine	Arginine
Leucine	Asparagine
Lysine	Aspartic Acid
Methionine	Cysteine
Phenylalanine	Cystine
Threonine	Glutamic Acid
Tryptophan	Glutamine
Valine	Glycine
	Hydroxyproline
	Proline
	Serine
	Tyrosine

˙In infants

nations, they must be eaten at the same meal in the right combinations.

There are two basic kinds of protein foods: animal protein and vegetable protein. The different protein foods do not all have the same combinations of the amino acids. Most animal proteins, such as eggs, fish, meat, milk, and dairy products, *do* have all the essential amino acids (EAA) in the right proportions. So these foods are already "complete proteins." The person who eats them will probably never need to worry about the protein in his food being well used. The body can easily use this protein.

Vegetable proteins are different. They are foods such as nuts, seeds, dry beans, dry peas, tofu (soybean curd), and grains such as wheat and corn and rice. These foods all contain most of the essential amino acids, but not in the best proportions for the body. Some are low in one or two amino acids; others may be low in different amino acids. The low or inadequate amino acid

Example 1: Egg

Complete Protein

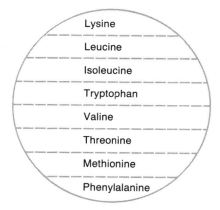

The eight essential amino acids (EAA) must be present in a protein in specific ratios. Egg protein has all eight in the ratio or proportions used most efficiently and completely by the body.

Example 2: Wheat germ

Incomplete Protein

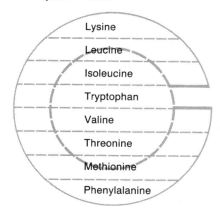

Wheat germ is not complete because it is deficient in tryptophan. As a result of this deficiency, less of the total protein (see inner dotted lines) can be used. The EAA present in the smallest proportion is called the "limiting amino acid" because it limits the amount of the other EAAs that may be used and thus the total availability of the protein.

Figure 3-1
Complete (animal) versus incomplete (vegetable) proteins.

is called the *limiting amino acid.* A vegetarian, who acquires most of his protein from the vegetable protein foods, may not be able to use the protein efficiently unless the foods eaten are combined in a certain way. This is illustrated in Figure 3-1.

COMPLEMENTARY PROTEINS

These protein foods must be combined (or complemented) to compensate for the limiting amino acid(s). For example, beans are deficient in sulfur-containing amino acids, but wheat has a high proportion of these acids. Wheat, though, is short in lysine, while certain dry beans have a high proportion of this amino acid. As a result of eating the two foods together, the final protein is of higher quality than that of each of them individually.

This is illustrated in more detail in Figure 3-2. The arrows designate foods that should be combined to ensure the best complemented proteins. This chart could be used to plan vegetarian meals or help a vegetarian to acquire high quality protein. *Complementary proteins* must be eaten together at the same meal.

PROTEIN KILOCALORIES

Each gram (1/28 of an ounce) of pure protein provides about 4 calories. Thus a 3-ounce portion of fish, which contains 21 grams of protein, provides 84 calories from protein. It also provides some calories from natural fats or oil as well.

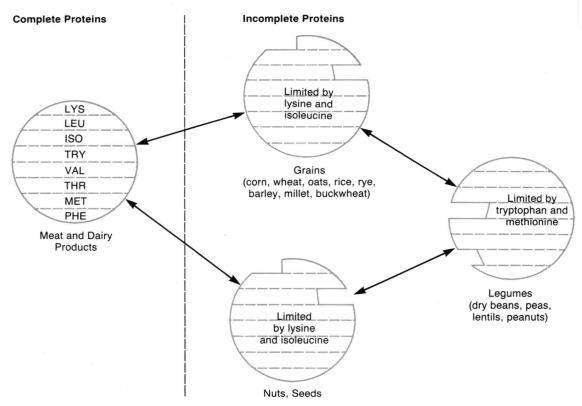

Complete Proteins

LYS
LEU
ISO
TRY
VAL
THR
MET
PHE

Meat and Dairy Products

Incomplete Proteins

Limited by lysine and isoleucine

Grains
(corn, wheat, oats, rice, rye, barley, millet, buckwheat)

Limited by tryptophan and methionine

Legumes
(dry beans, peas, lentils, peanuts)

Limited by lysine and isoleucine

Nuts, Seeds

Figure 3-2
Complementary proteins: foods to combine.

PROTEIN AND DISEASE

Marasmus and kwashiorkor, two diseases already mentioned, relate to a diet too low in protein. Adding protein foods to the diet under a doctor's careful supervision can have a very important role in bringing these victims back to health. Protein has an important role in other diseases, as well. They will be discussed in Chapter 23.

STUDY QUESTIONS

1. Why is protein important?

2. What are some of the products made by the body that contain protein?

3. What is the "recommended daily" amount of protein that a 50 kilogram person requires?

4. List six ways that nitrogen is lost from the body after protein breaks down.

5. How is the body's "protein balance" measurable? List three ways.

6. What are the basic building-blocks that make up proteins?

7. What do lysine, phenylalanine, and isoleucine have in common?

8. Is the body able to make the amino acid asparagine?

9. True or false: A complete protein is one that has the same amount of each of the 22 amino acids. Explain your answer.

10. True or false: If a protein food is short in one essential amino acid, it does not really matter because the body will make up the difference at another time.

11. What foods are the best sources of protein?

CHAPTER 4

Carbohydrates

OBJECTIVES

1. To differentiate between proteins and carbohydrates

2. To discuss the essential role of carbohydrates

3. To identify and define the different forms of carbohydrate and the food sources of each

4. To describe the different sweetening powers of various sugars

5. To list hidden and processed food sources of sugars, and alternate terms used

6. To describe the digestion and absorption of the various carbohydrates.

7. To discuss the energy and the nutrients in various carbohydrates

8. To introduce the concept of the ecological cost of carbohydrates compared to protein and fat, and the adequacy of a high carbohydrate diet

Carbohydrates are the most essential and usually the most digestible form of energy. The foods that are generally cheapest and most readily available throughout the world are foods high in carbohydrate. In some cultures, 80% or more of the body's energy comes from eating carbohydrate foods such as rice, wheat, and other grains or starchy vegetables. In contrast, 46% of the calories in the standard American diet come from carbohydrate.* The rest comes from protein (11%–12%) and fat (42%).

Carbohydrate differs from protein. It does not contain nitrogen. So when carbohydrate is digested, there is no "leftover" nitrogen to excrete. Carbohydrate is not able to manufacture antibodies against infection or heal damaged tissue in the body. Protein is needed to perform that function. But when infection or damaged tissue is present, the body does need a sufficient supply of carbohydrate in order to "spare" the protein so that it can do its job. The carbohydrate is then used for energy so the body can continue functioning well.

If there is not enough carbohydrate in the diet, fat and protein are broken down for energy and water is lost. The body responds as if it were "starving." Serious problems may develop if this state continues for long. Carbohydrate makes the difference between this condition and a balanced weight-loss diet. In a balanced diet, fat is also lost, but protein and water are "spared" because there is sufficient carbohydrate to meet basic needs. A sensible weight-loss diet should always contain sufficient carbohydrate. Carbohydrate foods are not necessarily "fattening" foods. However the carbohydrates chosen should be those rich in nutrients.

---

* Food and Nutrition Board, National Academy of Sciences: Recommended Dietary Allowances, 9th ed, p 31. Washington, National Research Council, 1980

TYPES OF CARBOHYDRATE

There are many different forms of carbohydrate. The terms "sugar," *"starch,"* and *"fiber"* are all general terms for the three major categories of carbohydrate.

Sugars

The sugars are the basic unit of carbohydrate. They are usually divided into two groups. The first group, the *monosaccharides,* comprises the very simplest sugars. The second group, the *disaccharides,* consists of sugars made from combinations of two monosaccharides.

The three monosaccharides important in normal nutrition are *glucose, fructose,* and *galactose.* Each is made of the same chemicals (carbon, hydrogen, and oxygen) in the same amounts. But each has a different shape or structure that gives it individual characteristics.

The three disaccharides are *sucrose* (1 glucose molecule plus 1 fructose molecule), *lactose* (1 glucose molecule plus 1 galactose molecule), and *maltose* (2 glucose molecules). Figure 4-1 illustrates the monosaccharides and the disaccharides, and lists the major food sources of each.

While both monosaccharides and disaccharides are sweet, some are much sweeter than others. On a scale of 1–10, fructose would rank 10, sucrose, 5.8, and glucose, 4.3; maltose, even though it is made of glucose units, would be 1.8. With a sweetening power of 0.9, lactose is the least sweet of all the naturally occurring sugars.†

---

† This numerical category of 1 to 10 is derived from an older numerical classification in which sucrose is 100. (See Guthrie HA: Introductory Nutrition, 3rd ed, p 24. St. Louis, CV Mosby, 1975

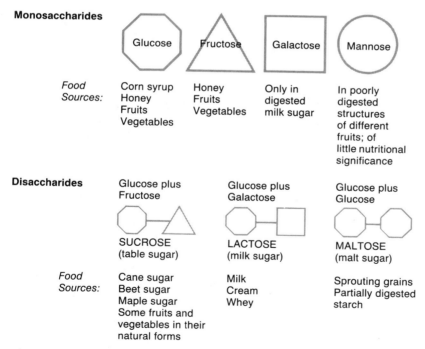

Figure 4-1
The sugars and their food sources. Shapes here help differentiate the monosaccharides but do not reflect their actual chemical structure. (Adapted from Howe PS: Basic Nutrition in Health and Disease, 7th ed, pp 44–45. Philadelphia, WB Saunders, 1981)

Of the six sugar units, glucose is the most important in nutrition. All digestible carbohydrates eventually break down into glucose in the blood. Blood sugar *is* glucose. The body's blood glucose level must stay within a certain range so that the individual can remain healthy. *Hyperglycemia* is the term used when blood glucose goes above the normal, safe level. *Hypoglycemia* means that the blood glucose is too low. Hyperglycemia and hypoglycemia are not diseases. They are symptoms of an abnormal blood sugar measurement.

The healthy body has a very elaborate alarm system that helps to keep the blood glucose level in its normal range. This system is vital, since blood glucose helps feed brain cells, nerves, and other body tissues. Carbohydrate, protein, and fats can all break down to form glucose. Even in a fasting state (where the individual is taking nothing but water), the normal, healthy person will be able to maintain a normal blood glucose level from body muscle stores, fat, and *glycogen.*

Sugar Alcohols

Sugar alcohols are products of the three monosaccharides that exist either naturally in small amounts in foods, or are commercially produced. They are not important sources of energy. The most common sugar alcohol is *sorbitol.* It is the sweetener generally used in sugarless gum. Sorbitol is made from glucose but is absorbed much more slowly into the bloodstream than glucose. It has a sweetening power of 3.4 and just as many calories as glucose — 4 per gram. Sugarless gum is not "low calorie." However, since the sweetener does not break down as quickly in the mouth, it is much less destructive to the teeth than regular gum. Chewing a large amount of sugarless gum in a short time may lead to a transient diarrhea, another effect of sorbitol.

Mannitol, the other common sugar alcohol, has a sweetening power of 2.9, but is of little known significance in normal nutrition.

Xylitol, the sweetest of the sugar alcohols, is not in common use because of questions about its safety.

Starches

Technically, starch is a *polysaccharide.* The polysaccharides are carbohydrates made of many units of monosaccharides or disaccharides. Starch is made of many units of glucose. The glucose is connected in long chains *(amyloses)* or in networklike structures (called *amylopectins*). Starch is the major digestible polysaccharide found in foods. Grains, root vegetables, and legumes (such as soybeans, lentils, and other dry beans and peas) are all primarily starch. They may contain enough protein to be very important in a vegetarian diet, but most of their energy comes from the carbohydrate they contain.

Other polysaccharides, such as *dextrin* and glycogen, do not occur naturally in foods. They are produced either by the metabolism or breakdown of other carbohydrates.

Fiber

Fiber is a broad term for all carbohydrates that are not completely digested by the human body. They will be discussed in more detail in another chapter. Most fibers are also polysaccharides.

CARBOHYDRATE DIGESTION, ABSORPTION, AND METABOLISM

Carbohydrates are broken down, or digested, by enzymes. The enzymes that digest carbohydrates are in the mouth and in the small intestine.

In the mouth, salivary amylase begins to break starch into dextrins and maltose. These partially digested products, together with all the other carbohydrates, pass through the stomach unchanged and on into the small intestine.

The pancreas produces the enzyme, *pancreatic amylase,* which flows into the duodenum and is used to break down the starches. The brushlike lining of the small intestine produces the remaining enzymes that break down the three disaccharides. The monosaccharides, glucose and galactose, are carried directly across the brush border into the blood *if* they enter the intestines in their pure form.

Figure 4-2 illustrates how these carbohy-

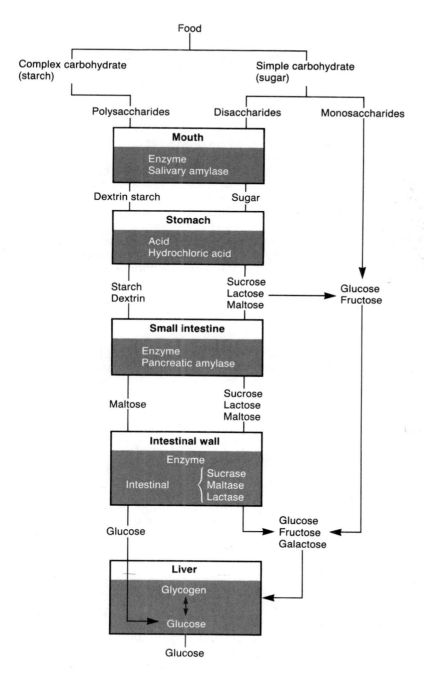

Figure 4-2
Summary of the digestion of carbohydrate. (From Guthrie HA:
Introductory Nutrition, 5th ed, p 31. St. Louis, CV Mosby, 1983)

drates are broken down or digested before they enter the bloodstream. Once the monosaccharides are in the blood, they are then carried to the liver. In the liver, galactose and fructose are converted into glucose. Glucose then enters the blood and travels to the cells, where it manufactures energy or is converted and stored as fat.

Not all of the carbohydrate that enters the liver is immediately sent out into the bloodstream. The liver is a "storehouse" for a small amount of reserve energy. This energy is stored in the form of the polysaccharide, glycogen. Glycogen is also stored in muscles. It is the first source of energy the body uses when blood glucose is low or inadequate. On the average, liver and muscles store about 600 kcals worth of glycogen.‡

The various monosaccharides are absorbed from the intestines into the bloodstream at different rates. Galactose is absorbed most quickly, and glucose follows closely. Fructose, however, takes over three times longer than glucose to be absorbed. Mannose is absorbed at one tenth the rate of glucose. While mannose is not usually present in an easily digestible form, the other monosaccharides eventually are completely absorbed. For example, if a meal providing 40 grams of glucose (or 160 calories, since carbohydrate, like protein, provides 4 calories per gram) is absorbed into the blood in 15 minutes, 40 grams of fructose may take almost an hour to be absorbed. But both meals provide exactly the same amount of energy in the long run.

In the cell, the glucose enters the common pathway for energy production that was discussed and illustrated in Figure 2-1.

Energy Costs of Carbohydrate

Carbohydrate foods in their natural state are, ecologically, the cheapest foods available because so little energy is required to produce them. Consequently, much of the world depends on them for survival. Animals must eat foods containing carbohydrate (such as grasses and grains) in order to manufacture protein and animal fat. Oils are pressed from foods high in

carbohydrate (corn, seeds, nuts, and olives). It takes a large quantity of these foods to produce a small amount of oil. Thus fats and proteins are, ecologically, much more "expensive" to produce. Highly processed foods, including highly processed carbohydrates, are usually more expensive than their less processed counterparts. Often carbohydrate foods that have experienced a good deal of processing have lost some of their nutrients. Refined white flour has less protein, fiber, and vitamins than does the wheat kernel. It is also less likely to spoil. Other processed foods may be high in sugar but not in other more nutrient-dense forms of carbohydrate. Grain products and dry beans and peas are always a more "nutritious" source of carbohydrate than sugars. In general, the closer a carbohydrate is to its "natural" form, the more nutrients it probably contains.

Most sugars, including the "natural" forms such as honey, contain very few vitamins or minerals. They provide energy but almost nothing else. Blackstrap molasses, a strong, dark, heavy by-product of sugar refining, is the only exception: it contains some iron. Sugars are frequently added to processed foods. Figure 4-1 lists terms that designate sugar, and foods that commonly contain them.

In summary, carbohydrates are essential to normal nutrition. Together with protein and fat they help meet the body's essential needs. Fat, the last of the three energy nutrients, will be discussed in the next chapter.

STUDY QUESTIONS

1. How does carbohydrate help the body to use protein?

2. List four major monosaccharides and at least one food source of each.

3. List three major disaccharides and at least two food sources of each. Have you eaten any foods containing these disaccharides in the past 24 hours?

4. What is the difference between disaccharides and monosaccharides? What do they have in common?

5. If one cold drink is sweetened with sucrose

‡ Stryer L: Biochemistry, p 378. New York, WH Freeman, 1975

and another with fructose, each to the same degree of sweetness, which drink will derive more calories from its sweetener? Explain your answer.

6. What sugar is commonly carried through the blood? Why is it important? If blood sugar reacher too low a level, what is this condition called? If the blood sugar level is too high, what correct term defines it?

7. Which is digested more slowly, sorbitol or glucose? List a food source of each.

8. True or false: Carbohydrates are broken down by enzymes in the stomach. Why or why not?

9. True or false: Monosaccharides, but not disaccharides or starches, can enter the blood in their original form. Why or why not?

10. You are a visiting nurse checking on a healthy, 80-year-old woman who lives alone. After she lets you in, you discover she ran out of food 2 days ago and has been drinking water only. Obviously this poses many problems, but you think her blood sugar level is probably safe for the moment. Why should you think this?

11. Based on what you know about carbohydrates and protein, which of the following has the most calories? How many does it have?

   ● A meal containing 30 grams of protein and 45 grams of carbohydrate

   ● A drink containing 20 grams of glucose, 10 grams of fructose, 12 grams of lactose, and 8 grams of protein

   ● A drink that tastes just as sweet as that in the example above but that contains no glucose.

CHAPTER 5

Fats

[handwritten: body temp / protect organs / insulation]

[handwritten: Saturated no room for H atom to be added]

OBJECTIVES

1. To define lipids
2. To explain the importance of fat in the diet
3. To describe how lipids may vary according to fatty acid content, fatty acid length, and saturation
4. To identify dietary sources of each of the major lipid types
5. To define and describe the importance of and dietary sources for essential fatty acids
6. To explain vegetable and animal sources of dietary lipids
7. To introduce the concept of lipids in the blood
8. To describe the contents of major blood lipids
9. To explain the role of fats in energy production and storage

Fats in the diet are more correctly called *lipids.* The body needs only a very small amount of fats or lipids from the diet to ensure good nutrition and health. The calories in foods all come either from the protein, the carbohydrate or the fat content in foods. Fat is a highly concentrated source of energy, providing over twice the energy found in the same amount of carbohydrate or protein. So, although only a small amount of

fat is needed in the diet, this small amount is very important for several reasons:

1. Lipids provide *essential fatty acids* (EFAs). EFAs help form part of the membrane around each cell in the body. They also help manufacture substances similar to hormones, and play a role in how *cholesterol* is used and excreted.
2. Lipids help carry vitamins A, D, E, and K into the body. These vitamins are dissolved in fats and stored in the fat cells of the body.
3. Lipids are the primary source of energy for the heart.
4. It is important to keep a small store of fat in the body. When food is not available, this "energy savings account" provides the needed extra energy. Fat stores can be maintained by extra carbohydrate and protein, not just dietary lipids. All healthy bodies, even the very muscular and the very thin, have some amount of fat stores.

TYPES OF LIPIDS

Lipids are composed of the same ingredients as carbohydrates: carbon, hydrogen, and oxygen. The differences are in the proportions (lipids have much less oxygen than carbohydrates) and in the way they are formed. Figure 5-1 illustrates the makeup of a typical lipid.

The typical simple lipid is called a *triglyceride* because it has three *fatty acids.* Other forms of lipids include *diglycerides* (two fatty acids), monoglycerides (one fatty acid), and *phospho-*

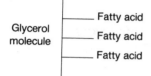

Figure 5-1
Lipid structure.

lipids (two fatty acids and a third molecule containing phosphate and some form of nitrogen.) *Cholesterol* also is a complex type of lipid that is regularly made by and stored in the liver. Cholesterol is also made and stored by animals and thus is present in all animal products. Foods that do not come from animals do not contain cholesterol. Plants cannot manufacture cholesterol even though they do contain fats. Food sources of cholesterol will be listed elsewhere in this chapter.

In addition to differences in the number of fatty acids they contain, lipids can differ in many other ways. The major difference among fats is the *types* of fatty acids and the way or degree in which these fatty acids are saturated.

A fatty acid is a chain or string of carbon atoms. Most fatty acid chains have an even number of carbons. But the chains may be short, medium, or long.

Short-chain fatty acids have between 2 carbons and 6 carbons. *Medium-chain fatty acids* have between 8 carbons and 12 carbons. A lipid molecule that has three fatty acids, each under 12 carbons long, is called a *medium-chain triglyceride,* or *MCT*. The body digests MCTs much more easily than it digests *long-chain triglycerides* (LCTs). People who cannot digest fat properly can usually digest and use oils made only of MCT. MCT oil is the only source of pure MCTs. Not available from food sources, it is laboratory-produced, is very expensive, and is essential for persons with certain problems of digestion or absorption.

Long-chain triglycerides have fatty acid chains between 14 carbons and 24 carbons long. Most naturally occurring fats contain long-chain fatty acids. The essential fatty acids (EFA)—*linoleic, linolenic* and *arachidonic acids*—are all long-chain fatty acids.

Fatty acids also differ in the way they are *saturated* with hydrogen. *Saturated fats* are those that are unable to absorb more hydrogen. They are usually stiff, hard fats. *Unsaturated fats* may have one point open to hydrogen (and thus are *monounsaturated*) or have several open points (and thus are *polyunsaturated*). Monounsaturated and polyunsaturated fats are usually in soft or liquid form. If a polyunsaturated oil has been *hydrogenated,* it has become

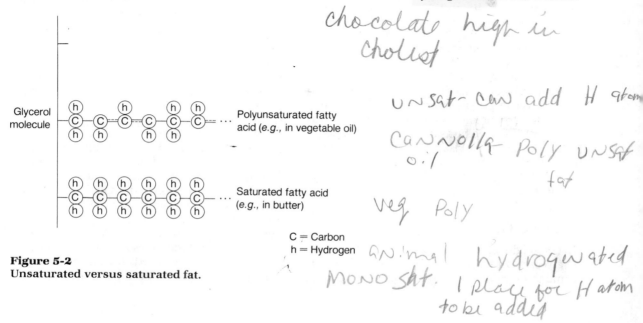

Glycerol molecule — Polyunsaturated fatty acid (*e.g.,* in vegetable oil)

Saturated fatty acid (*e.g.,* in butter)

C = Carbon
h = Hydrogen

Figure 5-2
Unsaturated versus saturated fat.

TABLE 5-1

Calculating P : S Ratio from a Margarine Label: One Example

"X" Brand of Margarine

Nutrition Information Per Serving

Serving size	14 g (1 tbsp)
Servings per 1 lb. container	32
Calories	70
Protein	0 g
Carbohydrate	0 g
Fat	7 g
Percentage calories from fat	99%
Polyunsaturated*	3 g
Saturated*	1 g
Cholesterol (0 mg per 100 g)*	0 mg
Sodium (510 mg per 100 g)	70 mg

← P : S ratio = 3 : 1 = 3.0

* This information relating to fat and cholesterol content is provided for persons who, on the advice of a physician, are modifying their total dietary intake of fat and cholesterol

more *saturated.* Many margarines are made of partially hydrogenated oils. See Figure 5-2 for an illustration of saturated versus unsaturated fats.

The *P : S ratio* is the proportion of *p*olyunsaturated fat to *s*aturated fat in a product. The higher the ratio, the more polyunsaturated fats are present in proportion to saturated fats. Most margarine labels list the grams of polyunsaturated and saturated fats in an average serving. A margarine that is high in polyunsaturates will probably have a softer consistency than a margarine—or other fat—that is proportionately lower in polyunsaturates. Table 5-1 illustrates how to calculate the P : S ratio on a margarine label. Since polyunsaturated fats may play a role in lowering the risk of heart disease, a margarine with a high P : S ratio may be preferred.

"PUFA" is a common abbreviation for *Poly*unsaturated *Fatty Acids.*

LIPIDS IN THE DIET

Ninety-eight percent of the lipids in foods are triglycerides of some kind. Exactly what percentage of calories in a healthful diet should come from fat is still a controversial issue. Currently the recommendations for a safe, adequate fat intake are that

1. Calories from fat should not exceed 30% of the total daily calories

2. Fat calories should not exceed 10% from polyunsaturates, 10% from monounsaturates, and 8% from saturated fats.[1]

These levels allow the body more than enough essential fatty acids and should be adequate to meet the body's other needs for fat. Food sources vary widely in the nature of their fat content.

Essential Fatty Acids

As mentioned, the EFAs are linoleic acid, linolenic acid, and arachidonic acid. Of these three, it is most important that a person acquire linoleic acid from the food in the diet. The other two fatty acids can be manufactured by the body. Linoleic is a long-chain, polyunsaturated fatty acid. Thus, foods high in PUFAs are likely to be high in EFAs. Since these foods also help the body meet its other needs for fats, good nutrition does not require fat in its saturated form.

An EFA deficiency is very rare in humans. In the USA it has occurred most frequently only in infants who were on infant formula that, by accident, did not include any EFAs. The signs of EFA deficiency in these infants included dry, flaky skin, and a decreased ability to use available energy. They did not grow as well as children who were receiving the necessary EFAs. When EFAs were added to their diets, they improved.[2]

The amount of fat a person needs in order to obtain the EFAs depends on the type of fat and its EFA content. A diet is adequate in EFAs if 1% to 2% of its calories in the adult and 3% in the infant come from linoleic acid.[1] However, foods vary widely in their content of linoleic acid. The foods that contain the highest linoleic acid in their lipid portion include safflower oil, corn oil, nuts, and wheat germ.

Depending on the mother's diet, breast milk may have up to 4 times to 5 times more linoleic acid than cow's milk.[3] Formulas now have EFAs added so that either of these sources is better for an infant than cow's milk.

Animal Sources of Fat

Figure 5-3 lists the fat components of various foods. Animal products are generally higher in fat than vegetable products. Animals store energy as fat, just as humans do, while most vegetables do not. Thus all animal foods usually contain some fat.

In animals, the fat is combined closely with the flesh. This is called "marbling." Beef, lamb,

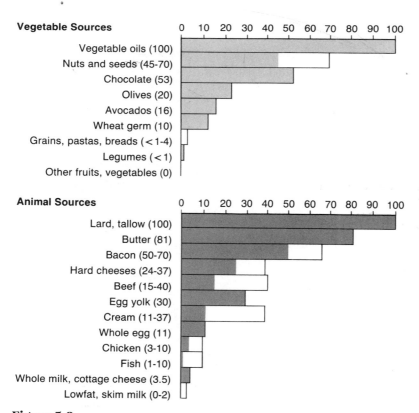

Figure 5-3
Vegetable and animal sources of fat. (From Composition of Foods. US Agriculture Handbook No. 8, 1975.)

and pork all contain fat even when the "visible" white chunks of fat are removed. Major sources of fat in chicken and turkey are the skin and the dark meat. Poultry is usually lower in fat than beef, lamb, or pork, although duck and goose may have as much or more fat than beef. Fats in these animals may be saturated or unsaturated,

and contain some cholesterol. The fat in eggs is all in the yolk and is high in cholesterol.

Fish vary widely in the fat content of their flesh. Mackerel and fresh salmon have almost 10% fat, while fresh tuna has 5%, canned salmon 6%, and cod, haddock, scallops, and canned tuna are all under 1% (before fat is added, as in

TABLE 5-2

Cholesterol in Foods: A Comparison

Food	Portion Size	Cholesterol (mg)
Beef, raw	3 1/2 oz	70
Brains, raw	3 1/2 oz	Over 2000
Butter	1 tbsp	36
Caviar	3 1/2 oz	Over 300
Clams*	3 1/2 oz	40–50
Cheese, cheddar	1 oz	30
cottage, creamed	1/2 cup	17
cream	1 tbsp	17
Chicken, raw	3 1/2 oz	60
Crab*	3 1/2 oz	60–75
Egg, white	1	None
Egg, yolk	1 large	315
Fish fillet	3 1/2 oz	70
Heart, raw	3 1/2 oz	150
Ice cream	1/2 cup	32
Kidney, raw	3 1/2 oz	375
Lamb	3 1/2 oz	70
Lard, animal fat	1 tbsp	14
Liver, raw	3 1/2 oz	300
Lobster*	3 1/2 oz	70–106
Margarine, all veg.	1 tbsp	None
Milk, whole	1 cup	25
Milk, skim	1 cup	7
Mutton	3 1/2 oz	65
Pork	3 1/2 oz	70
Shrimp*	3 1/2 oz	90
Sweetbreads	3 1/2 oz	250
Veal	3 1/2 oz	90

* Unpublished data on shellfish from National Marine Fisheries Service, Gloucester, MA, January 1985. At one time it was believed that all shellfish were high in cholesterol. Testing with new techniques detected differences and found that most shellfish have cholesterol levels very much like chicken, beef, and fish fillets.

(From: US Agriculture Handbook No. 8: Composition of Foods, 1975)

canning).[4] Fat in fish is usually in the form of an unsaturated oil. Cholesterol content is usually low.* Fish packed in oil (and usually vegetable oil, not fish oil) will obviously contain more fat and calories than fish packed in water.

Dairy products are also naturally high in fats, most are saturated and also contain cholesterol. Whole milk contains 3.5% fat. Other food products and their cholesterol content are listed in Table 5-2. Low fat and skim milk have had their natural butterfat partially or completely removed.

Vegetable Sources of Fat

The fat content of nonanimal foods varies widely as is illustrated in Figure 5-3. These foods would be the primary sources of fat for a vegetarian who ate no dairy products. Most vegetable fats are polyunsaturated, except for olive oil, which is monounsaturated and palm oil and coconut oil, which are saturated fats.

Cholesterol

Only animal products contain cholesterol. Vegetable products, regardless of fat content or saturation, do not. Table 5-2 lists the major sources of cholesterol.

The body needs cholesterol for brain and organ functions. The liver manufactures enough cholesterol daily to meet these needs. As a result, there is no dietary *need* for cholesterol.

For some people, too much cholesterol in the diet, when combined with other factors, may play a role in the development of *atherosclerosis.* The word "atherosclerosis" means that deposits of cholesterol have accumulated on the walls of the blood vessels. The walls become thicker and the passage becomes narrower. If the passage closes altogether, the person may have a heart attack or a stroke, and may die. Many doctors recommend a diet low in high cholesterol foods and high fat foods as part of their treatment for this condition.

---

* Fish oils are also high in a certain type of fatty acid called omega-3-fatty acid. This is the subject of much research and may actually be beneficial.[5]

LIPIDS IN DIGESTION

It is in the stomach that digestion of lipids begins. There, they are broken down, and fatty acids break off from their glycerol backbone. Complex lipids break down into diglycerides and triglycerides.

Fats remain in the stomach up to 3 1/2 hours after they are ingested (eaten). This is longer than carbohydrates and proteins remain in the stomach and may be why a meal containing some fat will satisfy hunger to a greater degree than will a fat-free meal.

While the pancreas manufactures the enzymes that break down carbohydrate, it is primarily the gallbladder that works on fat. The gallbladder manufactures bile, a yellow liquid that uses the same "channel" (the common bile duct) as the pancreatic enzymes to travel into the small intestine. Bile helps break down fat into small particles that can be easily absorbed. The pancreas and intestines also manufacture an enzyme, lipase, that helps break down lipids into their basic forms. Then they are all absorbed into the walls of the small intestine.

Short- and medium-chain fatty acids go directly into the blood and are carried to the liver through the portal vein. All other fatty acids are changed into a form in which they can be carried through the blood. When these fatty acids first enter the blood, it is in the form of *chylomicrons.* After the chylomicrons have entered the liver, their form is changed to that of more soluble fats such as *lipoproteins, cholesterol,* or *phospholipids.*

LIPIDS IN THE BLOOD

Most lipids are combined with proteins to become lipoproteins as they are carried through the blood. There are several distinct types of lipoproteins, depending on their density. Table 5-3 describes the most important characteristics of their makeup. The largest percentage (ingredient) is circled.

Premenopausal women usually carry a higher percentage of the lipids in their blood as high-density lipoproteins (HDLs) than do men. Persons at high risk for heart disease seem to carry a large fraction of their lipids in the form of

TABLE 5-3

Content of the Different Lipoproteins

Lipoprotein Type	% Make-up			
	Triglyceride	*Cholesterol*	*Phospholipid*	*Protein*
Chylomicrons	85	2–5	3–6	0.5–1
Very low-density lipoproteins (VLDL)	50–70	10–20	10–20	5–15
Low-density lipoproteins (LDL)	5–10	40–45	20–25	25
High-density lipoproteins (HDL)	2	18	30	45–55

Reproduced by permission from Thiele VF: Clinical Nutrition, 2nd ed, p 119. St. Louis: CV Mosby, 1980

low-density lipoproteins (LDLs). Regular aerobic exercise appears to change the way the blood carries lipids; the change results in lower LDL levels and higher HDL levels. This is one of several reasons why some medical authorities suggest that regular aerobic exercise may help prevent heart disease.

Triglycerides are another fat fraction that may cause health problems when they are found in excess in the blood. Dietary control goes beyond just exercise and limiting fat in the diet. Since blood lipids can be made from excessive intake of carbohydrates, and even alcohol as well as fat, treatment for high triglyceride levels may include diets low in simple sugars and alcohol.

LIPIDS IN STORAGE AND ENERGY

Fat is the storage form of energy in the body. If extra carbohydrate or protein is consumed, it turns into fat and is stored for later use. Then, when the body needs energy but cannot get it from food, the extra fat stores are burned instead. It does not matter from what form of food the fat stores originally came. They are all used or burned up by the same processes and there is only one way to get rid of them: energy needs must be greater than energy available in food.

Some fat is used for energy before it even reaches the cells. Some fat is used to maintain the liver's reserve energy stores of glycogen. The rest goes to the fat cells for storage.

All through the body there are pockets of "adipose cells" that specifically store fat. Their actual number is probably determined early in life and does not change with age. These cells change only in size, depending on the amount of fat to be stored. "Subcutaneous fat" is the fat stored beneath the surface of the skin. This fat

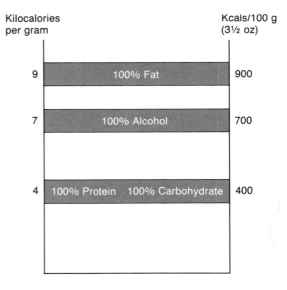

Figure 5-4
Food sources of energy, compared.

also acts as a protective "cushion" for the body. Fat called "cellulite" is nothing more or less than fat-filled adipose cells that are visible because they are immediately under the skin. They become less visible when the stores of fat are reduced through exercise and diet. There is no secret to "cellulite."

Fat is the most concentrated source of energy and Figure 5-4 illustrates this fact. The same amount of fat has more than twice the calories as carbohydrate or protein. This is why many weight loss diets are low in fat. Cutting down on fat is the easiest, safest way to cut down on calories.

STUDY QUESTIONS

1. List and explain three reasons fats are needed in the diet.

2. What is a typical lipid called?

3. People who have trouble digesting fat can usually digest which of the following?
   - Medium-chain fatty acids
   - Long-chain fatty acids

4. Are the essential fatty acids saturated or polyunsaturated?

5. What does PUFA mean?

6. The polyunsaturated fat and saturated fat content in two margarines is as follows:

	Margarine A	Margarine B
Polyunsaturated	1	4
Saturated	3	2

a. Which margarine is higher in saturated fats?

b. Which margarine is more likely to be recommended for someone who has had a heart attack?

7. In the normal diet, what percentage of calories should come from dietary lipids?

8. List all the foods you ate yesterday. Circle those that had any fat in or on them. Was it saturated or polyunsaturated?

9. Cholesterol is found in:
   - Peanut butter
   - Margarine
   - Coconut or palm oil
   - Avocados
   - All of the above
   - None of the above

10. What part of the body breaks down fat?

11. List four types of fat that may be found in the blood.

REFERENCES

1. Report of Intersociety Commission for Heart Disease Resources: Optimal Resources for Primary Prevention of Atherosclerotic Diseases. Circulation 70:191A, July 1984

2. Goodhart RS, Shils ME: Modern Nutrition in Health and Disease, 6th ed, p 134. Philadelphia, Lea & Febiger, 1980

3. Lawrence RA: Breastfeeding: A Guide for the Medical Profession, p 49. St. Louis, CV Mosby, 1980

4. National Fisheries Education and Resource Foundation, 1981

5. Glomset JA: Fish, fatty acids and human health. N Engl J Med 312:1253, May 9, 1985

CHAPTER 6

Fat-Soluble Vitamins

OBJECTIVES

1. To introduce and discuss the use and abuse of vitamins and minerals
2. To reinforce the importance of food as the major source of all vitamins and minerals
3. To introduce the fat-soluble vitamins: A, D, E, and K
4. To discuss briefly for each of the fat-soluble vitamins:
   a. Their importance in nutrition
   b. Their availability in food
   c. Symptoms of deficiency
   d. Potential for overdose
   e. Symptoms and dangers of overdoses
   f. Five major common food sources
5. To provide a list of the Recommended Dietary Allowances for each of these vitamins

Over the last few decades *vitamins* and *minerals* have all too often been promoted as the "common man's cure." Vitamins have been recommended to cure everything from chronic, debilitating diseases to impotency. The large amounts of each vitamin that are available in most stores may sometime be dangerous. This is especially true when some persons feel that if one vitamin is good, several vitamins must be even better.

It is true that vitamins and minerals are very important. But when the dosage is much higher than necessary, and the vitamins are taken in these doses without a doctor's specific recommendation, they are being abused. Vitamins and minerals should never be used as over-the-counter drugs for self-diagnosed illnesses. For one thing, they are not drugs. High doses may or may not be dangerous, but vitamins and minerals are nutrients, not medicine. The safest way to take vitamins in the small amounts the body needs is by eating them in foods. Even if the doctor does recommend vitamins or minerals, they should never take the place of foods, the "natural" sources of these nutrients, unless for some reason (e. g., lactose intolerance) the body cannot tolerate the major food sources of a vitamin or mineral.

Vitamins and minerals are used as "co-enzymes" in the body. That is, tiny bits of them are needed here and there to assist the body in its many functions. Each vitamin plays certain unique roles and each is needed only in very, very small amounts. The recommended amounts listed here, in fact, are already greater than many people need. Since each person varies in his physical makeup, needs may vary too. The RDAs have been developed to allow for almost all of these differences in healthy individuals. The amounts suggested by the RDAs are safe amounts. Higher amounts may or may not be safe, depending on the vitamin and on the individual.

There are 13 vitamins that we know man needs. Four are carried in fat. The rest are water soluble. *Fat-soluble* vitamins will be considered in this chapter. The *water-soluble* vitamins will be discussed in the next chapter.

The fat-soluble vitamins are A, D, E, and K. Because they are fat soluble, they are stored in the fat cells of the body. If the amount of a vitamin taken exceeds that which is needed, the extra amount is stored. As stores build up, especially stores of vitamins A and D, serious problems can develop. This is why it is not a good idea to take more than the recommended amount of these vitamins.

VITAMIN A

Vitamin A is absorbed from food in the duodenum and jejunum of the small intestine. It helps to maintain the health of the fatty membranes lining the body, including the mucous membranes of the gastrointestinal tract and the skin. Vitamin A is also part of the pigment (or coloring) that helps the eye to readjust to darkness after exposure to bright lights. Temporary deficiencies of vitamin A in Americans have led to *night blindness.* Long-term deficiencies, which occur frequently in the Third World when there is no vitamin A in the diet, lead to dry membranes, potential infection and eventually blindness. This is common today in South Asia and East Asia.[1]

Carotene, a chemical pigment in plants (which gives carrots their color), converts to vitamin A in the body. This is one dietary source of vitamin A. The other major source is retinol, the form of vitamin A found in animal products.

Both adults and children can overdose on this vitamin. Prolonged intake of 3000 Retinol Equivalents (RE), which equals 10,000 International Units, or IU, in children or 15,000 RE (equalling 25,000 IU) in adults daily may lead to toxic symptoms. Signs of vitamin A poisoning include headache (the most common symptom), fatigue, hair loss, skin lesions, joint and bone pain, irritability, and spleen and liver enlargement.

See Table 6-1 for the Recommended Dietary Allowances of vitamin A.

Five major common sources of vitamin A include beef liver, cantaloupe, carrots, sweet potatoes, and green leafy vegetables. One half of a large baked sweet potato contains all the vitamin A most adults need daily.

VITAMIN D

Cholecalciferol, or vitamin D, is absorbed in the distal (or lower) duodenum and proximal (or upper) jejunum. It is sometimes called a *hormone* or the sunshine vitamin. This is because the body can usually manufacture all of this vitamin it needs if exposed to enough sunlight. If sufficient vitamin D is not available to them, bones cannot harden or "calcify" properly. They become soft, cannot hold the body's weight without bending, and become infected easily. Teeth may rot more readily. *Rickets* in children and *osteomalacia* (a condition marked by softening of the bone) in adults is primarily due to a deficiency in this vitamin. Smog, smoke, dust, dark city streets, shade, clothing, extremely black skin color, and a largely indoor lifestyle are some of the factors that may prevent vitamin D absorption from the sun. These factors may lead to a deficiency unless vitamin D is found elsewhere in the person's diet.

Few foods contain natural vitamin D. Therefore some foods, such as milk, have been fortified. Milk is fortified so that one quart will provide 400 International Units (IU) of vitamin D or 10 micrograms (μg); 1 IU equals 0.025 μg of cholecalciferol. In addition, certain chemical sterols in plants and animal tissues are "precursors" of D. They help to manufacture it in the body.

Too much vitamin D can be toxic, since it is stored in fat cells. Overdoses of vitamin D usually result from supplemental capsules, not from food. Excess amounts build up in the body over time. Symptoms of toxicity may include nausea, vomiting, diarrhea, polyuria (excess urination), headaches, and renal (kidney) damage. Soft tissues, such as the heart, blood vessels, lungs, and stomach may harden. This is a result of too much calcium, which has been manufactured as a result of too much vitamin D. These symptoms have been reported to occur after a prolonged intake in an adult of over 2000 IU per day.

Occasionally, medical personnel may recommend vitamin D for certain conditions, and pa-

Table 6-1

Recommended Dietary Allowances of Fat-Soluble Vitamins

Age Group	Vitamin A (REs)[*]	Vitamin D (μg)[†]	Vitamin E (IU)[‡]	Vitamin K (μg)[§]
Infants				
0–6 mo	420	10	30	12
6–12 mo	400	10	40	10–20
Children				
1–3	400	10	50	15–30
4–6	500	10	60	20–40
7–10	700	10	70	30–60
Males				
11–14	1000	10	80	50–100
15–18	1000	10	100	50–100
19–22	1000	7.5	100	50–100
23–50	1000	5	100	70–140
Females				
11–14	800	10	80	50–100
15–18	800	10	80	50–100
19–22	800	7.5	80	50–100
23–50	800	5	80	70–140
Adults over 51	800	5	80	70–140
Pregnant women	Plus 200	Plus 5	Plus 20	No change
Lactating women	Plus 400	Plus 5	Plus 30	No change

[*]Retinol Equivalents. To determine approximate International Units, multiply RE by 3⅓.

[†]Micrograms. To determine approximate International Units, multiply μg by 40.

[‡]Vitamin E is more accurately described in terms of mg of the alpha form of tocopherol. To determine this, divide IU by 10.

[§]There is no RDA established for vitamin K. These figures are those estimated to be safe and adequate daily amounts. (From Food and Nutrition Board, National Academy of Sciences: Recommended Dietary Allowances, 9th ed. Washington, National Research Council, 1980)

tients should be warned of the toxic effects that could develop from high doses over time.

Five major common sources of vitamin D are sardines, cod liver oil, fresh water fish, fortified milk, and chicken livers. With the exception of milk, these are all natural sources of vitamin D. One half teaspoon of cod liver oil or two cups of vitamin D-fortified milk provide all the vitamin D an average adult needs daily.

VITAMIN E

A general term for several different forms of *tocopherol,* vitamin E is a vitamin less well understood than A or D. It is also fat soluble and is stored by the tissues. There are different forms of vitamin E and some forms are more "active" or potent than others.

Tocopherols seem to help stabilize the chemical makeup of the cell membrane. This stabilizing quality is demonstrated mainly by an ability to protect the cell from damage that potentially could be caused by too much oxygen. What this means for nutrition is not clear. But the vitamin is essential for good health.

Vitamin E is widely available in foods, so a deficiency is unlikely, although it can easily be lost in processing and in foods that are frozen. Oils are naturally high in E, but if the oil becomes rancid, the vitamin is destroyed. So oils should be kept in a cool place to help preserve their E content.

Hard to get deficiency

Overdoses can occur with a chronic intake of over 300 mg per day. Symptoms of toxicity include inadequate absorption of vitamin K, hemorrhage, diarrhea, high urine creatine levels, blurred vision, headaches, nausea, giddiness and, possibly, lowered gonadal function.

Five major common sources of vitamin E are nuts, seeds, wheat germ, vegetable oil, and fresh spinach. One and one half tablespoons of sunflower oil contain all the vitamin E an average adult needs each day.

VITAMIN K

Normally, bacteria in the gut (intestines) produce at least half the vitamin K needed by the normal person. Vitamin K is needed to help manufacture prothrombin. Prothrombin is essential to ensure proper blood clotting. Patients who hemorrhage may frequently receive medications containing vitamin K. Because it plays such an important role, an excessive intake can be very dangerous.

The vitamin is found in many foods, which usually provide all that is needed to meet the body's small requirement. However, premature infants whose gut is still sterile (contains no bacteria) are at risk of vitamin K deficiency. The greatest source of vitamin K is tobacco, but the vitamin is not well absorbed in smoke — only by those who chew tobacco!

Toxicity of this vitamin can occur since it, too, is fat soluble and stored by the tissues. Overdose can result in hyperbilirubinemia (which may result in jaundice) in infants, kernicterus (affecting the brain and spinal cord), jaundice, and mild hemolytic anemia.

Five major common sources of vitamin K (besides tobacco) are turnip greens, broccoli, lettuce, beef liver, and cabbage.

STUDY QUESTIONS

1. When may vitamins be dangerous?
2. Why are vitamins important?
3. What are the fat-soluble vitamins? What does "fat soluble" mean?
4. What does vitamin A do?
5. Describe two common results of vitamin A deficiency?
6. How much vitamin A does an adult, age 23–50, need?
7. What diseases are results of vitamin D deficiency?
8. What happens if a person takes too much vitamin D over a long period of time.
9. List three foods high in vitamin D.
10. Why is vitamin E important?
11. List four foods high in vitamin E.
12. What does vitamin K do?
13. List two foods high in vitamin K.

REFERENCES

1. Dwyer JT: International Aspects of Community and Public Health Nutrition, p 20. Boston, Frances Stern Nutrition Center, Tufts New England Medical Center, 1979

SUGGESTED READING

Sources and further references for information on vitamins and minerals include:

Kreutler P: Nutrition in Perspective, pp 226–357. Englewood Cliffs, NJ, Prentice–Hall, 1980

Marshall CW: Vitamins and Minerals: Help or Harm? Philadelphia, George F. Stickley 1985.

Food and Nutrition Board, National Academy of Sciences: Recommended Dietary Allowances, 9th ed. Washington, National Research Council, 1980

Roverton L et al: Laurel's Kitchen, pp 396–438. Petaluma, CA, Nilgiri Press, 1976

Brody J: Jane Brody's Nutrition Book. New York, Bantam Books, 1981

CHAPTER 7

Water-Soluble Vitamins

OBJECTIVES

1. To explain the differences between fat- and water-soluble vitamins
2. To introduce and name all of the water-soluble vitamins
3. To reinforce the importance of food as the major source of all vitamins
4. To discuss briefly, for each of the water-soluble vitamins:
   a. Its importance in nutrition
   b. Its availability in food
   c. Symptoms of deficiency
   d. Symptoms and dangers of overdoses
   e. Five major common food sources
5. To provide a list of the Recommended Dietary Allowances for each of these vitamins.

There are many more vitamins that are water soluble than there are fat-soluble vitamins. Most of them are members of the "B complex," that is, they have a designated number (B_1, B_2, B_3, B_6, B_{12}) in addition to their proper names. The numbers originated in the early days of vitamin research, when it was thought that there was one "B" vitamin. When several independent vitamins were determined to be part of "vitamin B," they were given numbers. Then, some of the numbered parts were discovered not to be vitamins at all. Today only the five listed above are accepted as genuine B vitamins, necessary for survival.

Besides the B vitamins, the other water-soluble vitamins include vitamin C, pantothenic acid, biotin and folacin (or folic acid).

In general, water-soluble vitamins are not as *toxic* as fat-soluble vitamins. They are readily excreted from the body and so stores do not build up to quite as dangerous a level. If taken in very large doses, some can have "bad" effects, but such doses are unlikely when food is the major source of these vitamins. Fat-soluble vitamins require at least a little fat in the diet in order to be absorbed properly. Water-soluble vitamins are not as dependent on dietary fat for proper utilization.

In this chapter, we will look at each of the water-soluble vitamins, and their major food sources.

THIAMIN

Thiamin, or vitamin B_1, is needed to metabolize carbohydrate properly. Thiamin deficiency is called *beriberi*. It is not a common disease and occurs most frequently in alcoholics and in kidney patients.[1] Symptoms of beriberi include fatigue, irritability, weight loss, atonic constipation, muscle cramps, nerve pains, and a weak, heavy feeling in the legs that can lead to paralysis. The cardiovascular, nervous, and gastrointestinal systems are all affected by beriberi.

This vitamin is easily lost from food by heat, prolonged cooking, or when baking soda has been added to the food. When foods high in thiamin are cooked in water, the vitamin may be lost in the water. Flour and many grain products are enriched with thiamin.

A thiamin toxicity is unlikely, since excess amounts are usually lost in the urine before any damage is done.

Thiamin is absorbed from the gastrointestinal tract into the blood along the jejunum and the proximal (or upper) ileum.

Five major common food sources of thiamin include whole wheat flour, cooked dry beans, pork chops, ham, and sunflower seeds. Five ounces of lean pork or 1 tablespoon of brewer's yeast contain all the thiamin an average adult needs daily.

Table 7-1 lists the Recommended Dietary Allowance (RDA) for thiamin and the other water-soluble vitamins.

Table 7-1

Recommended Dietary Allowances of the Water-Soluble Vitamins

Age Group	Thiamin (mg)	Riboflavin (mg)	Niacin (mg NE)	Vit. B_6 (mg)	Folacin (μg)	Vit. B_{12} (μg)	Vit. C (mg)	Pantothenate* (mg)	Biotin* (μg)
Infants									
0–6 mo	0.3	0.4	6	0.3	30	0.5	35	2	35
7–12 mo	0.5	0.6	8	0.6	45	1.5	35	3	50
Children									
1–3	0.7	0.8	9	0.9	100	2.0	45	3	65
4–6	0.9	1.0	11	1.3	200	2.5	45	3–4	85
7–10	1.2	1.4	16	1.6	300	3.0	45	4–5	120
Males									
11–14	1.4	1.6	18	1.8	400	3.0	50	4–7	100–200
15–18	1.4	1.7	18	2.0	400	3.0	60	4–7	100–200
19–22	1.5	1.7	19	2.2	400	3.0	60	4–7	100–200
23–50	1.4	1.6	18	2.2	400	3.0	60	4–7	100–200
51 and over	1.2	1.4	16	2.2	400	3.0	60	4–7	100–200
Females									
11–14	1.1	1.3	15	1.8	400	3.0	50	4–7	100–200
15–18	1.1	1.3	14	2.0	400	3.0	60	4–7	100–200
19–22	1.1	1.3	14	2.0	400	3.0	60	4–7	100–200
23–50	1.0	1.2	13	2.0	400	3.0	60	4–7	100–200
51 and over	1.0	1.2	13	2.0	400	3.0	60	4–7	100–200
Pregnant	+ 0.4	+ 0.3	+ 2	+ 0.6	+ 400	+ 1.0	+ 20	Same	Same
Lactating	+ 0.5	+ 0.5	+ 5	+ 0.5	+ 100	+ 1.0	+40	Same	Same

* These two vitamins do not have an RDA. The amounts listed here are estimated safe and adequate daily amounts. (From Food and Nutrition Board, National Academy of Sciences: Recommended Dietary Allowances, 9th ed. Washington, National Research Council, 1980)

Needed to break down protein

RIBOFLAVIN

Riboflavin, or B_2, is also needed to metabolize foods properly. It is a component of several enzymes and is used extensively by the body. *Cheilosis,* or cracking and sores at the corner of the mouth, are the key symptoms of deficiency.

Light destroys riboflavin easily. Milk products are a major source of the vitamin and, when exposed to light for several hours, such products may lose some of their riboflavin content. Foods enriched with thiamin are usually enriched with riboflavin, as well as niacin.

Riboflavin, like thiamin, is absorbed in the jejunum and proximal ileum.

Five major common food sources of riboflavin include milk products, calves' liver, kidneys, yeast, and fortified cereals. Three cups of milk or as little as one ounce of liver contain all the riboflavin an adult needs daily.

Light destroys Rib

NIACIN

"B_3," or niacin, is another vitamin that is rarely found to be deficient in the diet today. Like riboflavin, niacin is a co-enzyme, or partner to the enzymes, involved in most metabolic processes in the body.

Cooking does not destroy niacin, although the vitamin can partially dissolve, so that some might be lost in cooking water. A severe deficiency can lead to *pellagra.* This disease is more common in South America today than in North America, because the South American diet consists largely of corn and beans that have not been fortified with niacin. While corn and beans contain some of the vitamin, it is not in a form that can be easily utilized by the body. Also, the diet in South America may be low in the amino acid, tryptophan. The latter is plentiful in animal products and can convert (in the body) to niacin. Sixty milligrams (mg) of tryptophan convert to 1.0 mg of niacin or 1 Niacin Equivalent (NE).

Niacin is one water-soluble vitamin that can be toxic in high doses. A dosage of 3000 mg (which equals 3 grams) per day or more has been known to cause dilated blood vessels (with the skin becoming very warm and red), cardiac arrhythmias, increased uric acid levels, and an increased use of muscle glycogen stores.

Niacin is absorbed in the body at the jejunum and proximal ileum.

Five major common food sources of this vitamin include tofu (soybean curd), cooked dry beans, cottage cheese, steak, and chicken. Five ounces of tofu or chicken provide all the niacin an average adult needs daily.

PANTOTHENIC ACID

Widely available in food, this vitamin is stable in heat and was originally called B_3. It is found in every cell of the body and is vital for human metabolism. A deficiency is rare and usually occurs only when the diet is so poor that other vitamin deficiencies also become evident. Milling and freezing foods can result in lower pantothenic acid content than in corresponding fresh foods.

Deficiencies in rats (experimentally) have caused gray hair, but pantothenic acid in food or supplements for humans does not prevent hair from turning gray, contrary to some popular misconceptions.

This vitamin is absorbed in the jejunum and proximal ileum.

Five major common food sources of pantothenic acid include beef liver, eggs, mushrooms, chicken, and milk products. Three ounces of liver or four cups of milk fulfill all the average adult's daily needs.

VITAMIN B_6

Three different chemical substances — *pyridoxine, pyridoxal* and *pyridoxamine* — are the components of vitamin B_6. It is commonly called pyridoxine. B_6 is extremely important in protein metabolism, helping to convert tryptophan to niacin. Because of this relationship to protein, the body's need for B_6 depends on how much protein is in the normal diet.

Food processing easily destroys this vitamin. Brown rice and whole wheat flour contain much more natural B_6 than do polished rice or refined white flour. The vitamin is stable in heat but easily destroyed by light.

A deficiency of vitamin B_6 may resemble a niacin or riboflavin deficiency. Usually, a B_6

[handwritten: Pyridoxine - never give to someone who has Perkens diese]

deficiency occurs only with other vitamin deficiencies. Symptoms of such a deficiency include anemia, dizziness, irritability, confusion, kidney stones, and convulsions.

Women taking oral contraceptives may need extra vitamin B_6 in their diets. However, recent studies have been inconclusive, so there may be no reason for high levels of B_6 supplements. In addition, there have been significant side-effects to doses of vitamin B_6 greater than 200 mg per day, leading to peripheral neuropathy (difficulty feeling sensation in the hands and feet).[1]

Individuals receiving isoniazid (INH) as part of the treatment for tuberculosis may become deficient in vitamin B_6.

Five major common food sources of vitamin B_6 include bananas, spinach, avocados, cooked dry beans, and beef. An average adult may need to eat 1 pound of raw or cooked spinach, or 2 to 3 cups of cooked beans to obtain the RDA. This may indicate that most persons can function quite well on less than the RDA.

FOLACIN

[handwritten: Large Intestine]

Folacin may also be called "folic acid," "folate" or "pteroylglutamic acid," and is produced by bacteria that normally live in the gut (intestine). *[handwritten: LI]* It is needed in the diet because the bacteria cannot naturally produce enough for all needs.

Folacin helps synthesize (or make) and metabolize proteins. Because growth always involves protein, rapidly growing tissues may be harmed if the body is deficient in this vitamin. Since pregnancy places great growth demands on the body, pregnant women need twice the amount of folacin that nonpregnant women require.

Symptoms of folate deficiency include *macrocytic anemia,* diarrhea, and glossitis. Macrocytic anemia occurs when the young red blood cells (also called RBC or megaloblasts) are too large, too few, and are not carrying enough hemoglobin.

If a person is taking folate supplements and is also deficient in vitamin B_{12} (that is, he is developing pernicious anemia), he may not have any symptoms of pernicious anemia until it becomes severe, since folate supplementation masks, or hides, B_{12} deficiency.

[handwritten: Cemotherpy Need Folic A.]

Folate is absorbed in the jejunum and proximal ileum.

Five major common food sources of folate include beef liver, asparagus, green, leafy vegetables, orange juice, and dry cooked beans. Vegetables containing folate should be refrigerated to prevent loss of the vitamin. *[handwritten: lettuce, Whole wheat, spinach, lims bean, brol, Apples]*

VITAMIN B$_{12}$

Also known as *cobalamin,* vitamin B_{12} must be manufactured by fungi or bacteria, so it is only available in animal products or foodstuffs that have a bacterial culture. It is a co-enzyme for many metabolic functions and is stored very effectively by the body. When deficiencies *do* occur, which is rare, they take 3 or 4 years to develop, since it usually takes that long for the body to use up all its stores of vitamin B_{12}.

B_{12} is absorbed in the distal (or lower) ileum. In this part of the gut, there is a substance (called *intrinsic factor)* in the gastric secretions that is necessary for the absorption of B_{12}. When intrinsic factor is missing and B_{12} in food is not absorbed, the disease that results is called *pernicious anemia.* Old people frequently lose the ability to produce intrinsic factor, and the only effective treatment is B_{12} injections. These are usually given IM, that is, intramuscularly. These injections must be given on a regular basis.

If intrinsic factor is present, B_{12} deficiency is extremely unlikely. It has been known to occur in *vegans* (vegetarians who eat no animal products at all). Children who are raised from birth as vegans may be at a high risk of developing B_{12} deficiency unless their parents make a conscientious effort to plan menus containing certain foods. Most of the common soy-based infant formulas contain B_{12} supplement. Other sources of B_{12} for the vegan include B_{12}-fortified soy milk, yeast or soy products that have been grown or cultured in a B_{12}-rich medium, and vitamin B_{12} supplements. Regular yeast and most commercial soy milk contain no B_{12}.

Five common major food sources of this vitamin include fish, beef, lamb, milk, and egg yolk. Three and one half ounces of tuna or one and one half cups of cottage cheese contain all the B_{12} an average adult needs daily.

BIOTIN

Working together with other nutrients, biotin helps manufacture energy in the body.

Biotin is an extremely stable vitamin and no toxicity has ever been documented. The only practice that may cause biotin deficiency is the ingestion of a great amount of raw egg white. A protein in the egg white called *avidin* "binds" the vitamin so it cannot be absorbed by the gut.

Biotin is normally absorbed in the jejunum and proximal ileum.

Bacteria in the gut probably make all of the biotin required, but many foods also contain this vitamin. Five major common food sources of biotin include beef liver, oatmeal, clams, soybeans, and milk.

VITAMIN C

Bacteria is more likely to destroy than produce vitamin C, or *ascorbic acid,* so it must come from the diet. Vitamin C has many roles. It helps maintain the connective tissues; it helps increase absorption of iron and calcium from foods; it enhances red blood cell production in the bone marrow, and the production of the amino acids, phenylalanine and tyrosine. The body requires vitamin C for all these functions. But only 60 mg to 80 mg — or less — are necessary to meet the body's daily needs. This amount, the RDA, is much less than the amount commonly ingested. Refer to Table 7-1 in order to see just how much (or how little) vitamin C is actually needed by different categories of persons.

Ascorbic acid is the most easily destroyed vitamin, although proper processing can help preserve it. Acid foods, such as orange and lemon juices, retain the vitamin more successfully than other foods. The vitamin C in these products is a strong antioxidant, that is, it prevents oxidation or chemical changes produced by oxygen. When lemon juice is added to sliced apples, for example, it prevents them from turning brown.

Leaving cans or bottles open and/or unrefrigerated can result in a loss of vitamin C.

The role of ascorbic acid in preventing colds is still controversial, but it has never been substantially proved to do so. There is some inconclusive evidence that it may help shorten the length of a cold. Over a period of time overdoses can lead to kidney stones and gout in susceptible individuals. Overdoses may also lead to a burning sensation during urination and may confound urine tests of diabetics who take large amounts of the vitamin. Because the evidence is not all in, prolonged intake of more than the RDA of vitamin C is not recommended.

Vitamin C deficiency results in a disease called *scurvy.* Infants whose mothers had taken large amounts of this vitamin during their pregnancy have been known to have symptoms of "rebound scurvy" after birth, when they were no longer receiving the high doses of ascorbic acid. Symptoms of scurvy include bleeding gums, joint pain, and listlessness. Vitamin C is absorbed in the jejunum and distal ileum.

One small orange, one half cup of orange juice or one sweet green or red pepper provides all the vitamin C an average adult needs daily.

Common food sources include cranberries, kiwi fruit, other citrus fruits, broccoli, red and green peppers, and rose hips.

STUDY QUESTIONS

1. What are two ways in which water-soluble vitamins differ from fat-soluble vitamins?

2. Which three vitamins are usually added to enrich foods?

3. What foods are high in riboflavin?

4. Why may pellagra occur in South American countries?

5. Mushrooms are high in what vitamin?

6. What vitamin deficiency may occur in a person on INH (a drug used in tuberculosis treatment)? List three foods high in this vitamin.

7. What vitamin is especially important for pregnant women? What foods are high in this vitamin?

8. Describe two situations where a B_{12} deficiency might occur. In which situation can foods high in vitamin B_{12} help correct the deficiency? What foods would help?

9. A three-year-old who has pneumonia is being cared for by her grandmother. The caretaker thinks eggnog is good for any sickness, so she makes three or four large eggnogs each day for the child, using uncooked eggs. What vitamin deficiency could occur if this diet is continued for a long time?
10. List six foods high in vitamin C.

REFERENCES

1. Berger A, Schaumburg HH: More on neuropathy from pyridoxine abuse. Letter. N Engl J Med 311:986, October 11, 1984
2. Marshall CW: Vitamins and Minerals: Help or Harm?, p 87. Philadelphia, George F. Stickley, 1985

SUGGESTED READING

Sources and further references for information on vitamins and minerals include:

Brody J: Jane Brody's Nutrition Book. New York, Bantam Books, 1981

Food and Nutrition Board, National Academy of Sciences: Recommended Dietary Allowances, 9th ed. Washington, National Research Council, 1980

Kreutler P: Nutrition in Perspective, pp 226–357. Englewood Cliffs, NJ, Prentice–Hall, 1980

Roverton L et al: Laurel's Kitchen, pp 396–438. Petaluma, CA, Nilgiri Press, 1976

CHAPTER 8

Minerals and Trace Elements

OBJECTIVES

1. To identify the minerals and trace elements required in human nutrition
2. To introduce briefly those nutritional factors that affect good absorption of these elements
3. To discuss the minerals for which there is a Recommended Dietary Allowance, that is, calcium, phosphorus, magnesium, iron, zinc, and iodine, and to identify for each
   a. Its importance
   b. Likelihood and results of deficiency
   c. Likelihood and results of toxicity
   d. Its RDA
   e. Five major, common food sources
4. To discuss the minerals for which there is no established RDA, that is, copper, manganese, fluoride, chromium, selenium, and molybdenum, identifying for each:
   a. Known reasons for dietary need
   b. Likelihood and results of deficiency
   c. Likelihood and results of toxicity
   d. Estimated safe and adequate daily intake
   e. Sources for human nutrition

Minerals, like vitamins, are needed in small amounts for good health. Like vitamins, they play many roles in the body. And, as in the case of the fat-soluble vitamins, the body may not be able to rid itself of a high dose, so the minerals could build up in the body and cause serious problems.

In other ways, though, minerals are very different from vitamins. Their structure is much simpler; they originally come from the soil and are not destroyed by heat, light, or oxygen, and bacteria cannot manufacture them.

By nature, a mineral contains a "charge" within it. That is, each mineral has a positive or negative force that draws other elements to it, to combine with it. Minerals may combine with many other elements. Sometimes the elements attached to a mineral are in a combination that makes the whole complex indigestible. In certain forms, the mineral cannot be absorbed through the intestine (gut) into the blood. For instance, calcium may combine to become calcium lactate, calcium carbonate, or calcium gluconate. Calcium carbonate is not absorbed as readily as calcium lactate or calcium gluconate.

Minerals are usually carried in foods in this type of molecular combination. For example, many foods contain calcium in yet another form, calcium oxalate, and this form cannot be absorbed at all. _Oxalate_ is a substance naturally present in certain foods and calcium is naturally combined with it, but because the oxalate cannot be absorbed, all the calcium bound to the oxalate is excreted. Substances similar to oxalates are _phytates_. Phytates also are naturally present in some foods and inhibit mineral absorption. Listed opposite are those foods high in oxalates and those containing phytates.

It is important to remember that many of

FOOD SOURCES OF OXALATES AND PHYTATES*

Oxalates
Very High (over 100 mg/100 g)

Beets, boiled (109)
Cocoa, dry (623)
Coffee, instant dry powder (143)

Rhubarb, raw (537)
Rhubarb, stewed (447)
Spinach, boiled (571)

High (10–99 mg/100 g)

Beans, green, raw (43.7)
Beans, green, boiled (29.7)
Beets, raw (72.2)
Blackberries, raw (12.4)
Bread, whole wheat (20.9)

Carrots, boiled (14.5)
Gooseberries, raw (19.3)
Ovaltine powder (45.9)
Plums, raw (11.9)
Tea, brewed (12.5)

Low (2–10mg/100g)

Apples
Asparagus
Bananas
Beef
Blueberries
Butter
Cabbage
Cauliflower
Chicken
Chives
Coffee, brewed
Cucumbers
Eggs
Fish
Lamb

Leek
Lemon juice
Milk
Orange juice
Peaches
Pears, canned
Peas, green
Pepper, green
Pineapple, canned
Pork
Potato
Pumpkin
Radish
Rutabaga
Salsify

Phytates
Very High (over 900 mg/100 g)

All-Bran cereal (2425)
Almonds (1280)
Barley (970)
Brazil nuts (1799)
Bread, rye (940)
Flour, rye (919)
Grain, rye (970)
Gram beans, black, raw (1460)

Milo (990)
Oats, raw (943)
Peanut butter (1250)
Sesame seeds, raw (4710)
Soybeans, raw (1000–1470)
Wheat germ (4066)
Wheat, shredded (1482)
Wild rice, raw (2200)

High (500–899 mg/100 g)

Bran, crude wheat (843)
Corn, raw (890)

Corn chips (636)
Cornmeal (610)

(continued)

Flour, soy (660–705)
Flour, whole wheat (845)
Granola (625)
Gram beans, green, raw (660)
Hazelnuts (604)
Lima beans, raw (890)

Millet (750)
Navy beans, raw (615)
Peanuts (748)
Peas, split, raw (546)
Rice, brown, raw (890)
Walnuts (760)

Low (20 mg/100 g)

Broad beans, boiled
Blackberries, raw
Carrots

Coffee, brewed
Farina, cooked
Tomatoes, raw or canned

* Natural substances that may interfere with the absorption of minerals.
(Bowes and Church: Food Values of Portions Commonly Used, 14th ed. Philadelphia, JB Lippincott, 1985)

these foods also contain essential nutrients that are absorbed, and consequently these foods should be part of the diet, but they should not be used as the major food source for a mineral if they interfere with the absorption of that mineral.

Twelve minerals will be discussed in this chapter. Less than 4% of the body's mass is made of these minerals and, as far as most of them are concerned, only a very small amount is needed to meet the body's needs. Foods are the safest source of these minerals, since toxicities are possible, and can be dangerous.

Six of the minerals have established Recommended Dietary Allowances. These six are calcium, phosphorus, magnesium, iron, zinc, and iodine. They have been researched over many years and in more detail than the other six minerals. They are sufficiently understood so that an RDA was established and is listed in Table 8-1.

The other six, without an established RDA yet known to be necessary for health, include copper, manganese, fluoride, chromium, selenium, and molybdenum. Based on the research that has been done, the National Academy of Sciences has suggested the estimated safe and adequate ranges for them and these figures are listed in Table 8-2.

Sodium, potassium, and chloride are also minerals, but they will be discussed, together with fluid balance, in Chapter 9.

CALCIUM

Calcium is one of the most important factors in making and maintaining healthy bones and teeth, giving them the strength to resist damage. In this role, calcium works together with phosphorus and vitamin D, and the three must always be in balance. Other hormones and nutrients play a role in bone strength, but these three are the most important.

Deficiency in calcium can be a cause of osteoporosis, a common condition that occurs when the bone gradually loses calcium (demineralization) and becomes progressively thinner. It is most common in women who have passed menopause and frequently leads to broken bones at an age when healing is slow. Although each of these diseases differs in some respects, all have as one contributing factor an inadequate intake of calcium.

Calcium is important not only to bones. It is carried in other body fluids to help maintain muscles and nerves. When there is insufficient calcium in the diet, the calcium the body needs is taken from the bones and teeth. So it is apparent that calcium is important for all ages.

While too much vitamin D can lead to calcium deposits in soft tissues such as the heart (a very dangerous situation), there is no reason for a healthy person to worry about getting too much calcium from food. Calcium supplements, however, may be overused and in some forms, such as *dolomite*, may not be safe.

Table 8-1

The Recommended Dietary Allowances of Major Minerals

Mineral:	Calcium (mg)	Phosphorus (mg)	Magnesium (mg)	Iron (mg)	Zinc (mg)	Iodine (μg)*
Infants						
0–6 mo	360	240	50	10	3	40
7–12 mo	540	360	70	15	5	50
Children						
1–3	800	800	150	15	10	70
4–6	800	800	200	10	10	90
7–10	800	800	250	10	10	120
Males						
11–14	1200	1200	350	18	15	150
15–18	1200	1200	400	18	15	150
19–22	800	800	350	10	15	150
23–50	800	800	350	10	15	150
51 and over	800	800	350	10	15	150
Females						
11–14	1200	1200	300	18	15	150
15–18	1200	1200	300	18	15	150
19–22	800	800	300	18	15	150
23–50	800	800	300	18	15	150
51 and over	800	800	300	10	15	150
Pregnant	+400	+400	+150	+30–60	+5	+25
Lactating	+400	+400	+150	+30–60	+10	+50

*1 mg equals 1000 μg

Calcium is absorbed in the duodenum.

Dairy products (milk, buttermilk, cheese, and yogurt) are the best and most digestible sources of calcium. Even then, a teenager (under 19) needs 4 cups a day to meet the RDA. Adults, both men and women, require 3 cups. Other major sources of calcium include collard greens, sardines, salmon, figs, and sesame seeds.

PHOSPHORUS

The RDA for phosphorus is the same as for calcium. Widely used in the body, phosphorus helps carry fatty acids and provides energy. Although there is some phosphorus in every cell in the body, 90% of it is found in the bones and teeth.

A phosphorus deficiency is unlikely, because phosphorus is found in many foods. In fact phytate, or phytic acid, which binds calcium and other minerals so they cannot be used effectively, is a compound made of phosphorus. But these two minerals (phosphorus and calcium) should be present in equal proportions, since too much phosphorus may lead to calcium loss. In addition, the interaction of these two is affected by the quantity of vitamin D available.

As a rule, the seeds and flowers of plants have more phosphorus and the leaves, more calcium. Five major food sources of phosphorus include milk, fish, chicken, beef liver, and cooked dry beans.

MAGNESIUM

About 70% of the magnesium used by the body helps to "mineralize" the bones. The rest of the magnesium works in the muscles, the red blood cells, and also activates enzymes in carbohydrate metabolism.

Table 8-2

Estimated Safe and Adequate Daily Dietary Intakes of Trace Minerals

Mineral:	*Copper (mg)*	*Manganese (mg)*	*Fluoride (mg)*	*Chromium (mg)*	*Selenium (mg)*	*Molybdenum (mg)*
Infants						
0–6 mo	0.5–0.7	0.5–0.7	0.1–0.5	0.01–0.04	0.01–0.04	0.03–0.06
7–12 mo	0.7–1.0	0.7–1.0	0.2–1.0	0.02–0.06	0.02–0.06	0.04–0.08
Children						
1–3	1.0–1.5	1.0–1.5	0.5–1.5	0.02–0.08	0.02–0.08	0.05–0.10
4–6	1.5–2.0	1.5–2.0	1.0–2.5	0.03–0.12	0.03–0.12	0.06–0.15
7–10	2.0–2.5	2.0–3.0	1.5–2.5	0.05–0.20	0.05–0.20	0.10–0.30
Adolescents 11+	2.0–3.0	2.5–5.0	1.5–2.5	0.05–0.20	0.05–0.20	0.15–0.50
Adults	2.0–3.0	2.5–5.0	1.5–4.0	0.05–0.20	0.05–0.20	0.15–0.50

Magnesium deficiencies are very rare. They occur primarily in alcoholics and in the severe protein malnutrition of kwashiorkor. High doses of calcium may interfere with the effective absorption of magnesium.

Magnesium salts are a major ingredient in many laxatives.

Five common food sources for magnesium include cooked dry beans, beet greens, roasted peanuts, avocados, and bananas.

IRON

Iron is an extremely important mineral and is part of the hemoglobin in the blood. It helps carry oxygen from the lungs to the tissues. Lack of oxygen leads to exhaustion and lethargy, common symptoms of iron-deficiency anemia. Iron deficiency is one of the most common dietary deficiencies in the world, most of it due to needs that are higher than intake.[2]

For the premenopausal woman, iron needs are very high. A woman may follow an excellent diet, yet still may lack an adequate supply of iron. There are ways to help increase the absorption of the iron found in the diet. Usually only 10% of the iron in food may be absorbed. Three ways to increase this absorption include (1) eating foods high in vitamin C together with foods whose iron content is high; (2) eating animal protein along with them, or (3) doing both at the same meal. Cooking food in iron skillets and cookware increases the iron content of the food.

Pregnant women and infants need more iron than is usually available in their food. This is why iron supplements are recommended for pregnant women and why iron-fortified formulas are best for the formula-fed infant. (Breast-fed infants are also supplemented. Otherwise he or his counterpart on a noniron infant formula, who is not getting iron in some other form, may use up all the iron stores he had at birth by the age of 6 months.) Iron-deficiency anemia will be discussed in more detail in Chapter 27.

Too much iron in the diet can be dangerous. Iron toxicity is the fourth most common cause of poisoning in children under 5 years of age.[3] Consequently iron supplements should be kept with other medicines out of the reach of children. As with other vitamins and minerals, high iron supplements should only be taken with a physician's approval.

Like calcium and phosphorus, iron is absorbed in the duodenum.

Five major common food sources of iron include fortified cereals, beef liver, blackstrap molasses, red meats, and cooked dry beans.

ZINC

Helping to produce insulin and cell proteins, zinc is important for normal growth and wound healing. It also works to break down food into nutrients and energy, and to carry nutrients throughout the body. Although few supplements with iron also contain zinc, needs for zinc may increase with increased iron intake. High fiber foods can prevent zinc from being well absorbed. Symptoms of zinc deficiency may include taste changes, poor wound healing, poor appetite, and slightly retarded growth in children.

Although zinc supplements do help treat zinc deficiencies, they have no proven benefit when the supply of zinc in the body is adequate. They perform no additional special function and so there is no rationale for taking more than the RDA.

It is almost impossible to get *too much* zinc from food. All foods except oysters contain small amounts of the mineral. However, foods that are acidic and are stored in galvanized containers (that is, containers coated with zinc) can "leech" or drain toxic amounts of the mineral from the metal coating. This process can lead to severe gastrointestinal irritation and vomiting.

The average American diet may be low in zinc. A vegetarian diet may also be low in zinc, since seafood and animal products are the best sources of the mineral. Other major food sources include cooked dry beans, wheat and rice bran, and dairy products.

IODINE

Iodine is very important to the body, since those persons who do not absorb enough iodine over a long period of time may develop a *goiter* (a ring-like mass of flesh around the neck). Infants born to parents deficient in iodine may be "cretins," that is, mentally retarded for life.

Plants growing in soil that has enough iodine will absorb the iodine and become food sources of this mineral . Many areas of the world, including parts of the USA, have soil that is iodine-deficient. *Iodized salt* is salt that has been fortified with iodine and it is the major source of iodine for people in these areas of the world. Iodized salt provides 76 micrograms of iodine per gram of salt. That is about 290 micrograms per teaspoon of salt. One half teaspoon of salt daily is sufficient to meet the iodine needs of most people.

Thyrotoxicosis is the name for a disorder caused by too much iodine. Iodine's most im-

portant role is to help the thyroid gland function properly. Too much iodine affects the thyroid as seriously as too little iodine. The effects of the toxicity depend on the level of iodine. In Japan, too much iodine absorbed from seaweed led to goitrous conditions in a substantial percentage of the population. It has also led to death in experimental animals.

Seafoods and seaweeds are naturally very high in this mineral.

COPPER

A principal function of copper is to help incorporate iron into hemoglobin. Copper imbalances are rare, and generally are genetic imbalances, not related to diet. This deficiency in infants is usually detected early in life.

Copper also plays a role in forming bones and in keeping the lining of the nervous system intact. A copper deficiency due to diet has not been seen in humans.

Oysters, lobster, beef liver, fortified bran cereals, and avocados are five major sources of copper.

MANGANESE

Manganese is a trace mineral that is used as a co-enzyme in several metabolic functions. It is widely available in food and deficiency is extremely rare.

Toxicity usually cannot occur from diet alone. Manganese toxicities have been reported in towns where the mineral was being inhaled as dust during various mining activities.

Five major common food sources of manganese include tea, fruits, rice, spinach, and carrots.

FLUORIDE

Regular fluoride helps prevent tooth decay. Fluoride works together with calcium to make bones thicker and more resistant and there is some indication that it also helps to absorb iron and to heal wounds.

Both deficiency and excess are possible. The most common source of fluoride is *fluoridated water*. Current recommendations suggest that water be fluoridated at 1 part per million in order to provide 1.5 mg to 4 mg of the mineral per person per day. Individuals may learn about the fluoridation of their area water by contacting the local health department. With fluoridation, deficiencies are unlikely, unless a person drinks only bottled or spring water.

Fluorine (or fluoride) is also found in small amounts in many foods. As with iodine, the content varies according to location. Cooking foods in fluoridated water or in Teflon pans increases the fluoride content of the food. Aluminum pans reduce the fluoride content of whatever is cooked in them.

Over 50 mg of fluoride daily can cause mottled teeth and porous, (easily broken) bones; death has occurred with a dosage of over 2500 times the recommended level. Fluoridated water cannot cause toxicity. Its level of fluoride is much too low.

Common food sources of fluoride include tea, seafood, wheat germ, potatoes, and spinach.

CHROMIUM

A trace mineral involved in the metabolism of glucose, chromium in its natural form is known as glucose tolerance factor, or GTF. 10%–25% of this form of chromium is absorbed. However, only 1% of inorganic chromium (that is, the pure mineral or a tablet form) is absorbed. This mineral may play some very small role in certain glucose imbalances but this has not yet been established.

Processing can destroy the chromium content in foods. Some foods high in chromium are those also high in phytate (such as whole grain cereals, wheat germ, and bran), which would consequently interfere with chromium absorption.

Although no exact figures are available, the best dietary sources of chromium appear to be yeast, large amounts of black pepper, beer, beef, and some vegetables.

SELENIUM

Selenium is used to help protect the cells from damage. No human deficiency has ever been established. Those who live in the few parts of the world with levels low in selenium (that is, parts of New Zealand) have low serum levels but are otherwise quite healthy. Selenium is considered an essential nutrient because deficiency can cause harm in animals and thus, potentially, in humans.

Intake over 200 μg (or 0.2 mg) per day is not recommended, since long-term toxicity has been established in animals.

Common sources of selenium include whole wheat products, barley, garlic, oats, and mushrooms.

MOLYBDENUM

Like selenium, molybdenum is a trace element for which no deficiency has ever been established in humans. It works as a co-enzyme. It is more important to avoid taking too much of this element than too little. Toxicity has been established both in humans and in animals. In humans it has occurred among Russians who have worked at mining ore. High doses have led to copper loss. Symptoms of toxicity may include high serum uric acid, as well as high levels of molybdenum and xanthine oxidase in the blood.

Major food sources for this mineral include beef kidneys, natural cereals, buckwheat, lamb chops, and tomato sauce.

STUDY QUESTIONS

1. What, in general, is the function of minerals? Compare them with vitamins.

2. What are two substances in food that could prevent a mineral from being properly utilized by the body?

3. Which six minerals are understood well enough to have an RDA?

4. What happens if a person does not get enough calcium in his diet? What are the best food sources of this mineral?

5. From what mineral is phytate (phytic acid) made?

6. Describe three nutritional ways to help absorb as much iron as possible from foods.

7. Should infants take iron-fortified infant formula if they are not breast-fed? Why or why not?

8. List five foods high in iron.

9. True or false: Zinc supplements (that is, pills) help heal the wounds of a person who receives enough zinc in food to meet normal needs.

10. What problems develop after a long-term iodine deficiency?

11. How much iodized salt is sufficient to provide a healthy person with all the iodine he needs?

12. Why is fluoride important?

REFERENCES

1. Roberts HJ: (Letter) Dolomite as a source of toxic metals. N Engl J Med (304), p 423, 1981
2. Dwyer JT: International Aspects of Community and Public Health Nutrition, p 78. Boston, Frances Stern Nutrition Center, Tufts New England Medical Center, 1979
3. Howe PS: Basic Nutrition in Health and Disease, p 103. Philadelphia, WB Saunders, 1981

SUGGESTED READING

Sources and further references for information on vitamins and minerals include:
Brody J: Jane Brody's Nutrition Book. New York, Bantam Books, 1981
Food and Nutrition Board, National Academy of Sciences: Recommended Dietary Allowances, 9th ed. Washington, National Research Council, 1980
Kreutler P: Nutrition in Perspective, pp 226–357. Englewood Cliffs, NJ, Prentice–Hall, 1980
Marshall CW: Vitamins and Minerals: Help or Harm? Philadelphia, George F. Stickley, 1985

CHAPTER 9

Water and Electrolytes

*Can only live 3 days w/out O_2
to much to little of K can lead to cardac Irrithmics
musck weakness
flu like symp.*

OBJECTIVES

1. To discuss the importance of water and electrolyte balance
2. To explain the compartmentalization and uses of fluids in the body
3. To introduce the electrolytes and their role in fluid balance
4. To explain the role of water and channels of water loss
5. To describe the conserving function of the normal kidney
6. To explain and illustrate normal osmolarity and how it is affected by diet
7. To illustrate and list the normal dietary sources and requirements for water, sodium, potassium, and chloride.

Like vitamins and minerals, water and the *electrolytes* (sodium, potassium and chloride) do not contain any calories. They do not provide any energy. But the body cannot survive without them. In fact, the healthy body could go days or weeks without food energy and months or even years without certain vitamins or minerals before it would die or even show marked deficiencies. But three days is the limit that anyone could go without water.

Water makes up one half to three quarters of the body's weight. It is found in the cells, in blood, it bathes all the tissues, and carries food through the digestive tract. The body has complex ways of maintaining water balance within a narrow, safe range. Similar complex patterns help equalize the water balance in each of the areas where it is needed.

Water is separated and stored within two major compartments of the body: the extracellular space and the intracellular space. About 62% of the body's water is found in *intracellular fluid*. This is the fluid within each of the body's cells. 35% of the body's water is in *extracellular fluid* or fluid outside and around the cells.[1] Extracellular fluid includes:

Blood plasma

Circulating fluids around each cell (called interstitial fluid)

Fluids in the bone and the dense connective tissues

Protective compartments of fluid in, for example, the eye, body cavity, nerves, and joints

The job of keeping intracellular fluid separate from extracellular fluid falls to the electrolytes. Electrolytes are free particles that contain a charge or force. The most important electrolytes in body water are sodium (Na), potassium (K) and chloride (Cl). Intracellular fluid is high in potassium but low in sodium and chloride, while extracellular fluid is high in sodium and chloride but low in potassium. These differences between the two fluids help to separate them from each other. This balance is rarely affected

54

Norm Sodium level 137-142

by the consumption of foods high or low in these substances. Since sodium holds the body's water in balance, high sodium intake (from foods or from added sodium chloride, or table salt) may lead to water retention in some persons. This does not usually result in a noticeable weight change since other mechanisms are also at work. A person will not gain weight from drinking a great deal of water. The body flushes out all the water it does not need.

FLUID BALANCE

Each day an adult loses about 6% and the infant 15% of his body water. Thirst is the mechanism that helps an individual replace what has been lost.

Some of the ways that water can be lost from the body include:

Urination
Stools
Breathing
Perspiration
Vomiting
Oozing from wounds or burns
Breast-feeding

In the first three cases, electrolyte loss is not a problem, as long as the person is healthy. The kidneys, which are the water filters of the body, conserve electrolytes. They only excrete what is not needed. If a person drinks a great quantity of fluids, the resulting urine will be more dilute than that of someone who drinks less fluid.

Perspiration may be a result of exercise, a hot climate, or fever. Both sodium and potassium are lost in small amounts, and may need to be replenished. It takes a great deal of perspiration, however, to place a person in danger of an electrolyte imbalance.

Vomiting and fluid lost through injuries *can* result in dangerous electrolyte loss. Uncontrolled, these fluid losses can quickly change the body's electrolyte balance. Extensive wounds or burns result in huge losses of water, electrolytes, and protein and may lead to shock and even death if not treated promptly.

In breast-feeding, total fluid intake is more important than the maintenance of electrolyte balance. This is also one of the normal processes for which the body compensates.

Although any sudden electrolyte loss poses a risk, potassium imbalance is especially dangerous. Potassium may be lost with some diuretics and laxative use. The heart can stop if potassium levels are too low or too high.

While nutrition may play little or no role in actually causing an imbalance, diet is sometimes involved as part of the long-term plan for treatment. This will be discussed in more detail in the chapter on fluid and electrolyte-controlled diets.

High elevations (such as mountainous areas) and high protein diets also increase the body's need for water. Normal water requirements are currently set at 1 milliliter per calorie for adults and 1.5 ml/cal for infants. Figure 9-1 illustrates the major factors in the intake and output of water and the electrolytes.

Water is obtained from all liquids and most foods. A small amount of water is also produced in the process of metabolism. Water is not digested. It does not break down in the body into its elements but remains intact. Water from the diet is absorbed into the body from the stomach (see Fig. 1-2). From there, it diffuses freely throughout the body to maintain normal balance in all areas.

To maintain this delicate balance, many hormones also help regulate excretion of water through urination and defecation (excretion of the feces, or stools). The waste products of the stool absorb water as they travel through the large intestine. Water passes through the walls of the large intestine or colon to help make the stool, but the nutrients that may still be present in the undigested mass cannot be absorbed into the body at this point. The amount of water that is absorbed determines whether the stool will be soft or hard. The role that fiber may have in this water absorption will be discussed in Chapter 10.

Water loss through urination is more complex than through defecation. Before urination can occur, water and electrolytes must be filtered through the body's two kidneys. The kidneys may be compared to extensive filters with

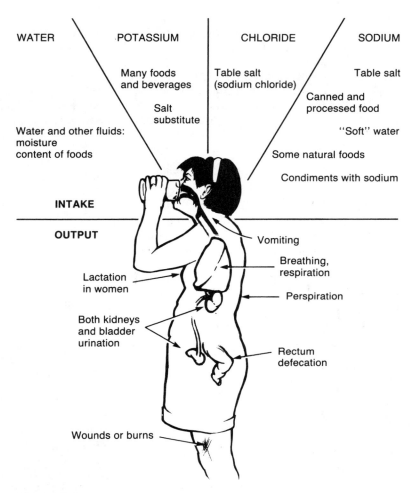

Figure 9-1
Routes of intake and output of water and the electrolytes. (Adapted from Nutrition Today: 5:22, 1970)

many channels. Blood vessels inside the kidneys are bridged by minute, maze-like filters called *nephrons.* The blood nourishes the kidney tissues and nephrons, and filters itself through them. This process is called *glomerular filtration,* and as it occurs, a liquid is formed that is composed of both the waste products and the vital substances. In the normal, healthy person, these vital substances return to the blood through the walls of the kidneys, and include some water, salts, glucose, and amino acids. Only what is truly extra waste and cannot be used is excreted. The vital salts, glucose, and amino acids return to the body again through the filtering channels and are not excreted. This conservation of substances is called *tubular resorption.*

The kidney does not always filter the same amounts of a substance. Hormones in the blood control how much water will be excreted and how much will be conserved. The amount of water lost depends on

Need

Intake

Diuretic and antidiuretic hormones

Blood pressure

Fluid losses by other routes

Total amount of filtered substances

Most of the waste products and excess water continue on "downstream" in the kidney, toward excretion. Trade-offs between charged particles (ions) such as hydrogen, sodium, and potassium, result in an acidic fluid. As this liquid moves out of the kidney and toward the bladder, still more water is absorbed back into the blood.

When cooking liquids such as syrup or soup, water is boiled off into the air, and the result is a more concentrated liquid than the original. The same is true in the kidneys, where filtration replaces boiling. As the water is drawn off into the surrounding tissue, the result is a more concentrated urine. The urine then travels into the bladder and, from there, leaves the body. The water and electrolytes have been conserved to circulate again through the blood. The average, healthy individual needs 1½ quarts to 2 quarts of water each day to replace what is lost.

OSMOLARITY

One of the factors that controls water loss is the number of substances filtered back into the blood. These substances attract or "pull" water with them. This force is called *osmolarity,* and it is extremely important in the role of water in nutrition.

Very simply, osmolarity is the concentration of particles in a certain amount of fluid. The osmolarity of body fluid is between 280 milliosmoles and 295 milliosmoles per liter of fluid (mOsm/L).[2] This normal osmolarity means that all the particles in the fluid together are creating a pressure of 280 milliosmoles to 295 milliosmoles for every liter of fluid.

Osmolarity is particularly relevant to nutrition in the intestinal fluids and in the blood.

The more particles a liquid contains, the greater its degree of osmolarity. If each of two liquids contains the same volume of particles, but one liquid has particles of glucose and the other has particles of amino acids, the osmolarities will differ. The glucose will register a higher osmolarity than the amino acids, because glucose particles are smaller than amino acids. Consequently, the total surface area of the glucose is larger, and the larger the total surface area of particles, the stronger the "pull" for water. One analogy to explain this is a comparison between a bucket of grapes and a bucket of oranges. There is more *total peel* on the grapes than on the oranges, because a larger percentage of each grape is its surface. It would take more water to make the grape skin:water ratio equal to the orange skin:water ratio. It is the same with osmolarity in body fluids.

Figure 9-2 illustrates the force of osmolarity (also called *osmolality*). Water works in the body to help maintain normal osmolarity in all of the fluids. It does this by diluting (or adding more water to) high-osmolarity liquids and concentrating (or removing water from) those with low osmolarity. If the osmolarity of the blood or intestinal fluids increased, water would diffuse into that area. The extra water would help dilute the liquid and make its osmolarity more equal to the osmolarity in the rest of the body.

When the osmolarity of the food in the intestines is extremely high, water may diffuse into that area very rapidly and result in diarrhea, or what is called the *dumping syndrome.* In this kind of massive fluid loss, many electrolytes are also lost. The loss might be so great that the body's electrolyte balance could be severely changed. The diarrhea should be stopped as quickly as possible, since both intra- and extracellular fluids have been lost. In the hospital patients with an *intravenous line* (a passage artificially made with a needle into the blood to administer medications) are constantly having a fluid consisting of water, dextrose, and sometimes sodium, "dripped" into their veins. This fluid keeps a stable concentration of particles in

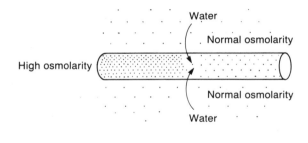

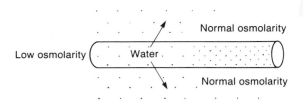

Figure 9-2
Osmolarity and water flow. In order to balance
the concentration of two adjoining fluid compartments, water flows through a filter into the
compartment with the highest concentration.
Tissue membranes between the compartments do
not allow the particles themselves to cross over.

the blood. Plain water would not help maintain
normal osmolarity. This is why the dextrose
and usually sodium are essential parts of this
fluid.

FOOD SOURCES

Figure 9-1 also lists the sources of water and the
major electrolytes, and how they are lost by the
body. As noted, almost all foods contain some
water. Fruits and vegetables have a higher percentage of water than fats, grains, and meats.
Fats contain almost no water unless they have
been artificially forced together by a stabilizing
ingredient as in salad dressings.

The major food source of chloride is table
salt, which is 40% sodium and 60% chloride.
Chloride is also present in most salt substitutes,
and in many foods. Deficiency in an otherwise
healthy individual is unlikely. There are no Rec-

ommended Dietary Allowances for the electrolytes, but a safe, adequate level of chloride in the
food supply is between 1700 mg and 5100 mg
for an adult.

Potassium is the major ingredient in salt substitutes. Table 9-1 lists the potassium content of
some high-potassium foods. Symptoms of deficiency include muscle weakness, apathy, difficulty breathing, irregular heart beat, and cardiac
arrest. Deficiency without unusual or induced
fluid loss (as in vomiting, laxative use, or use of
prescription diuretics that are low in potassium)
is unlikely. The average healthy adult probably
needs between 1875 mg and 5625 mg of potassium per day.

Sodium is also naturally present in many
foods, including milk and some vegetables. For
most people, a large percentage of their sodium
intake comes from the substances added to
foods, especially the sodium in table salt. Sodium is also present in condiments such as
Worcestershire sauce, steak sauce, monosodium glutamate, and ethnic sauces, such as soy
sauce, sofrito, and fish sauce. Spices and herbs
may contain sodium if salt has been added. For
example, onion salt, garlic salt, and celery salt
are each high in sodium. The corresponding
"powders" of these herbs contain almost no sodium. Many additives in processed foods have
"sodium" somewhere in their name ("sodium
bicarbonate"). Table salt is also added to canned
vegetables and soups. Table 9-2 contains a comparative list of some of these high-sodium food
sources. Medications may also contain sodium.

Infants receive all the sodium they need in
breast milk or infant formula. Cow's milk contains more sodium (and protein) than an infant
should ingest. Because of this and especially because of its high percentage of protein, cow's
milk may increase an infant's total fluid needs,
and is not recommended for infants in their first
year.

The normal adult should probably consume
between 1100 mg and 3300 mg of sodium per
day. This equals the amount of sodium in one
half a teaspoon to one and three quarters' teaspoons of table salt. Since there is natural sodium and chloride in foods, table salt is not necessary for the health of most persons.

Table 9-1

High-Potassium Foods: A Selection*

Suggested adult intake: 1875 – 5625 mg per day

Food	Amount	Potassium (mg)
Apricots, fresh	3	313
Avocados	½ medium (= 150 g)	600 – 750
Bananas	1 medium	451
Beans, kidney, cooked	100 g (3½ oz)	340
Cereals: All-Bran	1 oz	350
Bran Chex	1 oz	228
Most	1 oz	185
Oat flakes (fortif.)	1 oz	203
Chicken	100 g	200 – 250
Mushrooms, fresh	10 raw (100 g)	414
Milk, whole	1 cup	351
Orange juice, fresh	8 oz	496
Potato, baked	1 medium (100 g)	503
Salmon, broiled or baked	100 g	443
Scallops, steamed	100 g	476
Tomato	1 large (100 g)	488
Yogurt, plain	8 oz	351

* For more detailed information about fruits and vegetables high in potassium, see Table 28-3
(From Bowes & Church: Food Values of Portions Commonly Used, 14th ed. Philadelphia, JB Lippincott, 1985)

Table 9-2

High-Sodium Foods: A Selection*

Suggested adult intake: 1100 – 3300 mg per day

Food	Amount	Sodium (mg)
Baking soda	1 tsp	821
Cheese, Amer., past., process.	1 oz	406
Cheese, Feta	1 oz	316
Cheese, Velveeta	1 oz	430
Miso (fermented soybeans)	¼ cup	2100 – 3800
MSG	1 tsp	492
Peanuts, roasted, salted	½ cup	601
Potato chips	10	200
Salt, table	1 tsp	1938
Soy sauce	1tbsp	1029
Soup, reg. canned, diluted as directed	1 cup	800 – 1200
Tomato juice, canned	1 cup	878
Vegetables, reg. canned	1 cup	500 – 950
Worcestershire sauce	1 tbsp	206

* For a more detailed list, write for the booklet, The Sodium Content of Your Food. USDA Home & Garden Booklet #233, Superintendent of Documents, US Government Printing Office, Washington, DC 20402.

STUDY QUESTIONS

1. Into what two major body compartments is water separated?

2. What is the major electrolyte found in water in the cells?

3. Is there a higher or lower concentration of chloride in blood as compared to skin cells? Explain.

4. List six ways water may be lost from the body.

5. Why is it important to treat diarrhea and vomiting as quickly as possible?

6. Do the kidneys excrete all of the water and electrolytes that enter into them? Explain.

7. Explain osmolarity. Why may a solution of very high osmolarity be dangerous?

8. Why don't hospital patients receive plain water in their intravenous drip?

9. List seven foods high in sodium.

10. Does all the water in the diet come from beverages? Explain.

11. Is water fattening? Why or why not?

REFERENCES

1. McClintic JR: Basic Anatomy and Physiology of the Human Body, p 318. New York, JR Wiley & Sons, 1975.
2. Taber's Cyclopedic Medical Dictionary, 13th ed, App. 12. Philadelphia, FA Davis, 1977

CHAPTER 10

Fiber

1. To define fiber in general and by specific categories
2. To illustrate and explain the role of fiber in digestion and excretion
3. To describe the effects of fiber on other nutrients
4. To list the common food sources of fiber
5. To identify the terms used to define, describe, and quantify food fiber
6. To discuss briefly the dietary recommendations for fiber

Fiber, or *roughage,* has been important to the human diet for centuries. In ancient Greece, Hippocrates recommended bran in bread "for its salutary effect on the bowels."[1] In the last few years, however, fiber has assumed even greater importance. It first began to receive a good deal of public attention in the early 1970's, when reports were generated that there might be a connection between fiber and diverticular disease.[2] It was found that Africans, who had diets naturally high in fiber, had almost no incidence of the disease while Westerners, whose diet was much lower in fiber, had high rates of diverticular disease. Researchers thought a relationship might exist and began to search for other diseases where the action of fiber might assume

critical importance. Today, fiber is thought to have a possible role in the treatment of several diseases, such as diabetes,[3] diverticulosis, hyperlipidemia and, possibly, in prevention of cancer of the colon. [4,5] What role fiber plays in these diseases is, however, still quite controversial.

DEFINITION

In the strictest sense, fiber is not really a nutrient. It does not provide energy. The fibrous parts of foods may contain vitamins or minerals, but fiber itself is not a vitamin or a mineral. In fact, it is not even fully digestible. By definition fiber is "the sum of the indigestible carbohydrate and carbohydratelike components of food."[6] Fiber is the carbohydrate portion of food that cannot be fully digested. The acids in the stomach cannot break it down, nor can the enzymes in the mouth and small intestine. In fact, the part of the digestive tract where fiber is most important is in the colon, or large intestine. There, some of the fiber may be fermented or partially broken down to produce gas, water, and short-chain fatty acids.[7]

FIBER IN DIGESTION AND EXCRETION

The colon has no enzymes; rather, it has natural bacteria. It has no hairlike cilia covering its walls, but smooth, muscular walls that push through whatever comes along. Only water and electrolytes are absorbed in and from the walls of the colon.

It is in the colon that the stools are formed from water and undigested parts of food. As these come through the small intestine and into the colon, they are propelled along by the action of peristalsis (discussed in Chapter 1) toward the end of the colon and into the rectum. There, they are excreted.

Even though fiber cannot be digested, it is important in the colon because it can absorb water. The fiber in the colon draws water into the mass that is forming. Large particles of fiber absorb water better than many small particles of fiber. A stool that contains a good deal of water will be soft and easy to excrete, while a stool that contains very little water will be dry and usually painful to excrete. The muscles in the colon have to work harder to push along a dry mass. Fiber not only holds water, but also seems to trigger peristalsis, or muscle movement. If muscles are contracting quickly, waste is excreted quickly, giving food a short *transit time*. The latter is the time it takes for specific food to travel all the way through the alimentary tract, and for its waste to be excreted. Fiber seems to decrease transit time, pushing wastes through the colon more quickly. The benefits of this are discussed in greater detail in Chapter 24.

OTHER EFFECTS

As it travels through the digestive tract, fiber has an effect on those substances that can be digested. It has been discussed previously just how oxalates and phytates in food may prevent some minerals from being well absorbed. Fiber acts in the same way. A high-fiber food may interfere with the body's ability to absorb the minerals in that food (or others that were eaten along with it). The mineral may be only partially absorbed. Different forms of fiber have different effects on absorption. This is one reason why it is important to eat a variety of high-fiber foods, and not the same ones day after day. When fiber is included as part of a varied diet, nutrient absorption is not usually a problem, and high-fiber foods are frequently very high in many essential nutrients. A problem may develop, though, when the fiber is in the form of a medicine that is

taken regularly, such as a laxative. Table 10-1 lists the common ingredients in some of the gentle laxatives. All of them may interfere with good nutrition if they are used with meals on a regular basis.

Mineral oil, another foodlike substance, is not a fiber but is frequently used as an antidote to constipation. Mineral oil is made from petroleum products, and cannot be absorbed by the body. However, it also can interfere with good nutrition, and with the absorption of several important vitamins, if it is used daily.

Soluble fiber may also prevent fats from being completely absorbed. It may also carry some bile acids (produced by the gallbladder) into the stool. These effects are not dangerous; they may actually be healthful. As with vitamins and minerals, food sources of fiber are the best and safest sources.

TYPES OF FIBER

Just as there are different types of vitamins, there are different types of fiber, including *cellulose, hemicellulose, lignin, pectin, cutin* and *gum.* And just as some foods contain more than one vitamin, some foods contain more than one type of fiber.

There are other similarities between vitamins and fibers, which may be helpful in learning more about fiber. The various fibers can be divided into specific groups, illustrated in Table 10-2. The major groups of vitamins are fat-soluble and water-soluble, while the major groups of fibers are soluble and insoluble. Some foods contain both soluble and insoluble fibers.

Soluble fibers are the fibers that can be broken down by bacteria. They are usually broken down into acids, resulting in gas production. Both mature dry beans (such as kidney, soy, navy, and so forth) and cabbage-type vegetables contain a type of fiber that is broken down by bacteria into acids, with a gas by-product. Not all fiber foods cause gas. Soluble fibers, by definition, can be dissolved in water and may become "gummy" ; oat bran is an example. Hemicellulose, pectin, and gum are the soluble fibers.

Insoluble fibers do not absorb water well. They may soften and be broken down by heat,

Table 10-1

Common Ingredients in Laxatives

Bowel Effect	Laxative Type	Active Ingredients
Rapid, watery evacuation in 1–3 hours	Saline Cathartics	Sodium phosphates Magnesium sulfate Milk of magnesia
	Oil cathartic	Castor oil
Soft or semi-fluid stool in 6–8 hours	Diphenylmethane cathartics	Phenolphthalein Yellow phenolphthalein Bisacodyl
	Anthraquinone cathartics	Senna* Cascara sagrada* Danthron*
Softened feces in 1–3 days	Bulk formers	Agar Carboxymethylcellulose (synthetic made from cellulose) Chondrus (a plant gum) Guar gum (plant gum) Karaya gum (plant gum) Malt soup extract Bran Psyllium preparations (from plantago plant) Methylcellulose (synthetic made from cellulose) Prune powder Sodium alginate (from kelp) Tragacanth (plant gum)
	Fecal softeners	Dioctyl calcium sulfosuccinate (docusate calcium) Dioctyl sodium sulfosuccinate (docusate sodium) Dioctyl potassium glycerin Lactulose (an indigestible disaccharide) Mineral oil Mineral oil jelly (petroleum products) Polaxer Soft soap

* Not recommended for nursing mothers; substance known to be excreted into breast milk

as in a prolonged cooking process, but uncooked, they are insoluble and the body cannot do much with them. Cellulose, lignin, and cutin are insoluble.[7]

Just as vitamins may be made commercially, fiber is also commercially produced. This fiber is usually derived from food sources and used in industry. It may be added to processed foods, for example, as a thickener, it may be marketed as is, or in a laxative, or it may simply be left over and discarded after processing. Table 10-2 also lists by group some of the common derived fibers.

FOOD SOURCES

Foods that contain any undigestible parts have fiber. All high-fiber foods contain carbohydrate, but some high carbohydrate foods (such as sugars, syrups, honey, molasses, and refined flour) have had all of their fiber portion removed. Foods lose some or all of their fiber when they are

Processed, milled, or refined

Cooked

Hulled, peeled, or seeded

Table 10-2

Practical Sources of Fiber

	Natural Food Sources	Derived Sources*
Insoluble		
Cellulose	Soybean hulls Fruit membranes Legumes Carrots and other vegetables	Methylcellulose Carboxymethylcellulose Purified wood products
Lignin	Wheat straw Alfalfa stems Cottonseed hulls Tannins	Bagasse, the residue after sugar is extracted from sugarcane
Cutin	Apple peels Tomato peels Seeds in berries Peanut skins Almond skins Onion skins	
Soluble		
Hemicellulose	Corn hulls Barley hulls Oat hulls Wheat brans Corn brans	Soy fiber concentrate Brewer's grain residues Xylan, from xylose
Pectin	Citrus pulp Apple pulp Sugar beet pulp Cabbage and other "brassica" foods Legumes Alfalfa leaves Sunflower heads	
Gum	Oats	Agar (from red algae) Alginate (from kelp) Glycan (from yeast) Gum arabic (from locust beans) Gum tragacanth (from legumes) Guar gum (from legumes) Psyllium or fleaseed (from plantains) Xanthan (from prickly ash trees)

* These ingredients are listed here because they are frequently included in high fiber, processed foods, laxatives and other products.

(Adapted from Crosby L: Fiber: Standardized sources. Nutr Cancer 1:1, pp 15–25, 1978)

There are four major groups of foods that contain natural fiber. These are

1. Whole grains and grain products
2. Vegetables
3. Fruits
4. Nuts, seeds, and legumes.

Whole Grain Products

Whole grains are composed of three parts: The *germ* (high in protein and fat), the *endosperm* (high in starch), and the *bran,* chaff, or hull (pure, indigestible fiber).

When grains are milled for flour, the germ is usually removed, because it is high in fat and therefore spoils easily. De-germed grain products keep better in storage. The hull, or "chaff," of bran is usually removed to make a smooth, light, consistent meal. When wheat is milled into flour and these portions are removed, some vitamins and minerals are lost, so they are returned to the flour, artificially. "Enriched" flour or grain has had these nutrients restored. Enriched products are usually more nutritious than unenriched products.

Whole grain flour is heavier than refined white flour, because the bran and germ add bulk and slightly change the nature of its baking qualities. Whole grain bread has about eight times as much crude fiber (1.6%) as does white bread (0.2%).[9]

Beriberi (thiamin deficiency) has occurred in Oriental societies where white rice, the major food in the diet, has not been enriched. Brown rice is whole grain rice, with all the necessary thiamin contained in the bran portion. (The bran portion is the portion that is removed from brown rice to make white rice.) Because of this important vitamin, and because many societies depend on rice for survival, most white rice in the USA is enriched with several vitamins. In other countries, however, rice may not be fortified.

Fruits and Vegetables

Fruits and vegetables range in fiber content from between 0.5% to 1% crude fiber.[9] Many parts of fruits and vegetables are indigestible. Some of these parts include the stalks, threads, seeds, peels, and membranes. Pectin in apples and some other fruits is a form of fiber that is not visible, is more soluble, and is not measurable by crude fiber (see below).

These fibrous parts of fruits and vegetables may be softened by cooking. Heat may break down the fiber into digestible starches and sugars, so that cooked fruits and vegetables are often much lower in fiber content than are the same plants in their raw state.

Nuts, Seeds, and Legumes

Nuts usually have a thin, paperlike skin. These can easily be removed from peanuts, but not from almonds. This skin is one form of the fiber in these foods. The hulls of seeds are also indigestible, so that some seeds are excreted whole in the stool. The fiber in legumes is less visible. Legumes contain both the indigestible cellulose and soluble pectins. Legumes are an excellent source of fiber as well as protein, and of many vitamins and minerals.

CRUDE VERSUS DIETARY FIBER

The fiber in foods is hard to measure. It was at first measured by a rough, acid treatment that was designed to destroy all the food except the fiber portion. What was left was the *crude fiber,* primarily cellulose and lignin. Because the method was so harsh, all the soluble fiber was destroyed. Less than half the total fiber in a food could be measured this way.

Dietary fiber is the term used for ALL the fiber in a food. Dietary fiber includes crude fiber plus the soluble fibers. It is an accurate measure of how much fiber is actually contained in a food (Table 10-3).

REQUIREMENTS

There is no recommended intake for fiber in the diet, and there are few tables that measure dietary fibers in foods. We know fiber is essential to prevent chronic constipation and to keep stools soft, but the actual amounts needed have not yet been established. The amounts needed

Table 10-3

Comparative Sources of Dietary Fiber
*(Grams total dietary fiber/100 grams food)**

Raw, Dry, or Whole Grain Sources		Cooked &/or Refined Sources	
	g Dietary Fiber		**g Dietary Fiber**
Legumes and Nuts			
Coconut, fresh shredded	13.2	Beans, kidney, cooked	10.2
Cowpeas (blackeye), raw	12.8	Beans, white, canned	4.7
Fava beans, raw	24.99	Peanuts, dry roasted	7.7
Lentils, raw	19.3		
Peanuts, dry, raw	9.3		
Soy flour, defatted	10.8		
Fruit and Fruit Juices			
Apple, raw with peel	2.1	Apple juice	0.3
Avocado, raw	2.0	Applesauce	1.7
Banana, raw	2.3	Orange juice	0.4
Orange, raw	2.0	Peaches, canned, unswtnd	1.5
Peach, raw with skin	2.3	Prunes, canned, unswtnd	8.1
Prunes, dried	9.6	Rhubarb, cooked, unswtnd	2.4
Raisins	6.8		
Vegetables			
Beans, green, raw	2.7	Cabbage, boiled	2.8
Broccoli, raw	3.6	Carrots, fresh, cooked	3.7
Cabbage, raw	2.6	Corn, fresh, cooked	4.7
Carrots, raw	2.8	Onion, cooked	0.8
Celery, raw	1.0	Peas, canned	6.3
Green pepper, raw	1.6	Peas, frozen	4.8
Iceberg lettuce	1.3	Potato, boiled	1.1
Potato, baked with skin	2.0	Potato chips	11.9
Potato, raw with skin	2.8	Spinach, cooked	8.5
Spinach, raw	1.8	Tomato, canned, drained	0.8
Tomato, raw	1.7		
Cereals, Grains, and Baked Products			
Bran chex cereal	16.1	Bread, white	2.7
Bran, wheat, dry	39.6	Crackers, saltines (24 squares)	3.3
Bran, oat, dry	27.8	Flour, white	2.8
Bread, whole wheat	11.3	Rice chex cereal	0
Bread, rye	6.6	Rice, white, cooked	2.3
Crackers, graham (7 squares)	10.0	Shredded wheat cereal	12.3
Flour, whole wheat	12.6	Spaghetti, cooked, enriched	3.3
Oats, rolled dry	11.2		
Popcorn, popped (7 cups)	7.1		
Rice, brown cooked	5.6		

* 100 grams = 3½ ounces

Sources: Anderson JW: Plant Fiber Source Book, Lexington, KY, HCF Diabetes Research Foundation, © 1980. U.S. Dept. of Agriculture, Human Nutrition Information Service (USDA — HNIS): Unpublished compilation of fiber content in foods, Hyattsville, MD, USDA/HNIS, March 1985

may also depend on what role fiber has in preventing certain diseases. Again, this has not yet been established.

How much fiber persons actually consume varies greatly, depending, of course, on how they eat. Vegetarians may consume 12 g to 24 g of crude fiber each day, while the typical American who eats meat may consume 8 g to 11 g per day.[9] A person who eats only highly processed and cooked foods may consume much less fiber.

From what is known about fiber, it is probably better for the healthy person to eat high-fiber carbohydrate foods than to eat low-fiber foods. High-fiber carbohydrate foods are usually less processed and contain more vitamins and minerals than low-fiber foods. When fiber from the legumes is increased in the diet, it should be increased *gradually*. Otherwise problems with gas may be severe. A very high-fiber diet may lead to excess gas and also inhibit the absorption of certain minerals. Fiber may not be a nutrient, but it is an important part of the normal, nutritious diet.

STUDY QUESTIONS

1. What is fiber?

2. In what part of the digestive tract is fiber most important?

3. What does fiber do?

4. Different types of fiber are divided into two general groups. List and explain these groups.

5. Which is more effective, wheat bran in large particles or wheat bran ground up into smaller particles?

6. List three groups of foods naturally high in fiber. What parts of these foods contain fiber?

7. Which contains the least fiber in each of the following examples:
- A raw whole tomato, a raw, peeled tomato, or a cooked, peeled tomato?
- Bread labelled "100% whole grain" or dark rye bread with no seeds?
- White bread or oatmeal bread?
- Grapefruit juice, strained, or prune juice labelled "with pulp added?"

8. Is it harmful to eat a high fiber diet? Why or why not?

REFERENCES

1. Facts about Fiber, available from the Washington County (ME) Cooperative Extension Service, 1982
2. Burkitt DP, Walker ARP, Painter NS: Effect of dietary fibre on stools and transit-times, and its role in the causation of disease. Lancet Vol 2, p 1408, 1972
3. Diabetes Care and Education Practice Group: Fiber and the Patient with Diabetes Mellitus: An Annotated Bibliography. American Dietetic Association, 430 N. Michigan Ave., Chicago 60611, © 1980
4. Trowell H: Definition of dietary fiber and hypothesis that it is a protective factor in certain diseases. Am J Clin Nutr 29:417–427, 1976
5. Burkitt D: Fiber as a protective against gastrointestinal diseases. Am J Gastroenter 79(4):249–252, 1984
6. Food and Nutrition Board, National Academy of Sciences: Recommended Dietary Allowances, p 32. Washington, National Research Council, 1980
7. Dietary Fiber: An Overview for Physicians, p 3. Chicago, Searle Consumer Products Inc., 1985
8. Dwyer J et al: Drug therapy reviews: Dietary fiber and fiber supplements in the therapy of gastrointestinal disorders. Am J Hosp Pharm 35:278–287, March, 1978
9. Thiele VF: Clinical Nutrition, p 62. St. Louis, CV Mosby, 1976

CHAPTER 11

Alcohol, Caffeine, and Artificial Sweeteners

OBJECTIVES

1. To describe the absorption and metabolism of alcohol, its nature as a drug, and its role in the diet

2. To identify energy values in common alcoholic beverages

3. To discuss the nutritional implications of long-term alcohol abuse

4. To discuss briefly the moderate and safe use of alcohol

5. To discuss the use, physiologic effects, and safety of caffeine, and to illustrate the caffeine content of specific beverages.

6. To describe the history of, and controversies surrounding the three most common artificial sweeteners: cyclamate, saccharin, and aspartame

Alcohol and caffeine have been a part of almost every culture for centuries, both socially and as drugs. Artificial sweeteners are a more recent development of technology. The three are discussed together in this chapter because they are all "social" substances, although alcohol may technically be called a nutrient because it provides calories (seven per gram). None of the three have any nutritional benefits. None are essential in any way. To varying degrees, all three may, in excess, be harmful.

ALCOHOL USE

The fermentation of grain or berries into an alcoholic liquid is probably one of the oldest methods of producing naturally "processed" foods. Alcoholic beverages have long been used as the common drink of many diverse cultures. They have been used as medicinal drugs, and as intoxicants. This has not changed today.

Alcohol is used in cooking as well as in beverages. In cooking, the calories from alcohol evaporate. Foods cooked in a liquor or wine will retain the flavor but none of the alcohol in the liquid used. Vanilla extract is a common example of a substance used in cooking that contains alcohol. When the alcohol from wine or extracts for example, evaporates, it leaves the flavor but no calories.

If the food is not cooked, the alcohol and its calories remain. Some desserts use liquors or liqueurs and are not cooked, but refrigerated. They will keep their alcohol content, as well as the extra calories provided by the alcohol.

In the digestive tract, alcohol enters the blood rapidly. It is directly absorbed through the walls of the stomach. Food that is in the stomach at the same time can slow down the rate of absorption, but it cannot prevent it.

Once alcohol is in the blood, it stays there until it is gradually broken down by the liver. The liver works to lower blood levels, and it can only handle a certain amount of alcohol at one time. The liver of a large person can handle more alcohol than the liver of a smaller person. If alcohol is taken with a meal, it usually enters the blood more slowly, giving the liver time to break it down. This is one reason a meal is always recommended when alcohol is ingested. The other reason a person should eat when drinking is because alcohol is a depressant, not a stimulant. It can depress, or lower, the blood sugar levels. However, with its ability to raise blood sugar levels, food helps prevent this from happening.

Table 11-1 list the calorie and alcoholic content of some common alcoholic beverages. Many of them contain ingredients other than alcohol, and these ingredients (such as sugar, milk, and so forth) usually provide added calories from carbohydrates, making mixed drinks usually higher in calories than the pure distilled or fermented liquor.

Even though some ales, beers, and wines may contain traces of vitamins or minerals derived from their original ingredients, the amounts are usually insignificant. So alcoholic beverages may be important socially, or may be acceptable beverages when water supplies are not reliable, but they should never be used as a source of good nutrition. They are extras, not essentials.

ALCOHOL ABUSE

People who abuse alcohol may have other problems long before their liver wears out from too much alcohol.

By nature, alcohol is similar to a drug rather than to a food, and this makes dependence easily acquired in some persons. Nutritionally, a chronic use of alcohol can quickly add up to a lot of "empty" calories. In this way, alcohol is akin to junk food: most people can afford the calories sometimes, but something (protein, vitamins, minerals) will probably get short-changed if alcohol becomes a major, daily part

Table 11-1

Energy Content of Common Alcoholic Beverages

Beverage	Size	Calories	Grams alcohol
Ale, mild	8 oz	98	9
Beer, regular	12 oz	148	13
	8 oz	99	9
Creme de menthe	20 g (Cordial glass)	67	7
Daiquiri	100 g (approx. ½ cup)	122	15
Eggnog, Christmas	4 oz	335	15
Gin, rum, brandy, whiskey, or vodka:			
*80 Proof**			
Jigger (1½ oz or 44 ml)		97	14
Fluid ounce (29.6 ml)		65	7
*100 Proof**			
Jigger		124	18
Fluid ounce		83	10
Wines:			
Champagne	4 oz	84	11
Port	4 oz	200	16
Sherry, dry	2 oz	84	9
Vermouth, dry	4 oz	120	17
Vermouth, sweet	4 oz	126	18

* Another way to calculate calories in pure alcoholic beverages is: $0.8 \times proof \times ounces$.

Bowes & Church: Food Values of Portions Commonly Used, 14th ed, pp 196–197. Philadelphia, JB Lippincott, 1985

of life. For a normal, healthy adult, an occasional one or two drinks may not be harmful as long as the person has calories to spare.

However, alcohol is almost never recommended in pregnancy. The fetus is extremely sensitive to alcohol in the blood, and its tiny body cannot handle what seems to be a proportionately enormous drink, even when the mother feels no negative effects. Children born to women who are chronic alcohol abusers may be severely affected. Their symptoms characterize the "fetal alcohol syndrome," and have a negative effect on the child's lifelong ability to learn and grow. However, the level of alcohol that causes fetal alcohol syndrome has never been clearly established. The studies done on alcohol in pregnancy certainly show that a large dose of alcohol may be harmful if it affects the fetus at certain crucial times in development. It is not clear what those crucial times are, or how much alcohol is too much alcohol. Consequently, it seems wisest for a pregnant woman simply to avoid alcohol during her pregnancy.

When alcohol is abused to the point of intoxication, the person involved may not merely pass out. With an extremely high intake (or low tolerance), death is even possible. This is partly because alcohol is a depressant on the system.

It is a myth that coffee can sober an intoxicated person. Nothing but time can do that. What coffee can do, though, is help keep a person awake, countering the depression of the system. Alcohol will lower the blood sugar. Coffee, though a stimulant, may also lead to lower blood sugar. So, again, it is important to accompany alcoholic beverages with food, and to provide for those persons who are intoxicated. The effects of alcohol are much quicker and greater on an empty stomach than on a full one.

Alcohol is abused when its user begins to depend on it, even for social purposes. There is no universally established lower limit of drinking that can be pinpointed as the beginning of "abuse." Some persons may abuse alcohol when they have just one drink. Others can drink regularly without any indication of abuse. The definition of alcoholism and alcohol abuse is a complex one, beyond the realm of this text. Nutritional damage is only a small part of the complex effects of alcohol abuse.

Since alcohol contains lots of calories, it is easy to gain weight with just a few extra drinks daily. Too much alcohol can also harm the lining of the stomach and intestines, and make it more difficult for them to absorb other nutrients. Some vitamin deficiencies, such as thiamin deficiency and niacin deficiency are common in alcoholics. Older, chronic alcoholics, who may develop these diseases, do not acquire them just because they drink. They develop them because they eat very poorly, if at all. The chronic alcoholic may actually become thin, as a result of eating very little for many years. The older alcoholic may also be socially isolated, and have little ability, resources, or interest in preparing good food. He may minimize or deny intake of alcohol, and may be honestly unaware of how little he is eating. What can be done to help, nutritionally, depends to a great extent on the family and community resources available, and the individual's willingness to use or accept these resources.

HOW MUCH ALCOHOL IS OK?

It is hard to define how much alcohol is too much alcohol, just as it is hard to define how much "junk food" a person can eat. How many calories does the person need? How many vitamins, minerals, protein, and other essential nutrients are provided in the usual diet? How many calories does he have to spare after all his other essential needs are met? How much can he consume without gaining weight? Unfortunately, alcohol is so closely related to social practices that this type of rational calculation is usually unrealistic.

As a result, the government guidelines for this substance, while vague, are the most specific general guidelines available. They simply say, "For many individuals, a reduction in alcohol consumption would also assist in achieving proper calorie balance,"[1] and "If you drink alcohol, do so in moderation."[2]

WHAT ABOUT CAFFEINE?

Caffeine is the name for the active stimulant in coffee, chocolate, and many carbonated beverages. Its "relative," theobromine, is the active stimulant in tea. Caffeine has been used for centuries. Cultivation of coffee started in southern Arabia and it became a popular stimulant and social drink in the Muslim world (where alcohol is forbidden). Constantinople is said to be the home of the first coffee house, the Kiva Han which flourished around 1475 A.D. Over the next two hundred years, the coffee rage quickly spread into Europe.[3]

Lately, however, coffee has become more controversial. Some researchers believe that high large amounts of coffee consumed on a regular basis may play a role in causing cancer. Others say the evidence for this is shaky. To date, no one really knows and nothing has been proven, conclusively, one way or the other. If coffee is harmful, the levels drunk may need to be very high over a long period of time.

However, caffeine is a drug. It stimulates the nervous system, and can pass through the placenta into unborn children. Many obstetricians recommend that pregnant women limit the amount of caffeinated beverages they drink while they are pregnant.

Coffee, tea, and chocolate beverages are a basic part of many cultures. And though fewer people in the USA today drink coffee, more persons drink colas and other caffeinated soft drinks.[4] So the form in which persons ingest caffeine may be changing, but the total amount they ingest may not. Cola beverages sometimes have a lower concentration of caffeine than perked coffee, but many people drink very large quantities of them.

Is caffeine "bad?" True, it may not be recommended for some persons. Because caffeine stimulates the nervous system, it makes the heart work harder. It can also stimulate the pancreas to manufacture more insulin, which will affect blood sugar. Coffee products may also stimulate the stomach to produce more acid. So some doctors advise certain individuals to limit their intake of caffeine. But there is no evidence to date that caffeine is harmful to the average, healthy person. Even a pregnant woman may be told that she can have 2 or 3 cups of a caffeine beverage each day, if she likes.

Table 11-2 lists the caffeine content for some common beverages. These figures may change, however, since many soft drinks are now being

Table 11-2

Caffeine-Containing Beverages

Beverage	Caffeine Content (per fluid oz or 30 ml)
Instant, dry tea	32/tsp
Drip coffee	27.4
Perked coffee	23.4
Instant coffee	12
Black tea, 5 min	10.8
Tea bag, 5 min	9.2
Green Japanese tea, 5 min	6.2
Teabag, 1 min	5.6
Diet Mr. Pibb	4.8
Mountain Dew	4.5
Mello Yellow	4.4
Coke	3.8
Tab	3.8
Dr. Pepper (diet, regular)	3.3
Pepsi	3.2
RC Cola (diet, regular)	3.0
Decaffeinated coffee	0.4 – 1.0
Cocoa	0.8
Root beer, ginger ale	0
Ovaltine	0

From Bowes & Church: Food Values of Portions Commonly Used, 14th ed. Philadelphia, JB Lippincott, 1985

"decaffeinated," in response to concerned consumers. Coffee and tea are both available in decaffeinated forms.

While caffeine may not be harmful, neither is it high in any necessary nutrient. Any person who thinks that perhaps he should not drink it, because of certain symptoms or problems that seem related to caffeine, should let his physician be the judge.

This discussion is based on a "moderate" intake of 2 or 3 daily servings of caffeine. As with any druglike substance, caffeine in massive doses can be fatal, and even very heavy coffee drinkers, whose intake is still far below a fatal dose, sometimes have health problems that improve when the daily caffeine intake is lowered.

WHAT ABOUT ARTIFICIAL SWEETENERS?

The main appeal of artificial sweeteners is obvious: they attract people who love sweets but feel they cannot afford the calories. Artificial sweeteners promise calorie-free flavor. They promise "pleasure without plumpness." Weight-conscious North Americans have stocked up on these sweeteners for decades instead of—or in addition to—regular sugars.

Saccharin, cyclamates, and *aspartame* are the three artificial sweeteners that have dominated the market in this century. Saccharin was discovered in 1879 and became popular just after the turn of the century. However, persons experienced a bitter aftertaste, making it undesirable. Cyclamate, a better tasting sweetener without an aftertaste, was discovered in 1937 and was the more popular of the two between the years 1950 and 1970, when it was banned. Aspartame, which also has no aftertaste, was discovered in 1965 and was approved for public use in 1981.[5]

Currently, the safety of all three sweeteners is being questioned. Cyclamates were banned because they were found to cause cancer and genetic damage in test animals. Then studies on saccharin showed that it caused bladder cancer in animals, although additional saccharin studies in humans have not yet clearly proved it would cause cancer in humans.[5] Saccharin is now banned in Canada (though cyclamates may be sold.) In the USA foods with saccharin must be labeled with the statement: "Use of this product may be hazardous to your health: this product contains saccharin which has been determined to cause cancer in laboratory animals."

Aspartame appeared in the midst of the saccharin controversy and seemed to be the ideal solution. It was acceptable to those who found saccharin bitter. Although it decomposed easily and would not retain its sweetness during cooking, it seemed ideal as a replacement for saccharin, and is now common in soda, powdered beverages, toppings, gums, desserts, and individual packets for coffee and tea.

However, by late 1983, persons began to report problems they believed were connected to their use of aspartame. Headaches, mood changes, menstrual changes, convulsions, blurred vision, dizziness and worsened memory were a few complaints.[6] Complaints began to be filed at the Food and Drug Administration.* Some consumers began to wonder if this sweetener, too, was a health hazard. The industry marketing the sweetener defended its safety, citing studies that had been conducted, and certain groups of concerned nutritionists and scientists countered that there were serious faults inherent in the studies.

The primary problem with aspartame is that is breaks down after several days' exposure to heat, the heat of a warm room, or the heat of a summer day. It breaks down into particles of phynylalanine (an amino acid) and methanol. High levels of phenylalanine in the blood can cause severe problems and lead to mental retardation for those who have phynylketonuria (PKU), a genetic disease that is diagnosed at birth and controlled by diet throughout life. It is discussed in Chapters 23 and 34. No one knows what effect (if any) temporary high levels of phenylalanine may have in the blood of normal individuals. Methanol, or methyl alcohol, the other product of aspartame's decomposition, is a form of alcohol that is considered a cumulative poison by the FDA.[7] It also is present naturally in many common foods.

Since all the problems that may occur with aspartame seem related to its breakdown, it may be harmless if it does not have the time to break down. Powdered aspartame may be alright. It sometimes has been combined with saccharin, in carbonated beverages, in order to cut down the bitter aftertaste of the saccharin. This means the beverage contains both artificial sweeteners.

The final word is not yet in. Although artificial sweeteners contain fewer calories than natural sweeteners, they are not calorie free†. North

---

*This government bureau officially "polices" the marketing of foods and beverages (and drugs) and makes the final decisions about what is safe, what is not and what will legally be allowed on the market.

†Aspartame has just as many calories per gram as sugar; but it is 180 times sweeter. Since much less is needed to provide the same sweetness, the total calories are much less. Other substances with calories may also be added to give volume and texture.

Americans as a group do not seem to be thinner, even after more than 80 years of using available artificial sweeteners. And the substances may carry a good deal of risk. In the meantime, while the evidence for all three is being reevaluated and debated, moderate use of the natural sweeteners (honey, molasses, fruit juices and corn syrups) is still safe.

STUDY QUESTIONS

1. How much alcohol does the average, healthy adult need for good nutrition?
2. What is the alcohol content of foods that have been sautéed one hour in wine?
3. What are two factors that affect how much alcohol a person can handle at one time?
4. Does caffeine help to "sober up a person"? Why or why not?
5. True or false: Alcohol is a stimulant. Explain your answer.
6. True or false: A person who drinks too much will usually be thin, because he won't eat properly. Explain your answer.
7. Describe some nutritional problems that may result after years of alcohol abuse.
8. A 19-year old woman is trying to limit her daily intake to 1700 calories. Her boyfriend can easily eat 2500. The two go to a party, after a day during which she ate 1500 calories and he ate 2200 calories.
    - How much beer can each drink, without going over their limits?
    - Popcorn (at 50 calories per cup) and pretzels (about 30 calories each) are also available. Should the woman eat some? Why or why not?
9. List three beverages high in caffeine. Can you think of low-caffeine alternatives to each?
10. Why would some people want to limit their caffeine intake? What level is often recommended?
11. List the three most popular artificial sweeteners. Why is each one controversial?
12. From what is aspartame made? People should avoid its use if they have what disease?
13. List all the beverages you consumed yesterday. Which ones contained caffeine? Artificial sweeteners? Alcohol?

REFERENCES

1. Food and Nutrition Board, National Academy of Sciences: Recommended Dietary Allowances, 9th ed, p 37. Washington, National Research Council, 1980
2. US Department of Agriculture: Dietary Guidelines for Americans. Washington, 1980
3. Coyle LP: The World Encyclopedia of Food, pp 184–185. New York, Facts on File, 1982
4. Zuckerman S: Coffee drinking takes a tumble. Nutrition Action, Vol II (3), April 1984
5. Lecos C: The sweet and sour history of saccharin, cyclamate, aspartame. HHS Publ. No. (FDA) 81–2156 FDA Consumer, September 1981
6. Community Nutrition Institute: Nutrition Week, Vol XIV 13:3, March 29, 1984
7. Community Nutrition Institute: Nutrition Week, Vol XIII: 50, December 22, 1983

UNIT 2

Designing an Adequate Diet for the Individual

CHAPTER 12

Standards for an Adequate Diet

OBJECTIVES

1. To introduce the concept of national standards for good nutrition

2. To define and illustrate energy standards, and ways to determine caloric needs

3. To explain and illustrate the current weight-for-height standards and their history

4. To explain and illustrate the Recommended Dietary Allowances and the US RDA as standards for nutrients

5. To explain and illustrate the Basic Four Food Groups

6. To introduce the use of food composition tables to assess nutrient adequacy

7. To discuss the use of the Dietary Guidelines as standards for health

8. To introduce the concept of anthropometrics to assess health in the USA and in underdeveloped nations

A standard is an established reference point. A dietary standard is a guide that can be used to help a person decide whether or not he is getting the nutrients he needs. Many countries have created dietary standards for their populations. Canada and Sweden are two countries that are similar to the USA and have developed their own national standards. The World Health Organization (WHO) has also developed standards used to assess nutrition and to plan programs in underdeveloped nations.

These standards may all vary somewhat, but the differences are usually small. They are not different because the nutrient needs of each culture are different, but because it is impossible to determine exactly how much each person should weigh, how many calories each person needs, or exactly how much of a nutrient is enough. Dietary guidelines are developed to help a person determine approximately how many of these essentials he needs. Guidelines can also help a person prevent deficiencies as well as overdoses of a nutrient. Some standards (for example, in Canada) are guidelines to the needs of an *average* person. Others (for example, in the USA) have higher figures for some nutrients because they are guidelines meant to cover the needs of *all* persons in a group. When this is understood, the differences between standards are small. This chapter will discuss the dietary standards that have been developed in the USA.

STANDARDS FOR ENERGY

How many calories does an adult need to maintain his weight? How many calories does an infant, child, or teenager need to grow well? The standards for energy help answer these questions.

The RDA

The Recommended Dietary Allowances, discussed in other chapters, includes standards for energy. (The RDA will be discussed in more detail below, under "Standards for Nutrients.") Because so many factors can influence energy needs (see Chapter 2), the RDA gives both upper and lower limits of the average ranges (Table 12-1). These ranges vary, depending on age and sex, and are based on average height and weight for each group. An extremely active person may need the higher number of calories in his range. A person who is not very active, or who weighs less than the average for his range, may need to limit intake to the lowest figures to keep from gaining weight.

Because energy needs depend partly on just how active a person is, the RDA includes guide-lines to help persons determine the energy used in certain activities. These are illustrated in Table 12-2.

Basal Energy Needs

The body needs energy, even during sleep and rest. Some standards exist that help determine basal energy needs. One common standard for this basic, minimum energy requirement is the *Harris-Benedict Equation,*[1] which includes both an equation developed for men and one developed for women. This equation considers weight, height, and age, and is shown in Figure 12-1.

Other Methods

There are a few quick ways to estimate how many calories a person needs to keep, lose, or

Table 12-1

Average Heights, Weights, and Energy Needs

	Age	Weight		Height		Energy Needs (Kilocalories*)	
Category	(Years)	(kg)	(lb)	(cm)	(in)	(Average)	(Range)
Infants	0.0–0.5	6	13	60	24	kg × 115	(95–145)
	0.5–1.0	9	20	71	28	kg × 105	(80–135)
Children	1–3	13	29	90	35	1300	900–1800
	4–6	20	44	112	44	1700	1300–2300
	7–10	28	62	132	52	2400	1650–3300
Males	11–14	45	99	157	62	2700	2000–3700
	15–18	66	145	176	69	2800	2100–3900
	19–22	70	154	177	70	2900	2500–3300
	23–50	70	154	178	70	2700	2300–3100
	51–75	70	154	178	70	2400	2000–2800
	76+	70	154	178	70	2050	1650–2450
Females	11–14	46	101	157	62	2200	1500–3000
	15–18	55	120	163	64	2100	1200–3000
	19–22	55	120	163	64	2100	1700–2500
	23–50	55	120	163	64	2000	1600–2400
	51–75	55	120	163	64	1800	1400–2200
	76+	55	120	163	64	1600	1200–2000
Pregnancy						+300	
Lactation						+500	

* Kilocalorie is the technical term for what is commonly known as a "calorie." Although technically incorrect, the two terms are used interchangeably throughout this text.

(From Food and Nutrition Board, National Academy of Sciences: Recommended Dietary Allowances, p 23. Washington, National Research Council, 1980.)

Table 12-2

*Approximate Energy Use of Various Activities**

	Kilocalories/ minute for:	
Activity	**70 Kg Man**	**58 Kg Woman**
1. *At Rest* Sleeping, reclining	1.0–1.2	0.9–1.1
2. *Very light* Seated Truck driving Typing Sewing Standing	up to 2.5	up to 2.0
3. *Light* Walking 2½ to 3 mph Reaching Carpentry Restaurant work Washing clothes Sailing Volleyball	2.5–4.9	2.0–3.9
4. *Moderate* Walking 3½ to 4 mph Gardening Farmwork Scrubbing floors Biking, skiing Tennis Dancing	5.0–7.4	4.0–5.9
5. *Heavy* Walking with load Basketball Football Swimming Climbing	7.5–12	6–10

* Adapted from information from Food and Nutrition board, National Academy of Sciences: Recommended Dietary Allowances, p 24. Washington, National Research Council, 1980.

Men

$$66 + (13.7 \times W) + (5 \times H) - (6.8 \times A)$$

Women

$$655 + (9.6 \times W) + (1.7 \times H) - (4.7 \times A)$$

Key: W = Weight in kilograms
H = Height in centimeters
A = Age in years

Figure 12-1
Basal energy needs: the Harris-Benedict equation. (From Benedict FG: Lectures on Nutrition, Mayo Foundation Lectures. Philadelphia, WB Saunders, 1925)

gain weight. The simplest of these multiplies a person's desired body weight (DBW in pounds) $\times$ 13, 14, or 15 (depending on activity). This equals calories necessary to maintain one's current weight. Desired Body Weight $\times$ 10 yields a figure low (and yet safe) enough to permit an individual to lose weight, at the rate of about 1 pound per week.

STANDARDS FOR WEIGHT

A person's health and the quality of his diet (eating habits) are more important than body weight. Weight does not indicate a person's degree of health, the bodily percentage of fat, or the body's muscle strength. Still, some diseases are more likely to occur if a person is overweight, and his body is enduring some degree of stress. Severe underweight (20% or more below recommended weight for height) can also lead to serious stress and disease.[2] Because of these factors, weight standards have been designed. These standards help persons compare their weight to the rest of the population and make decisions about changes.

Height/weight tables have been developed since the 19th century, usually for insurance companies. The most popular weight standard for adults is one prepared by the Metropolitan Life Insurance Company. These tables were first published in 1959, and were revised in 1983. Both sets of tables were based on the average reported weights of healthy persons who owned life insurance. They are divided by sex, height, and frame size, although there is no adjustment for older ages. Frame size has been calculated by using wrist circumference or elbow breadth

FINDING BODY FRAME BY ELBOW BREADTH

To make a simple approximation of your frame size:

Extend your arm and bend the forearm upwards at a 90-degree angle. Keep the fingers straight and turn the inside of your wrist toward the body. Place the thumb and index finger of your other hand on the two prominent bones on either side of your elbow. Measure the space between your fingers against a ruler or a tape measure. Compare this measurement with the measurements shown below.

These tables list the elbow measurements for men and women of medium frame at various heights. Measurements lower than those listed indicate that you have a small frame, while higher measurements indicate a large frame.

Height (in 1-in heels)	Elbow Breadth	Height (in 2.5-cm heels)	Elbow Breadth
	in	←——— cm ———→	
Men			
5′ 2″ – 5′ 3″	2 1/2 – 2 7/8	158 – 161	6.4 – 7.2
5′ 4″ – 5′ 7″	2 5/8 – 2 7/8	162 – 171	6.7 – 7.4
5′ 8″ – 5′ 11″	2 3/4 – 3	172 – 181	6.9 – 7.6
6′ 0″ – 6′ 3″	2 3/4 – 3 1/8	182 – 191	7.1 – 7.8
6′ 4″	2 7/8 – 3 1/4	192 – 193	7.4 – 8.1
Women			
4′ 10″ – 4′ 11″	2 1/4 – 2 1/2	148 – 151	5.6 – 6.4
5′ 0″ – 5′ 3″	2 1/4 – 2 1/2	152 – 161	5.8 – 6.5
5′ 4″ – 5′ 7″	2 3/8 – 2 5/8	162 – 171	5.9 – 6.6
5′ 8″ – 5′ 11″	2 3/8 – 2 5/8	172 – 181	6.1 – 6.8
6′ 0″	2 1/2 – 2 3/4	182 – 183	6.2 – 6.9

* Source of basic data: Data tape, HANES I.

Courtesy of Metropolitan Life Insurance Company.

1983 Metropolitan height and weight tables. Statistical Bull Metropolitan Life Insurance Co. 64(Jan. – June):3, 1983

(From J Am Diet Assoc 84(4):423)

---

measures. The two methods of determining body frame are illustrated above and on page 80, while Table 12-3 illustrates current weight standards.

Children's height and weight standards are very useful in assessing the health of a child. A child whose diet is poor—lacking the needed nutrients—may not grow as fast as other children of the same age. Healthy children grow and gain weight at predictable rates, although these rates vary among individuals.

Two standards commonly used in the USA to follow a child's growth are (1) the Harvard Growth Charts and (2) those of the National Center for Health Statistics (NCHS). The latter's growth chart is illustrated in Figure 12-2. Both standards are divided by age and sex. Normal growth usually falls between the 5th and 95th percentile for the child's age. A child who is in the 25th percentile for age and for height is taller and heavier than 25% of the other children his age. The child may continue to grow and stay

FINDING BODY FRAME BY WRIST CIRCUMFERENCE

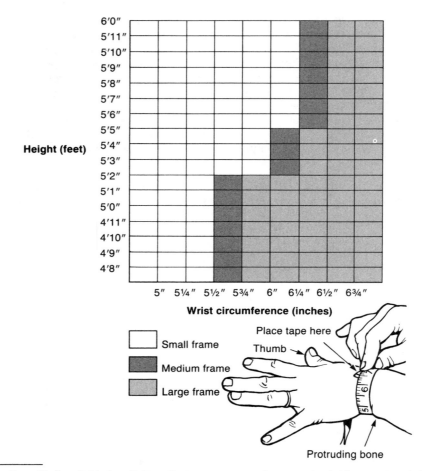

From Sindner P, Lindner D: How To Assess Degrees of Fatness. Cambridge, MD, Cambridge Scientific Industries

at this percentile curve. If he becomes ill and remains so for a long period of time, growth may slow down and the child may "fall" into a lower percentile. Most children can catch up again, after they recover. Some, who have many illnesses, cannot do so. Following a child's growth curve is one indirect way to check on his health and nutrition. In some countries, where most persons are small in stature, there are very different growth charts. Children may grow more slowly. When these children come to the USA and are measured on USA standards, it is hard to tell if they are genetically small, or small because they have been poorly nourished. It is impossible to determine if their parents are small genetically or because their ancestors may also have been poorly nourished. It may not matter that these children are small, if they are completely healthy. But often they are not, and this puzzle — how to interpret their growth chart — is a common problem among health providers who work with recent immigrants and refugee

Table 12-3

1983 Height and Weight Tables*

Height (inches)	Weight (pounds)			Height (cm)	Weight (kilograms)		
Men	Small frame	Medium frame	Large frame	**Men**	Small frame	Medium frame	Large frame
5'1"	128–134	131–141	138–150	154	58–61	59–64	63–68
5'2"	130–136	133–143	140–153	157	59–62	60–65	64–69
5'3"	132–138	135–145	142–156	159	60–63	61–66	64–71
5'4"	134–140	137–148	144–160	162	61–64	62–67	65–73
5'5"	136–142	139–151	146–164	164	62–64	63–69	66–74
5'6"	138–145	142–154	149–168	167	63–66	64–70	68–76
5'7"	140–148	145–157	152–172	170	64–67	66–71	69–78
5'8"	142–151	148–160	155–176	172	64–69	67–73	70–80
5'9"	144–154	151–163	158–180	175	65–70	69–74	72–82
5'10"	146–157	154–166	161–184	177	66–71	70–75	73–84
5'11"	149–160	157–170	164–188	180	68–73	71–77	74–85
6'0"	152–164	160–174	168–192	182	69–74	73–79	76–87
6'1"	155–168	164–178	172–197	185	70–76	74–81	78–89
6'2"	158–172	167–182	176–202	187	72–78	76–83	80–92
6'3"	162–176	171–187	181–207	190	74–80	78–85	82–94
Women				**Women**			
4'9"	102–111	109–121	118–131	145	46–50	49–55	54–59
4'10"	103–113	111–123	120–134	147	47–51	50–56	54–61
4'11"	104–115	113–126	122–137	150	47–52	51–57	55–62
5'0"	106–118	115–129	125–140	152	48–54	52–59	57–64
5'1"	108–121	118–132	128–143	154	49–55	54–60	58–65
5'2"	111–124	121–135	131–147	157	50–56	55–61	59–67
5'3"	114–127	124–138	134–151	159	52–58	56–63	61–69
5'4"	117–130	127–141	137–155	162	53–59	58–64	62–70
5'5"	120–133	130–144	140–159	164	54–60	59–65	64–72
5'6"	123–136	133–147	143–163	167	56–62	60–67	65–74
5'7"	126–139	136–150	146–167	170	57–63	62–68	66–76
5'8"	129–142	139–153	149–170	172	59–64	63–69	68–77
5'9"	132–145	142–156	152–173	175	60–66	64–71	69–79
5'10"	135–148	145–159	155–176	177	61–67	66–72	70–80
5'11"	138–151	148–162	158–179	180	63–69	67–74	72–81

* Based on lowest mortality, ages 25 to 59. From Metropolitan Life Insurance Co. Adjusted for height in bare feet. Figures allow 5 lb (2kg) of clothing for men, 3 lb (1kg) of clothing for women.

children. Simple guidelines for weighing and measuring young children are shown on page 83.

A child is usually considered too small if height-for-age is below the 5th percentile (that is, 95% of all children that age are taller). A small height-for-age may mean that, over a long period of time, poor nutrition has caused the child to grow too slowly. A child is too skinny if weight-for-height is below the 5th percentile,

measuring recent poor nutrition. Many providers become concerned if a child does not gain any weight or height for 6 months or more. Very young children who fit most of these categories are often called "failure-to-thrive" children. This is a diagnosis that only a physician can make, and one that demands a great deal of attention, since it sometimes implies a poor social environment, and not just poor nutrition. It will be discussed in Chapter 33. On page 83

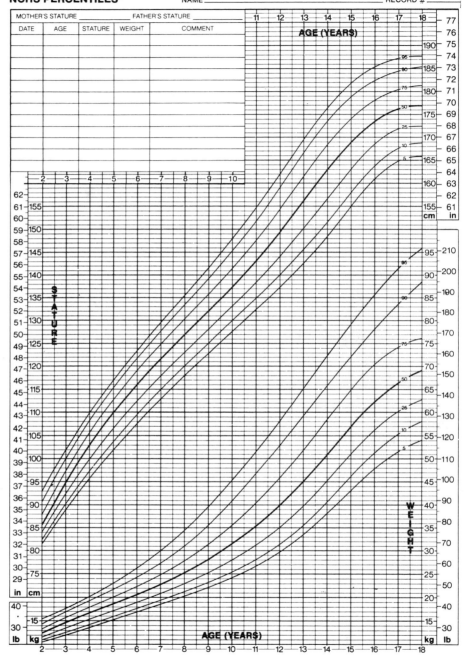

Figure 12-2

Sample NCHS growth chart. (Adapted from Hamill PVV, Drizd TA, Johnson CL, Reed RB et al: Physical growth: National Center for Health Statistics percentiles. Am J Clin Nutr 32:607–629, 1979. Data from the National Center for Health Statistics [NCHS], Hyattsville, Maryland. © 1982 Ross Laboratories)

GUIDELINES FOR WEIGHING AND MEASURING YOUNG CHILDREN

Weighing. Make sure:

1. The scale is standardized (calibrated) before each weight is taken. It must begin at zero.

2. The scale is safe and in good working order.

3. The child cannot hold onto the wall or touch the floor. These will change the results.

4. The child is wearing as little as possible. Infants in diapers should be weighed naked (on a dry diaper for comfort, if the weight of each dry diaper is known). Older children should be in their underwear. If it is too cold for this, the child should wear exactly the same minimal clothing at each weigh-in.

5. The child's mother is nearby.

6. To balance a beam scale, move the weights until they are slightly *more* than the child's weight. Then slowly go backward until the beam balances.

7. If the child is weighed once a month or less, record weight to the nearest 250 g or 1/2 pound. If weight is taken more often, record to nearest 100 g or 1/4 pound.

Length/Height. Make sure:

1. There are two people to measure. One can be the mother.

2. The numbers on the board or stick are easy to read.

3. The child's head and feet are pressing against right angles. One may be the floor or wall and another a movable block or wooden triangle.

4. The child is barefoot and wearing no hat or headgear.

5. Heels are down, knees are straight, and body is as still as possible. The mother can help with this.

6. The child is in the correct position for the growth chart being used. NCHS growth charts for 0 to 36 months are designed for children lying down; charts for ages 2 to 18 are designed for standing children.

7. One end of the child is at zero.

8. Read measures to the nearest 1/2 cm or 1/8 inch.

(Adapted from Griffiths M: Growth Monitoring, pp 69–70. Washington, International Health Programs, American Public Health Association, October 1981)

---

there are basic guidelines for obtaining accurate, consistent measures when weighing young children.

STANDARDS FOR NUTRIENTS

The RDAs

The most reputable, well-established, and thoroughly researched standard available for nutrient needs in the USA is the Recommended Dietary Allowances, or RDA. The first RDAs were used during World War II, and the data is reviewed approximately every 5 years or as changes are indicated from new research. Each

RDA uses the most recent research to help determine how much of each nutrient Americans need.

The RDAs are not minimums; they are maximums. They list the amount of a nutrient that (as far as can be carefully estimated) is almost certainly enough to cover the needs of most healthy people. Appendix 1 is a complete list of the RDAs for each nutrient for which there is an established human need.

US RDA

Another standard for nutrients is the *US RDA* or US Recommended Daily Allowances, which

Table 12-4

U.S. Recommended Daily Allowances

	Protein (g)	Vitamin A (iu)	Vitamin D (iu)	Vitamin E (iu)	Vitamin C (mg)	Folic acid (mg)	Thiamin (mg)	Ribo-flavin (mg)	Niacin (mg)
*Infants**	18† 25	1,500	400	5	35	0.1	0.5	0.6	8
Children under 4 yrs.	20‡ 28	2,500	400	10	40	0.2	0.7	0.8	9
Adults & children 4 or more years of age	45§ 65	5,000	400	30	60	0.4	1.5	1.7	20
Pregnant or lactating women	5[11]	8,000	400	30	60	0.8	1.7	2.0	20

* Infant less than 1 year
† 18 g if quality equal to or greater than casein; 25 g if quality less than casein
‡ 20 g if quality equal to or greater than casein; 28 g if quality less than casein
§ 45 g if quality equal to or greater than casein; 65 g if quality less than casein
[11] No protein stipulation provided for pregnant or lactating women (NAS/NRC RDA suggests +30 g for pregnant and +20 g for lactating women).

differs from the RDA. It is more general, since it does not consider sex differences, has only a few age categories, and is used exclusively for food labelling. Grocery products frequently list their nutrient content in percentages of the US RDA.

Table 12-4 defines the current US RDA. Since the US RDA uses the *highest figures within each age group,* many persons will be well nourished on *less than* 100% of this standard. However, these rough approximations can be useful to consumers. They are helpful in comparing the nutritive value of various supermarket foods, which is exactly why they were designed. They are too general to be used in planning individual menus. The RDAs and the "basic four" are more appropriate for that purpose.

The Basic Four

The *Basic Four Food Groups* is another set of standards that can be used to check for good nutrition. This method is easy, practical, and is a help in teaching persons how to eat, because it is fairly easy to learn.

The "basic four" are food groups into which can be categorized all foods that naturally contain needed vitamins, minerals, and other essential nutrients. Foods that provide only energy and/or fat are considered "low nutrient density" foods and do not belong in any of the four groups. This method will be described in detail and will be used throughout the rest of this section. The basic four is presented in brochure form from the American Dairy Council, and is partially illustrated in Table 12-5.

The four food groups are (1) Milk/Dairy, (2) Meat and Protein Sources, (3) Fruits and Vegetables, and (4) Grains. A person needs to eat a certain number of servings each day from each of the four groups to obtain most of the essential nutrients he needs. Each group contains foods with similar nutrients.

For example, the milk group does not contain just milk alone. It also includes cheese, ice cream, pudding, and yogurt. These are the foods that contain large amounts of calcium. Eating from this group each day helps a person obtain the required amount of calcium. Other nutrients in this group include protein, riboflavin, and thiamin.

The meat group is important for protein, niacin, and iron. Again, it contains more than meat. Eggs, cheese, peanut butter, tofu, nuts, seeds, and legumes also provide protein, so they belong in this group, along with fish and poultry.

Table 12-4

U.S. Recommended Daily Allowances

Vitamin B_6 (mg)	Vitamin B_{12} (μg)	Biotin (mg)	Panto-thenic Acid (mg)	Calcium (g)	Phos-phorus (g)	Iodine (μg)	Iron (mg)	Mag-nesium (mg)	Copper (mg)	Zinc (mg)
0.4	2	0.15	3	0.6	0.5	45	15	70	0.6	5
0.7	3	0.15	5	0.8	0.8	70	10	200	1.0	8
2.0	6	0.30	10	1.0	1.0	150	18	400	2.0	15
2.5	8	0.30	10	1.3	1.3	150	18	450	2.0	15

Fruits and vegetables are combined into one group because the key vitamins, A and C, are found in many fruits and vegetables. Citrus fruits (such as oranges, grapefruit, kiwi, lemons, and limes) are important members because they are extremely high in vitamin C. Green and orange vegetables (such as greens, squash, carrots, and sweet potatoes) are important because they are rich in vitamin A. Other fruits and vegetables provide fiber and many trace minerals.

The grain group provides carbohydrate, thiamin, niacin, and some iron. Breads and cereals fit into this group, but pastries, cookies, and cakes do not. Those sweets contain carbohydrate, but few essential vitamins or minerals, and are usually high in fat and sugar. These foods, together with other common snack foods, such as potato chips, candy, pie, and soft drinks, are not necessary for good health. The four food groups serve as a guideline to *good* nutrition. The "junk foods" listed above may fill calorie needs without providing other nutrients that are essential to a balanced diet.

The four food groups does not consider minor (trace) vitamins and minerals, nor does it consider the body's need for a small amount of fat. But a person who, each day, chooses foods according to this guideline, and uses some fat or oil in cooking, will probably obtain enough of almost all the necessary vitamins and minerals. This is why choosing a variety of foods within each of the groups is so important.

The four food groups can be a useful system in menu planning. It will be used as a guide for this purpose in Chapters 13 through 19. More information on menu planning using the four food groups is usually available at local County Cooperative Extension or Dairy Council office's.

Food Composition Tables

Other helps in meeting nutrient standards are food composition tables. These are books that list most foods available in the USA and exactly how much of each major nutrient can be found in them. Three common food composition tables are available and are listed at the end of this chapter.[3,4,5]

STANDARDS FOR HEALTH

Dietary Guidelines

Good eating habits can help a person acquire and maintain good health. A proper diet is not the answer to every ill, but it is important. Some

Table 12-5

*The Four Food Groups — a Recommended Daily Pattern**

| | Recommended Number of Servings† | | | | |
Food Group	Child	Teenager	Adult	Pregnant Woman	Lactating Woman

Milk
 1 cup milk, yogurt, OR calcium equivalent:
   1½ slices (1½ oz) cheddar cheese‡
   1 cup pudding
   1¾ cups ice cream
   2 cups cottage cheese‡
	3	4	2	4	4

Meat
 2 ounces cooked lean meat, fish, poultry, OR protein equivalent:
   2 eggs
   2 slices (2 oz) cheddar cheese‡
   1 cup dried beans, peas
   4 tbsp peanut butter
	2	2	2	3	2

Fruit-vegetable ½ cup cooked or juice 1 cup raw Portion commonly served such as a medium-size apple or banana	4	4	4	4	4
Grain Whole grain, fortified, enriched 1 slice bread 1 cup ready-to-eat cereal ½ cup cooked cereal, pasta, grits	4	4	4	4	4

Others

Sweets, oils, condiments and other foods high in sugar and/or fat sould not replace foods from the Four Food Groups. Amounts should depend on individual energy needs, since they have very few essential nutrients and are often high in calories.

* The recommended daily pattern provides the foundation for a nutritious, healthful diet.

† The recommended servings from the Basic Four Food Groups for adults supply about 1200 calories. This chart gives recommendations for the number and size of servings for several categories of people.

‡ Count cheese as serving of milk OR meat, not both simultaneously.

"Others" complement but do not replace foods from the Basic Four Food Groups. Amounts should be determined by individual caloric needs.

(Courtesy of National Dairy Council, Rosemont IL 60018. Copyright © 1977. All rights reserved.)

eating—or drinking—habits are not healthful, and every person has a right to know what those habits are and so to make appropriate, informed choices.

The "Dietary Guidelines for Americans," first issued by the US government in 1980, include recommendations in seven areas relating to nutrition. Each of the seven guidelines covers an area in which eating or drinking may affect health. These guidelines do not recommend specific foods or vitamins; they simply recommend moderation.

The seven guidelines are:

1. Eat a variety of foods
2. Maintain ideal weight
3. Avoid too much fat, saturated fat, and cholesterol
4. Eat foods with adequate starch and fiber
5. Avoid too much sugar
6. Avoid too much sodium
7. If you drink alcohol, do so in moderation

Some critics feel that the guidelines are too general; each person must determine what is "too much" for him. But the guidelines can be a basis for further teaching. They are explained in detail in a booklet called "Nutrition and Your Health: Dietary Guidelines for Americans", available from the US Department of Agriculture and from most local county extension agencies. Booklets with recipes to help incorporate the guidelines into daily life are also available.[6]

Anthropometrics

Other standards used to assess nutrition and health involve measuring body fat and muscle. There are many ways of doing this. Any measurement of the body is an anthropometric measure. Most include height and weight, as well as other measures, such as upper arm fat stores. The most popular is the triceps skinfold thickness measurement (TSF).

A person's upper arm usually contains fat measurable by "pinching". In the TSF method, this fat measure is compared to certain standards.* The result tells whether the person has

more or less fat than the rest of the population. Specially designed "calipers" are the instruments used to help measure arm fat stores and, indirectly, muscle. Too little muscle, or a loss of muscle mass, can be a sign of poor nutrition. A person may not look thin because he has stores of fat, but he may be poorly nourished and need medical attention.

This method is not widely used, because it is difficult to obtain consistent results. Health professionals who do use this method successfully are those who use this method in combination with other, more precise methods. Usually quicker methods, or laboratory tests, are used to assess poor nutrition.

Another form of *anthropometrics* is sometimes used in poorer, underdeveloped nations to evaluate food programs. Some may use a tape measure or strip of colored cloth around the upper arm. The parents or health workers learn that a child needs extra food if the tape shows a measurement below a certain number, or within a certain color range. Growth charts are also commonly used in underdeveloped countries. Although the parents may be unable to read them, they may highly value this bit of paper that belongs to *their* child.

These are the common standards used to determine nutrition and health. They are general, and often involve approximations and ranges of numbers. The human body is unique, and can adapt to many different health and nutrient conditions. This is one reason the guidelines must be general in order to be practical. Yet there is a great deal of research behind each standard, so that advice based on these standards can certainly help prevent malnutrition, nutrient toxicities, and many other nutrient related health problems.

STUDY QUESTIONS

1. What types of nutrition and health-related standards are used in the USA?

2. How do the energy and nutrient standards of other countries differ from USA standards? Is this difference due to differences in the population of these countries? Why or why not?

---

* Am J Clin Nutr 34:2540–2545, November 1981

3. A 58-year-old woman weighs 53 kg and is 154 cm tall. How many calories does she need
   - According to the RDA?
   - According to the Harris-Benedict Equation?

4. How many calories do *you* need according to each of these standards?

5. What are the Recommended Dietary Allowances? Do most people need more than they recommend? Why or why not?

6. Does the US RDA differ from the RDA? If so, in what way?

7. A Southeast Asian boy, age three, has just arrived in the US from a refugee camp. His parents bring him to see a doctor in a local clinic because he has had a fever for three days. The child is weighed and measured. He is below the 5th percentile of height for his age.
   a. Describe at least three reasons why he might be so small.
   b. What standards might be used in the US to compare his height and weight?

8. What are the Basic Four Food Groups? List at least two foods in each group.

9. Where in the Basic Four do chocolate bars, cookies, and jelly beans belong? Why?

10. What are the major advantages and disadvantages of the "Basic Four" guidelines?

11. List at least four of the seven dietary guidelines.

12. Make a list of all the foods and beverages (including snacks) that you ate yesterday.
    - Next to each food, write where it fits in the Basic Four.
    - Compare your intake to the Dietary Guidelines. How does it meet or not meet them?

13. What are anthropometrics? How are they useful as nutrition and health standards?

REFERENCES

1. Benedict FG: Lectures on Nutrition. Mayo Foundation Lectures. Philadelphia, WB Saunders, 1925
2. Weighley ES: Average? Ideal? Desirable? A brief overview of height–weight tables in the United States. J Am Diet Assoc 84(4):417–423
3. Bowes & Church: Food Values of Portions Commonly Used. Philadelphia, JB Lippincott, 1984
4. Nutritive Value of American Foods in Common Units (Handbook 456), 1975. Repr. 1981*
5. Composition of Foods: A revision of Handbook 8 with sections by food types*
6. Ideas for Better Eating: Menus and Recipes to Make Use of the Dietary Guidelines. US Department of Agriculture, 1981

———————

* Copies are available from the Superintendent of Documents, US Government Printing Office, Washington, DC 20402

CHAPTER 13

Nutrition in Pregnancy

OBJECTIVES

1. To create an awareness of the vital role of maternal nutrition during pregnancy

2. To explain in simple terms how a fetus is nourished

3. To explain weight gain during pregnancy

4. To list, quantify, and describe the increased needs a pregnant woman has for
   a. energy
   b. protein
   c. calcium
   d. iron
   e. folic acid

5. To illustrate these increased needs by a specific eating plan and sample menu

6. To explain physical issues, problems, and social considerations that may affect the nutrition of mother and child

7. To encourage health providers to be aware of other community resources available to a pregnant woman

8. To provide simple, educational graphs and illustrations that may be used in counseling pregnant women

G ood nutrition is always important, but it has the greatest long-term influence on life during the prenatal (before birth) period. During the first 9 months — in the womb — the body experiences more changes than it does throughout the rest of its life. It grows from a single, fertilized egg cell into a complete and complex system. During most of this womb life, the unborn child is called a *fetus* (latin for "young one") and this is the term that will be used throughout this chapter.

The fetus is not a parasite. He cannot take everything needed from the mother, regardless of her health. Studies have shown that if the mother's health or nutrition is poor, the fetus may suffer, too.[1,2,3] Growth in the womb occurs so rapidly that the fetus might not be able to compensate later for these deficiencies.

The guidelines used in this chapter are designed to help the pregnant woman eat the foods she needs for good nutrition. What she needs will depend on her reserves, her health before pregnancy, her weight, and the demands of pregnancy itself. These vary according to each individual and are hard to measure. Because of this, it is better for the mother to acquire a little more rather than a little less of the essential nutrients. It is not wise to try and "get by" with the minimum during pregnancy, because the minimum is not really known to science. Nor is pregnancy the time to diet. The mother may be able to live from her excess fat stores, but the fetus cannot. Fat stores do not contain needed vitamins, minerals, and protein. Nor is pregnancy the time to gorge on sweets and fats. Every food counts, and every nutrient counts.

Nutrition is important even before a woman *knows* she is pregnant. It is important even before the woman *becomes* pregnant, because a healthy body will probably handle the stress of pregnancy better than could a body in poor condition from faulty nutrition or illness. The healthy, well-nourished woman will provide the fetus with a good chance for developing his own good health and nutrition.

Some women going through pregnancy eat poorly, gain very little weight, and have apparently healthy babies. In such cases, the mother's reserves have helped the fetus to survive and thrive, but this is never an ideal situation. The mother's health may suffer. She is utilizing more nutrients than she is acquiring in order to nourish the growing child. And the infant may not always thrive.

Studies of pregnant women who lived in Holland and Russia under famine conditions during World War II are good examples of what may happen if a pregnant woman compromises her nutrition.[4] Since the brain and spinal cord are formed in the first few weeks of pregnancy more babies whose mothers were starved early in their pregnancies were born with brain or spinal cord defects. And since babies usually gain protective fat stores during the last few weeks in the womb, the infants born to mothers who starved during these weeks were born lighter than average. They were more likely to be low-birth-weight babies (*i.e.,* under 5½ lb or 2.5 kg). This is dangerous because such infants have many more health problems early in life than heavier infants. They are also more likely to die in the first four weeks of life (the neonatal period). This is illustrated in Figure 13-1.

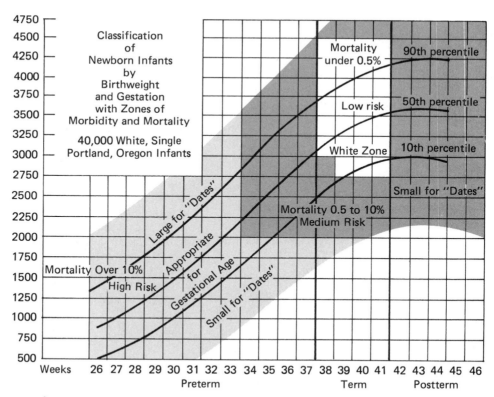

Figure 13-1
Mortality risk in newborns by gestational age and birthweight. (From Babson SG, Benson RC, Pernoll ML, Benda GI: Management of High-Risk Pregnancy and Intensive Care of the Neonate. St Louis, CV Mosby, 1975)

These are only a few reasons why nutrition is extremely important during pregnancy. Good nutrition never guarantees a healthy baby, but it makes the birth of one more likely. The guidelines in the following pages can be used to help a pregnant woman build a "margin of safety" into the nutrition and health of herself and her growing child.

FETAL NUTRITION

A fetus receives its food and oxygen directly from its mother's blood. Her blood flows into the *placenta* (a mass of blood vessels attached to the wall of the uterus; the placenta becomes the "afterbirth"). Nutrients and oxygen in the placenta pass into vessels (veins) that travel through the umbilical cord (attached to the placenta) to the fetus. Waste products and blood that requires new oxygen then travel from the infant, through the cord, back to the placenta. The wastes are passed into the mother's blood (and from there to her kidneys) and new oxygen is absorbed. The process repeats itself constantly, and so the fetus constantly requires more nutrients for growth. If a pregnant woman smokes, less oxygen may be available for the fetus. If a woman does not eat over a long period of time, less nutrients may be available. Whatever happens in the mother's life has some influence on the fetus.

THE MOTHER'S INCREASED NEEDS

Weight

Most physicians today believe a woman should gain between 24 lb and 27 lb during her pregnancy. This helps ensure good health for both mother and fetus. Figure 13-2 illustrates where this extra weight is usually needed, and these areas are outlined below.

The *breasts* are being prepared for lactation.

The *placenta* is the organ (described above) that allows the infant to receive food and oxygen from the mother's blood.

Amniotic fluid surrounds the fetus in the uterus at all times. The fetus "swims" in this fluid

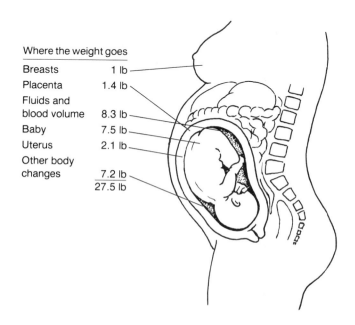

Where the weight goes	
Breasts	1 lb
Placenta	1.4 lb
Fluids and blood volume	8.3 lb
Baby	7.5 lb
Uterus	2.1 lb
Other body changes	7.2 lb
	27.5 lb

Figure 13-2
Weight gain during pregnancy.

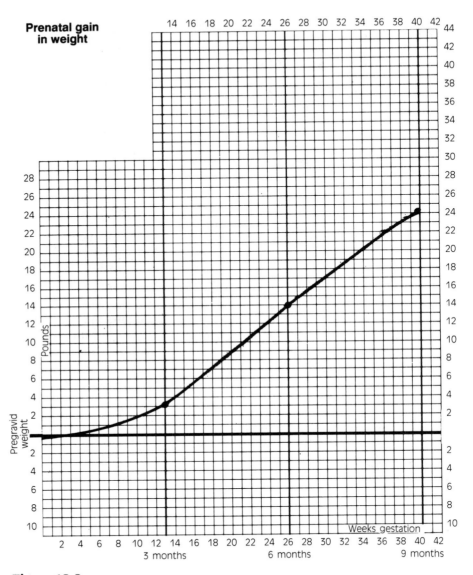

Figure 13-3
Recommended prenatal weight gain by weeks. (From Nutrition During Pregnancy and Lactation. Maternal and Child Health Unit, California Department of Health, 1975)

until birth. This is the "bag of waters" that breaks at the beginning of labor.

Extracellular, extravascular fluid is deposited throughout the body. When there is too much of this fluid, the condition is called *edema* and is not healthy for the woman. However, some extra fluid is normal.

Blood is needed to nourish the fetus and all the new cells in the body. The blood may contain a slightly higher proportion of water than did the woman's blood supply before her pregnancy. "Hemodilution" (diluted blood) is the term for this condition.

Fetus or infants under 5½ lb at birth are at a high risk for complications and neonatal death. Premature infants are frequently below this weight, and their lungs may not be sufficiently developed for proper breathing. An average, healthy birth weight is 6–8 lb.

The *uterus* grows as the fetus grows.

Maternal stores are extra stores of fat. Some extra stores are usually helpful for a breast-feeding woman, since breast-feeding may use more energy than pregnancy.

Figure 13-3 illustrates the rate at which weight should be gained during pregnancy. This graph can help a woman plot her own weight gain. Some women may not even begin to gain weight until the third month, but a 2 lb to a 4 lb gain during this period is recommended.

During the final 6 months, women should gain between three quarters of a pound and 1 pound each week. The healthiest rate of gain is one that falls somewhere within the dotted lines on the graph (Fig. 13-3). If weight gain goes above these lines, it may be a sign of extra fat or too much fluid. Weight gain below the grid is a sign that the mother's (or the fetus') nutrition is being shortchanged.

Women with severe nausea and vomiting often lose weight early in their pregnancy. This condition is never recommended, but sometimes seems unavoidable. A woman who is losing weight and has trouble "keeping food down" (or eating at all) *must* talk to her doctor about this problem. Some measures that can keep nausea and vomiting to a minimum for many women are listed below.

Energy

Another increased need in pregnancy is energy. Almost everyone knows that a woman should eat more food during pregnancy. Often, however, the amount is exaggerated so that it is easy for many women to gain too much weight. Sometimes energy needs are emphasized and other nutrient needs are ignored.

NAUSEA/VOMITING

Nausea and/or vomiting may occur in the early months of pregnancy. Some suggestions for relief:

Before getting out of bed, have plain toast or crackers and then get up slowly. Wait several hours before brushing your teeth.

Eat when you feel hungry; try 5 or 6 *small* meals rather than 2 or 3 large meals.

Eat slowly.

Avoid greasy, fried, or spicy foods.

Drink fluids between meals rather than with meals.

Drink a small amount of 100% fruit juice (apple, grape, or cranberry may settle best) every 1–2 hours.

If severe vomiting continues, see your physician.

From Prenatal Feeding Guide, Form 75, Massachusetts WIC Program.

A pregnant woman needs (on the average) only 300 more calories each day over and above her normal, nonpregnant energy needs. This increase is small compared to the great increase in her needs for certain nutrients. So she should choose her foods carefully.

Nutrients

Pregnancy increases a women's need for *every* nutrient, not just the four nutrients that will be discussed in detail below. This is one reason most obstetricians routinely prescribe prenatal vitamins. Vitamins do not provide all the nutrients the women needs, but they can give a "margin of safety" to help provide mother and child with some of the essential vitamins and minerals.

The four most important nutrients in pregnancy (other than energy) are (1) protein, (2) calcium, (3) iron, and (4) folacin. The needs for these four nutrients increase tremendously in pregnancy, and they may be hard to obtain. Figure 13-4 illustrates the increased needs for these four nutrients.

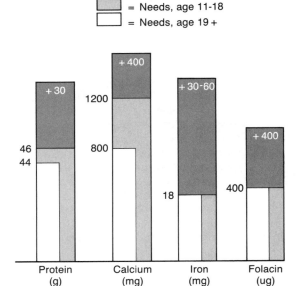

= Increased needs in pregnancy
= Needs, age 11-18
= Needs, age 19 +

Figure 13-4
Increased needs for four key nutrients during pregnancy. (Adapted from information from Food and Nutrition Board, National Academy of Sciences: Recommended Dietary Allowances. Washington, National Research Council, 1980)

Iron and folacin help prevent anemias. Low-iron levels are common in pregnancy, and this is a time when the body's demands for iron are high. Iron levels low enough to create *iron deficiency anemia* make the heart work harder to provide oxygen, and consequently the pregnant woman feels short of breath, weary, weak, and listless. Extreme folic acid deficiency is called *megaloblastic* or *macrocytic anemia.* In this type of anemia, red blood cells become enlarged and die more quickly. Women deficient in folacin are often iron-deficient at the same time. If the mother does not have enough iron, the fetus may not be receiving a sufficient quantity. The pregnant woman needs twice as much of these nutrients as she did before her pregnancy. Chapters 7 and 8, and Table 13-1 outline foods high in these nutrients, which are also contained in most prenatal supplements.

Prenatal prescriptions, however, do not pro-vide the extra protein or calcium a pregnant woman needs. These must come from food. The foods the woman eats can also provide the vitamins and minerals that might not be adequately supplied in her prenatal supplements.

FOOD GUIDE

Table 13-1 illustrates a guideline that can be used in planning meals for a pregnant woman. It is based on the four food groups, and does not include oils, fats, or sugars. If weight gain is normal, they can be added to what is needed, as desired. The chart also list foods high in the four key nutrients discussed above.

Women who only eat foods selected from this

SAMPLE MENU PLAN FOR A PREGNANT WOMAN*

Breakfast:
　2-egg omelet
　1 cup milk
　2 slices toast
Lunch:
　½ cup orange juice
　open-faced grilled cheese, using 1½ oz cheese
　1 cup salad greens
Aft. Snack:
　1 cup yogurt
Dinner:
　1 cup milk
　4 oz broiled chicken
　½ cup rice
　½ cup broccoli
Bed. Snack:
　1 banana
　1 cup milk

*This is an example of how the recommended foods might be distributed throughout the day. Most pregnant women will need more calories for proper weight gain than this menu provides. A woman might have a larger snack, more whole-grain breads and cereals, or butter, mayonnaise, or oil in foods to acquire the calories she needs.

Table 13-1

Food Guide for Pregnancy and Lactation

Food Group (nutrients)	Recommended Daily Servings	Sample Serving		Why Is This Important?
Milk (calcium, protein)	4–5	1 cup milk, yogurt, buttermilk 1½-2 oz hard cheese 1½ cups ice cream 1 cup pudding with milk 1 cup cream soup (with milk) 1 cup calcium—fortified soy milk 2 cups cottage cheese	*Other high calcium foods:* 3 oz sardines 4 oz canned mackerel 1 cup macaroni and cheese 3 cups leafy green vegetables (mustard or collard greens, broccoli)	*calcium* helps strengthen forming bones and teeth
Protein Foods (protein, iron)	3–4	2 oz cooked lean meat, fish, poultry 2 eggs 2 oz hard cheese ½ cup cottage cheese 1 cup cooked dry beans/peas 4 tbsp peanut butter 5 oz tofu (soybean curd)	*Other high iron foods:* iron-fortified cereals liver from beef, pork, poultry, or lamb dried prunes other dried fruits	*iron* keeps blood healthy *protein* helps form muscles, bones, organs, tissues, and blood.
Fruits, Vegetables (folacin, vitamins, fiber)	4	1 med. size fruit or vegetable ½ cup cooked 1 cup raw ½ cup juice	*To get ≈100 µg folacin*[*] 1 cup leafy green vegetables ¼ cup wheat germ 1 cup cooked dry beans/peas 6 oz fresh or frozen reconst. orange juice 1 avocado 3 oz liver 2 raw tomatoes	*folacin* keeps blood healthy *vitamin C* helps body use iron, helps skin *vitamin A* is needed for eyes and skin *fiber* keeps bowels soft. *carbohydrates* and *B vitamins* help body make and use energy
Breads, Cereals (iron, B vitamins, fiber, carbohydrate)	4	1 slice bread, tortilla 1 cup ready-to-eat cereal ½ cup hot cooked cereal, pasta ½ cup rice or other grains 5 crackers 1 medium pancake ½ English muffin or bagel		

[*]J Am Diet Assoc 70:161, 1977. (Adapted from Dairy Council, Guide to Good Eating and Prenatal Feeding, Form #75, Massachusetts WIC program.)

guide will not gain excess fat. If weight is already a problem, a pregnant woman may choose lower fat milk and protein products, but should not choose less than the recommended number of servings. Illustrated on page 94 is a sample menu plan, using only the foods listed in the guide. It is an example that can be modified and changed according to a woman's preference. "Extras" a woman might use with this example include margarine, jelly, peanut butter, or salad dressings. She may want to choose more than the suggested number of servings in each group, and may need more to ensure enough calories. If she is eating everything recommended and is not gaining weight at all she should consult her doctor.

Few pregnant women eat exactly according to a food guide each day. Some feel that this is a time when they can finally eat all the "junk food" they want. Some women do not like milk or are unable to drink it. Some eat only food they crave. It is not essential to follow the guide *exactly* each day, in order to ensure a healthy pregnancy. Regardless of cravings and preferences, however, it is important to acquire as much as possible of these necessary nutrients from foods each day.

COMMON ISSUES IN PREGNANCY

Certain complaints, practices, or problems may recur in pregnancy. Some are discussed below. Health professionals must be able to respond to each of these, and to know how to respond to a pregnant woman's beliefs concerning folklore or home remedies, especially if they influence good nutrition.

Cravings and Appetite Changes

A craving is a strong desire for a particular food. Popular cravings in pregnancy include cravings for pickles, pizza, and for ice cream. Many women believe the craving comes from the baby and must be satisfied, since the baby is asking for it. Cravings per se are not harmful, but a woman who eats only foods she craves may be neglecting major nutrients. Feelings alone are not an adequate criterion for deciding how and what to eat.

Some women suddenly develop tremendous appetites during pregnancy. If they are eating the proper foods and want more, the fetus will probably not be harmed. But the woman may gain too much weight.

Some substances may not be healthful for the pregnant woman. Caffeine, tobacco, alcohol, and large quantities of foods high in sodium may all be potentially harmful.

Body Aches

Aches and pains and cramps are common in pregnancy, and may or may not be related to nutrition. The growing fetus places a strain on the woman's back, frequently causing backaches. As the shape of the woman's body changes, so does her center of gravity. All activities require more exertion. Hormonal changes often result in leg cramps. Good posture, low-heeled shoes, and plenty of rest are usually the only solutions to these problems.

Constipation

This common problem is usually related to three changes in the body:

1. Slower muscle movement (motility) in the intestinal wall during pregnancy. This is probably related to hormonal changes.

2. The growing fetus presses against the rectum, making the opening narrower. This makes it harder for the woman to excrete waste products.

3. Iron supplements frequently seem to cause constipation.

Just as there are three contributing factors in constipation, there are also three steps that may help to relieve the condition:

1. Regular exercise, such as walking

2. Lots of fluids, including water and juices; a large cup of hot liquid on an empty stomach may help

3. Foods high in fiber such as prunes, raw vegetables and whole grain or bran products. See Chapter 10 for specific high fiber foods.

Heartburn

Heartburn is also related to hormonal changes and fetal growth. Some persons believe that heartburn is a sign the baby has lots of hair. It would not be possible for a baby's hair to cause heartburn in his mother. The baby's *entire body* is causing the heartburn, usually by pushing up against the stomach. The muscle that keeps the stomach contents inside the stomach opens and the fluid in the stomach (which is quite acidic) is "splashed up" into the esophagus, where it causes a burning sensation. Heartburn may be especially severe in women who are short in stature, because the baby has less space in which to grow and stretch. Some suggestions that may relieve heartburn are listed below.[5]

Nausea

The most common complaint during the first 3 months of pregnancy is nausea, or "morning sickness." If it is accompanied by vomiting, or if it lasts more than a few hours each day, a woman

HEARTBURN

Heartburn may occur as the baby grows and pushes on the stomach. Some suggestions for relief:

Eat small, frequent meals.

Decrease coffee and tonic.

Avoid taking antacids; try plain crackers between meals.

Avoid bothersome foods (fried, fatty, spicy foods, coffee, and tonic).

Eat 2 – 3 hours before bed rather than immediately before bedtime.

Sleep in elevated position.

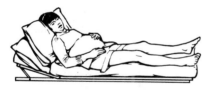

Adapted from Prenatal Feeding Guide, Form 75, Massachusetts WIC Program.

may lose weight and lose her appetite as well. Women who suffer severe or extended vomiting are sometimes placed in the hospital and fed intravenously. Severe vomiting can cause dehydration and can be a serious problem, unless it is controlled.

Nausea seems to be related to:

- Increased levels of certain hormones in the early weeks of pregnancy
- Low blood sugar, which can occur rather quickly in the pregnancy, because the mother is also feeding the fetus with her blood sugar
- A slower motility rate along the digestive tract.[5]

Of these three, only blood sugar may be controlled by the pregnant woman. Suggestions for this, as well as other recommendations that may help alleviate the other side effects, are listed on page 93.

When nausea and vomiting are a problem, it may be impossible to eat according to the recommended guidelines. It may be impossible to eat much at all! When this is the case, and the woman's doctor is aware of the problem, a pregnant woman may find it helps to eat only the foods she feels she can eat without discomfort. In this situation, any food that will stay down is more important than a balanced meal. A woman should keep trying to eat small amounts of foods from the recommended groups, since nausea and vomiting often pass by the end of the third month.

Pica

Pica is the practice of eating clay, dirt, laundry starch, or other nonfoods, and is common in some cultures. It is not a problem in itself (in the same way that cravings may not be a problem), if the substance is harmless. But it may affect the amount of nutritious foods a woman eats. Pica is sometimes a sign of iron – deficiency anemia.[8]

SOCIAL ISSUES

Teenage Pregnancies

Pregnant teens are a mixed group. As Figure 13-4 illustrates, their nutritional needs during pregnancy are higher than those of adults. This is because they are still growing in height and physical maturation. The way in which a teen eats during her pregnancy will depend on many attitudes, as well as on her physical health. These attitudes include

1. Her attitude toward the pregnancy. She may try to ignore the pregnancy, tell no one, and keep her weight down to avoid "showing."

2. Her peers' attitude toward the pregnancy. If her friends have been or are pregnant, and if pregnancy for teens is an accepted part of her culture, she may view her pregnancy more positively.

3. Her attitude toward weight gain. She may feel great pressure to maintain a thin body and so choose low calorie foods during her pregnancy to gain as little weight as possible. Teens should always receive prenatal education appropriate to their age and concerns. Teens frequently have low-birth-weight babies who develop problems in the first few weeks of life. Low weight may be directly related to the mother's beliefs and attitudes about weight gain, and is usually not related to her age.

Often, nothing can be done until the teen admits she is pregnant. But then sensitive counseling and supplemental foods (if finances are a problem) may help her through a healthy pregnancy.

Proscribed Foods

Some cultures, particularly in underdeveloped nations, may forbid certain foods during pregnancy. This proscription is usually related to cultural beliefs about the specific food. For example, Vietnamese traditionally may avoid oranges and lemons during the first trimester.[7] This is because they believe the food has qualities that would create an imbalance in the mother's body. This theory will be discussed in more detail in Chapter 20.

If a certain food is not permitted by a certain culture, a health care provider should inquire about other foods in the same food group. The pregnant woman may be able to receive the nutrients she needs from another food in the same group that does not have the same perceived "risks."

Religious Practices

Few religions include dietary practices that harm or endanger a fetus. However, in some Muslim cultures, a pregnant woman may choose to fast during the month of Ramadan. This month is a time when Muslims are instructed neither to eat nor to drink anything from dawn to sunset. Pregnant women are exempt but may be required to make up later (after delivery) the fasting period they missed. So some women choose to fast during the month of Ramadan, along with everyone else. These women do not eat or drink anything for the 12 hours to 15 hours of daylight, and may be quite active during this time. Their blood sugar is often lower than recommended, which suggests that the fetus may also be "going hungry" at a time when he needs constant nourishment.[8] A Muslim woman and her husband should be told that this is a risk to the fetus and it is wisest to use the exemption their religion allows during pregnancy.

Economic Problems

Another situation in which a woman may not eat enough or eat the right foods is when money is very limited. The woman may have a large family with other children who need available food. Or she may be single and lose her job because of the problems of her pregnancy. This is a time when health providers should be aware of the woman's needs, and of the many resources available, including emergency food stamps, housing if necessary, and the federally funded Aid to Families with Dependent Children and the Women, Infants, and Children's (WIC) programs. Physicians and nurses can make referrals to the WIC program and a social worker should be able to direct a woman to other available community resources, when family support is not adequate or does not exist. (Some such resources are listed at the end of this chapter.) Many communities also have private organizations that offer free support and resources.

Alcohol, Tobacco and Drugs

Alcohol is *never* recommended during pregnancy. Birth defects are more likely to occur when a woman drinks regularly during her pregnancy.[9] The fetus is very sensitive to alcohol, and even occasional moderate drinking may be harmful. Research in this area is still unclear regarding how much alcohol is too much alcohol during pregnancy.

Heavy smoking may deprive the fetus of the oxygen it needs in order to develop fully. Women who are heavy smokers have lower birth-weight babies than women who do not smoke. For these reasons, doctors often recommend that pregnant woman quit smoking and drinking, even in moderation, during their pregnancy.

During the 1950s, many infants were born with missing limbs because their mothers had taken a drug called thalidomide during their pregnancy. This was a vivid, tragic example of how sensitive a fetus is to drugs. This is true of narcotics, "street drugs," high potency prescription drugs, as well as the more "common" aspirin, laxatives, and antibiotics. A pregnant woman should check with her doctor before taking *any* medicine, even if it is a "home remedy."

Coffee

Caffeine, contained in coffee, is a type of drug. Studies have shown birth defects in rats whose mothers were fed high doses of caffeine during their pregnancy.[10] However, this has not yet proved true in humans. We do know caffeine enters the blood of the fetus. It is also in breast milk of women who drink beverages high in caffeine. Many drugs also contain caffeine, so it probably would be wise for a pregnant woman to limit herself to two or less servings of these beverages each day. Beverages high in caffeine are outlined in Chapter 11.

DISEASES IN PREGNANCY

Pregnant women with diabetes, Grave's Disease, or other chronic conditions will be closely followed by their physician. They should also be counseled by a dietitian concerning the special nutrient needs of their pregnancy. Their needs are highly individual, and often are closely followed by the entire health care team.

STUDY QUESTIONS

1. Why is good nutrition especially important in pregnancy? List at least two problems that may occur if an infant does not obtain enough nutrition at critical periods.

2. True or false? Explain your answer:
   - The fetal blood supply is the same as the mother's blood supply.
   - The organ that helps the fetus receive food and oxygen from the mother is called the uterus.
   - A woman can eat as many calories as she wants during pregnancy, as long as she gets the right foods. She need not worry about gaining too much weight.
   - A woman's needs for some vitamins and minerals double or more than double while she is pregnant.

3. How much weight should a woman gain during pregnancy? Where the weight distributed?

4. A pregnant woman needs how many more calories than she did before she was pregnant?

5. What are four of the most important nutrients required in pregnancy? How much more of each does a woman need?

6. List two foods high in each of these four nutrients.

7. Which of these four is not provided in prenatal vitamins?

8. List four common physical issues or complaints during pregnancy.

9. What foods may help constipation?

10. L.G. is 15-weeks pregnant with her first child. She has had nausea and vomiting ever since she perfomed a home pregnancy test and learned that she was pregnant. She lives alone with her husband and has not yet seen a doctor. She has lost about ten

pounds. The most important thing for her to do is (choose one)

- Begin to eat small, frequent meals and crackers every morning.
- See a doctor immediately.
- Consult a nutritionist.
- Take medicine to stop her nausea and vomiting

11. How much milk should a pregnant teen drink? What are some reasons she might not be interested in eating all the foods recommended and in gaining 27 pounds?

12. How much alcohol is permissible for a woman who is pregnant?

13. Should she smoke? Why or why not?

14. Can she keep on drinking lots of Coke, as long as she drinks enough milk? Explain your answer.

15. What resources are available in your community to help a woman during her normal pregnancy?

COMMUNITY RESOURCES

The WIC Program

The Women, Infants, and Children's program is a government-funded supplemental food program for pregnant and breast-feeding women and for infants, and children under the age of 5 years. There are moderate income restrictions, but many working women are eligible. Pregnant women are a high priority. Referral forms must be from a doctor, nurse, or nutritionist and appropriate referrals can be made as soon as a woman knows she is pregnant and sees her doctor.

The WIC program is staffed by qualified nutritionists and provides vouchers that can be used in grocery stores to obtain milk, eggs, cereal, peanut butter, dry beans, and fruity juices. For more information, contact individual state WIC offices.

Prenatal Classes

Many health centers, hospitals, Red Cross, or community centers offer prenatal classes, usually conducted by nurses. Their content varies. Such classes provide films, speakers, educational materials, and often tours of a hospital's labor and delivery rooms to help women prepare for preg-

nancy, delivery, and infant care. Providers who work with pregnant women would be aware of all local resources.

REFERENCES

1. Burke BS et al: The influence of nutrition upon the condition of the infant at birth. J Nutr 26:569, 1943
2. Balfour MJ: Supplemental feeding in pregnancy. Lancet 1:208, 1944
3. Food and Nutrition Board, National Academy of Sciences: Maternal Malnutrition and the Course of Pregnancy. Washington, National Research Council, 1970
4. Stein Z et al: Famine and Human Development: The Dutch Hunger Winter, 1944–45. New York, Oxford University Press, 1975
5. Butman M (ed): Prenatal Nutrition: A Clinical Manual. Boston, Department of Public Health, March 1982
6. Goodhart RE, Shils, ME: Modern Nutrition in Health and Disease, p 748. Philadelphia, Lea & Febiger, 1980
7. Manderson L, Mathews M: Vietnamese attitudes toward maternal and infant health. Med J Aust 1:69–72, 1981
8. Prentice AM et al: Metabolic consequences of fasting during Ramadan in pregnant and lactating women. Human Nutr: Clin Nutr 37C:283–294, 1983
9. March of Dimes, Birth Defect Foundation: Drugs, Alcohol, Tobacco Abuse During Pregnancy. Publication No. 9–0029, October 1980. Available from 1275 Mamaroneck Ave., White Plains, NY 10605
10. Food and Drug Administration, US Department of Health and Human Services: Caffeine and Pregnancy. HHS Publication No. (FDA) 81–1081. Available from Office of Public Affairs, 5600 Fisher Lane, Rockville, MD 20857

SUGGESTED READING

Bing E; Moving Through Pregnancy, 8th prtg. New York, Bobs–Merrill, 1975
Erick M: Pregnancy and Nutrition: The Complete Guide and Calendar for D. I. E. T. During Pregnancy. Brookline, MA, Grinnen-Barrett, updated annually
Worthington-Roberts BS, Vermeersch J, Williams SR: Nutrition in Pregnancy and Lactation, 3rd ed. St. Louis, Times Mirror/Mosley College, 1985

CHAPTER 14

Breast-Feeding

OBJECTIVES

1. To introduce the importance of attitude in successful lactation
2. To explain advantages for both mother and infant
3. To list and dispel common misconceptions about breast-feeding
4. To define and explain nutrient needs during lactation, and how these needs compare with those of pregnancy
5. To provide specific guidelines for meal planning
6. To provide detailed instruction on how to initiate and maintain success in breast-feeding
7. To illustrate and define the differences between colostrum, human milk, and cow's milk
8. To explain weaning
9. To introduce infant nutrition needs

Breast-feeding (or *lactation*) is the oldest, most natural way to feed a baby. It has many advantages, even today, over bottle-feeding, and a woman should know as much as possible about it in order to help her decide how she will feed her baby. Since many health providers may not be familiar with breast-feeding information and the practical details that will help a woman start lactation successfully, this chapter will outline these guidelines and provide further resources that can be used to help a woman think through and act on a decision to breast-feed.

Almost every woman is physically able to produce enough milk, no matter how many children she has had, or how small her breasts. Success does not necessarily begin with her body; it begins with her attitude. And her attitudes about breast-feeding are influenced, long before she is pregnant, by many persons in her life. Did her mother breast-feed? What does the infant's father feel about it? Her friends? Her culture? These persons all have a strong influence, as does her attitude toward her own pregnancy.[1]

But a medical provider can also influence the woman. The medical provider can listen, explain, provide materials, show films, and/or refer to programs that will support breast-feeding. The Women, Infants and Children (WIC) program is highly supportive of women who choose to breast-feed. Many communities also have Nursing Mother's Councils and/or chapters of the La Leche League. These organizations are supportive and also provide answers to many practical questions.

So, why breast-feed? There are benefits for both woman and infant.

Benefits for the Woman

1. *Breast milk is inexpensive.* Even when the mother's extra food is considered, breast milk is still cheaper than infant formula.[2]

101

2. *It is convenient.* A woman who breast-feeds does not need to warm bottles in the middle of the night. Many women "express" (or squeeze) their milk into bottles and leave these bottles at home whenever they must leave the baby with someone else. After she becomes used to nursing, a woman's milk will "come" on the schedule her infant needs, usually every 2 or 3 hours. Breast milk is always ready and at the right temperature; it is sterile and no bottles need be washed after the infant has finished feeding. Few women feel comfortable breast-feeding in public, but for those who do, the milk is always ready.

3. *It may make weight loss easier.* Breast-feeding utilizes even more energy than pregnancy, about 500 extra calories per day for the mother of an infant who is solely breast-fed. The mother may eat high-quality foods, drink the recommended milk, juices and water, and still lose weight because her intake of nutrients may not match her output. It is not harmful to lose weight, slowly and steadily, while nursing. Sensible dieting (losing 1 lb to 2 lb per week) will not affect the quantity or quality of the milk, as long as the mother gets enough liquids and enough rest. But if she loses weight too quickly, or if she feels unusually tired or weak, she may not be eating enough or properly. Unfortunately, though, breast-feeding is not a guaranteed way to lose weight! But it may help.

4. *It helps flatten the stomach.* Actually, it helps the uterus shrink back ("involute") to its prepregnancy size. This makes the stomach look flatter. The uterus involutes more quickly if a woman is breast-feeding than if she is not doing so, because nursing stimulates the hormones that perform this function. In fact some breast-feeding women have cramps during the first few days they breast-feed, because the uterus is changing shape and size so quickly.

5. *Breast-feeding acts as a contraceptive.* Warning: It is not 100% effective! But many women who totally breast-feed do not begin to ovulate for several months after giving birth. Until a woman ovulates, she cannot become pregnant. However, there is no way to know when ovulation occurs until after it has actually happened and menstruation (or pregnancy!) occurs. It is best to use another contraceptive during breast-feeding—one that is safe, effective, and will not interfere with the supply of milk.

Benefits for the Infant

1. *Breast-milk is "custom-made" for the infant's needs. Colostrum,* the yellow fluid that is secreted *before* the breast milk, is very different from the breast milk. It is less likely than formula to cause problems if the infant accidentally aspirates it (swallows it into the lungs). It is very high in antibodies that can help protect the infant from infections. Its other unique characteristics and nutrient composition (see Table 14-1) seem to make it the ideal food for an infant in the first 3 or 4 days of life.

Women who have premature infants also produce a breast milk that is a little different from the breast milk of mothers of full-term infants. The differences seem ideally suited for the needs of the premie.[1]

2. *It helps prevent disease and infection.* Many of the ingredients in breast milk cannot be put into formula, since they cannot be produced artificially. These are the substances that help the infant fight viruses and infections. Both colostrum and breast milk contain these essentials.

3. *Breast-fed babies may develop fewer allergies than formula-fed infants.* An allergy occurs when the body responds to something it identifies as "foreign" or not of itself, just as antibodies fight "foreign" infections. There is still some controversial indication that breast milk may keep an infant from developing allergies as long as he is breast-fed.[3] These studies recommend that infants be breast-fed completely for 6 months before starting formula.

4. *Bonding.* Many people believe that breast-feeding benefits both mother and infant because it encourages close emotional ties. This is called "bonding" and occurs as a

Table 14-1

The Nutrient Composition of Colostrum, Human Milk and Cow's Milk

Composition	Colostrum*	Human Milk*	Cow's Milk*
Energy, Kcals	60	70–75	66
Protein, g	3.2	1.1	3.5
Fat, g	2.5	3.8–4.5	3.7
Lactose, g	5.7	6.8–7.0	4.9
Protein breakdown:			
casein, % protein	47	40	82
whey, % protein	53	60	18
Calcium, mg	27	34	117
Phosphorus, mg	15	14	92
Sodium, mg	47	0.7	2.2
Potassium, mg	74	1.3	3.5
Chloride, mg	88	1.1	2.9
Magnesium, g	3	4	12
Sulfur, mg	20	14	30
Vit. A, μg	54–161	190	102–169
Vit. C, mg	1.4–7.2	4.3	1.1–2.1
Vit. K		1.5	6
Zinc	0.57	0.3–0.5	0.3–0.5
Iodine	12.2	3	4.7
Iron, mg	0.1	0.05	0.05

Adapted largely from Worthington-Roberts BS, Vermeersch J, Williams SR: Nutrition in Pregnancy and Lactation, 3rd ed, p 143. St. Louis, Times Mirror/Mosby College Publishing, 1985
* Except for protein, all figures are stated in units per 100 ml of liquid (1000 ml = 1 liter).

mother gets to know and care about her infant as an individual. Bottle-fed babies can certainly be given just as much love, closeness, and maternal attention as breast-fed infants. This argument should not be used to make a woman feel guilty if she chooses to formula-feed her infant.

Common Misconceptions

There are many false beliefs and misconceptions about breast-feeding. For example, some women feel they will "lose their figure" if they breast-feed. Others think they must either breast- or bottle-feed, but should never do both. Listed on page 104 are some misconceptions concerning breast-feeding, and responses to them.

Diet and the Breast-Feeding Woman

The breast-feeding woman *does* need, on average, 500 calories more than before she became pregnant, or 200 calories more than during her pregnancy. If she keeps on breast-feeding, after the baby is 6-months-old, the baby will need even more calories. So, consequently, will she.

The breast-feeding mother needs more than just extra calories. She still needs high levels of protein, calcium, folacin, iron, and even more vitamins A, C, and zinc than when she was pregnant. Most doctors recommend that breast-feeding women stay on vitamin/mineral supplements, but the supplements themselves may not have all these necessary nutrients. Food continues to be important. However, if a postpartum, breast-feeding woman does not eat enough of these essentials, it is she, and not the baby,

COMMON MISCONCEPTIONS ABOUT BREAST-FEEDING

Some women hesitate to breast-feed because of things they have been told, which are not true. A few of the more common misconceptions are listed below, with appropriate responses.

"It Makes You Lose Your Figure."

It is pregnancy, not breast-feeding, that causes the physical changes in the breasts and nipples. Pregnancy stretches the breasts and may cause them to "sag." Breast-feeding has no effect on this, and it actually helps the abdomen regain its shape more quickly.

"It Will Tie Me Down Too Much."

It is true that a breast-feeding woman may feel "chained" to her infant for the first month. But those first few weeks are very demanding for all new mothers, whether they breast-feed or not. Breast-feeding may help save time that would otherwise be spent preparing formula. After the first month, bottles may be introduced to give the mother more freedom to go out or to get some extra sleep. Many mothers work, giving formula or breast milk in bottles during the day and nursing in evenings, night, and mornings.

I'm Too Modest."

This is a common feeling. Most women need privacy for breast-feeding, especially in the early weeks. The woman needs a place where she can relax, comfortably. Many women who feel this way breast-feed at home and give their infants a bottle when they are in public.

However, breast-feeding can be done modestly in public. Clothing should be loose. Blouses can be unbuttoned from the bottom and sweaters pulled up from the waist. Extra cardigans or a diaper over the shoulder provide complete coverage. It is also possible to adapt some clothes so that they open with slats at the breast during feeding, and close with Velcro or snaps.

"I Don't Eat Well Enough to Breast-Feed."

Breast-feeding women do not need a nutrient-perfect diet for successful nursing. A woman needs lots of fluids, a regular source of calcium for her own nutrition, and as much rest as possible and practical. The quality of the breast milk is always the same, regardless of her diet. If her diet is poor, she is hurt more than the baby. Women in underdeveloped nations are sometimes malnourished, but they breast-feed successfully. A nutritious diet is important for the lactating woman, but a poor diet should not be an excuse for deciding not to breast-feed.

---

who suffers. Eating well can help her develop sufficient energy to deal with an active, demanding infant, as well as help her body repair and restore itself after delivery.

A lactating woman needs one more serving of dairy products than when she was pregnant. She could still use the sample menu plan shown in the preceding chapter. However, another plan for a day's menu is shown on the opposite page. These charts do not consider the high fluid needs of the lactating woman. Breast-feeding women should drink at least 2 quarts of fluid every day, and more, if necessary, to satisfy thirst.

BREAST-FEEDING: HOW TO BEGIN

1. Preparation

Breast-feeding may be natural, but breast-feeding techniques do not come automatically. They have to be learned. A woman should be prepared. Even while she is still pregnant, she should learn how to initiate breast-feeding, how to care for lactating breasts, and how to make enough milk. She should know what to expect during the first few days, and she should know where to turn if she has questions or problems. She should know how the hospital is going to

*SAMPLE MENU PLAN FOR A BREAST-FEEDING WOMAN**

Breakfast:
1½ cups iron fortified bran cereal
6 oz juice
1 cup milk
Snack:
1 cup plain, lowfat yogurt
Lunch:
Tuna salad, made with 3 oz tuna
2 slices raisin toast
raw carrot sticks
6 oz orange juice
Snack:
1 oz cheese with crackers
ice water
Dinner:
1 cup brown rice
1 cup cooked, dry beans
salad, made with 1 cup raw, washed spinach, tomato
1 cup milk
Snack:
1 oz cheese with crackers
6 oz orange juice

---

* The Sample Menu Plan shown in the preceding chapter could also be used as a model for the breast-feeding woman. Add 1 cup milk to that Menu Plan. (All sample menus in this text are suggestive, based on known nutrient needs. They should never be used as diet *prescriptions.* Diets should be adapted individually to the guidelines. Physicians can make referrals to a registered dietitian if detailed diet counseling is necessary.)

---

help her start breast-feeding. Will she be able to place the baby on the breast for feeding immediately after delivery? Will the hospital feed the baby glucose water if it seems hungry between "feeding times" in the nursery, or will the infant be brought to the mother on demand? Can she keep the baby in her room during the hospital stay? If a woman is prepared, she should feel comfortable, confident, and relaxed when breast-feeding does begin. She will know what to say to friends and relatives who might not approve of her decision.

A woman should examine her nipples during the last month or two of pregnancy. Some nipples are *inverted.* When the breast is squeezed behind the areola (the brown area surrounding the nipple), as the baby takes the breast to nurse, the inverted nipple recedes backwards into the breast. Normal nipples protrude forward and out, becoming more prominent. Inverted nipples make frustrated infants, because the infant will have difficulty getting milk from them. If nipples are found to be inverted, special shields (see the "Resources" section at the end of this chapter) can be worn over the nipple, under the bra, during the last few months of pregnancy, to help force the nipple outward. If shields are not available, it sometimes helps to massage the breast daily, beginning outward around the nipple, as illustrated in Figure 14-1. This may help

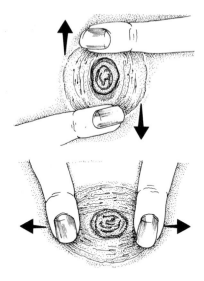

Figure 14-1
Inverted nipples can be treated by placing the thumbs close to the inverted nipple, pressing firmly into the breast tissue, then gradually pushing away from the areola. The strokes should be directed vertically *(top)* and horizontally *(bottom)* and done four or five times in succession. (From Reeder SJ, Mastroianni L, Martin LL: Maternity Nursing, 15th ed, p 424. Philadelphia, JB Lippincott, 1983)

to stretch out the muscles and fibers that keep the nipple "inverted."

Some manuals recommend "nipple preparation," an exercise intended to "toughen" the nipples. However, there is little evidence that it is effective and it may be very uncomfortable and stimulate early production of colostrum.

Breasts must be kept as clean and dry as possible, because too much moisture may lead to infections. For this reason, nursing bras should *not* have plastic liners. If they do, the liners should be removed. This is also why breast shields should not be used during nursing. (However, breast shields are sometimes worn, with a large hole cut out of the center, as another mechanism to encourage inverted nipples to come "out" during pregnancy.) Breast shields are often more uncomfortable for a mother than is a vigorously sucking infant, and they invite

infections. When leaking is a problem between nursings (and it usually *is* during the first month), breast pads or clean handkerchiefs are helpful.

2. The First Few Days

When the placenta (or afterbirth) is delivered, it triggers the brain to "tell" the breasts to begin lactation. This happens regardless of the mother's plans to breast-feed or not to breast-feed. Colostrum begins to flow, and the body is ready for the message that will cause it to begin making more and more milk.

That message is the action of the baby nursing. The way in which to build an adequate supply of milk is to nurse frequently, and thus nursing should begin as soon as possible after delivery.

An infant has to work hard to get milk from the breast. This act of sucking actually signals the mother's body to make more milk. If a baby does not breast feed, or is full of formula when he* begins to nurse, the body will not get the message. There will not be enough stimulation to send the "signal" (controlled, again, by hormones). See Figure 14-2 for an illustration of breast-feeding reflexes.

When first taking her baby to nurse, the mother should be in a comfortable position. She should have enough privacy to feel relaxed. Many women lie on their side in bed or use pillows in an armchair. The infant will not need help learning to suck, but he will need help finding the nipple. If he is stroked on one cheek, he will automatically turn in that direction and open his mouth. This is called the "rooting reflex" and can be used to help him start nursing.

Once his mouth is open, the mother's hand should guide the whole nipple into his mouth, together with as much of the areola (the brown area) as possible. His head should face directly into the breast; if he pulls up, down, or to one side, his nursing may become uncomfortable or even painful to the mother. She can press in on her breast beneath his nose if breathing seems to be a problem.

---

* For the sake of clarity, "he" is used to refer to the infant and "she" to the mother throughout this and the next few chapters.

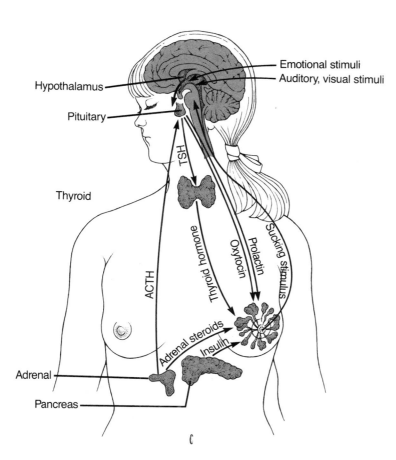

Emotional stimuli
Auditory, visual stimuli
Hypothalamus
Pituitary
TSH
Thyroid
Thyroid hormone
ACTH
Oxytocin
Prolactin
Sucking stimulus
Adrenal steroids
Insulin
Adrenal
Pancreas

Figure 14-2
Breast-feeding reflexes. (From Reeder SJ, Mastroianni L, Martin LL: Maternity Nursing, 15th ed, p 609. Philadelphia, JB Lippincott, 1983. Redrawn from Hytten FE, Leitch I: The Physiology of Human Pregnancy, 2nd ed. Oxford, Blackwell Scientific Publications, 1971)

Once he begins, he need only take each breast for 7 minutes to 10 minutes. Every baby has slightly different sucking patterns, and the mother will begin to learn what these are, and how to work with them. After 7 minutes to 10 minutes, the mother can put her finger gently into the baby's mouth, breaking the suction with the nipple, burp the baby, and then offer the other breast. If she wants to let the baby suck longer at the breast, there is no harm in this, but he has probably taken all the available milk after 10 minutes.

When breast-feeding is over, the breasts should be washed gently with plain water and allowed to air dry for about 15 minutes. This helps prevent infections and helps to "toughen" the breast.

Soreness is a common discomfort during the first few days of nursing. The mother's body is still holding fluid from pregnancy, and going through many changes. Often the best relief is to take milk from the breasts. This can be done with a warm, wet washcloth, or by hand, not only by putting the baby to the breasts. Soreness is usually gone by the end of the fifth or sixth day after delivery.

Starting a breast-fed baby on a bottle during the first week or two is not recommended. Babies suck on bottles in a different way than they take the breast (see Figure 14-3). Taking the breast is more work for the infant. It helps his mother make enough milk, and helps his own jaw muscle development. It is better to wait until both milk supply and breast-feeding schedule are well established before introducing a bottle. Supplementing breast-feeding with bottle-feeding will be discussed in more detail below.

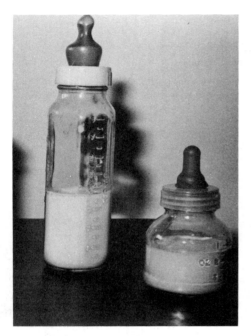

Figure 14-3
Nuk nipple (left) designed to imitate the shape of
the human nipple during breast-feeding versus
the standard bottle nipple (right). Liquid from the
standard nipple flows so quickly that some
infants use their tongue to stop the flow. Getting
milk from the breast requires more jaw work,
controlled flow, and different tongue action.
(From Reeder SJ, Mastroianni L, Martin LL:
Maternity Nursing, 15th ed, p 729. Philadelphia,
JB Lippincott, 1983)

To have enough milk for her baby, a woman
must (1) make it and (2) release it. Delivery of
the child and the action of hormones help to
make milk in the glands at the back of the breast.
The reflex that moves it out of the glands and
into the nipple is called the *let-down reflex*. Once
breast-feeding is well established, this reflex may
work so well that milk will be "let down" simply
as a result of the baby's cry. Breast-feeding will
become a comforting part of life for both
mother and child (see Figure 14-4).

The first few days are a time of trial and error.
During these days, the mother's support system
is very important. These are the days when she
will have the most questions, and when she will
be deciding whether and how long to continue
breast-feeding this and any future children.

3. When the Milk Comes In

On or about the fourth or fifth day after delivery,
the mature or "full" milk replaces colostrum.
This milk looks different. It is thin and bluish in
color, but it is adequate to meet all the baby's
needs for its first four months of life.

Sore, rigid, "engorged" breasts are common
when the milk comes. The best relief for this is
breast-feeding. If the breasts are so swollen that
the baby cannot grasp the nipple, or if he cannot
breathe when he is nursing, some milk should be
expressed by hand or with a warm washcloth
before each nursing. This swelling is a natural
result of the postpartum period, and will disappear within a day or two.

Women express milk for other reasons, too.
Many working mothers express their breast
milk into bottles during their work hours. Fathers or babysitters use this milk to feed the baby
during the next day. Some women express at
each breast-feeding because their infant will
take only one breast per feeding. This milk can
be stored in the refrigerator for 24 hours to 48
hours. If it is frozen, it should be defrosted by
running hot water over the bottle and not by
placing the bottle in the refrigerator to thaw.
Both formula and breast milk can grow bacteria
very quickly.

Many women use breast pumps to express
milk. The quality of these pumps varies widely.
Turn to the end of this chapter for more information on breast pumps. They should be adaptable to nipples of different sizes and should be
easy to clean.

4. Breast Care at Home

Breast care at home is similar to breast care in
the hospital. Breasts must be kept clean and dry
between nursings. Leaking is common until a
schedule is well established, so pads, cloths, or
towels used should be absorbent.

Just as an open cut heals better if it is exposed
to air, sore nipples become less sore through
regular contact with the air, when the breasts are
drying. Some women leave the "flaps" down on
their nursing bras for a short time after nursing.
If cracking still becomes a problem, it can be

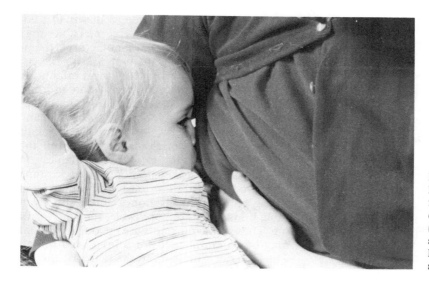

Figure 14-4
Breast-feeding can be both modest for the mother and comforting for the infant. (Photo courtesy Massachusetts Department of Public Health. Used with permission.)

resolved by exposing the breasts to the heat of a 60 watt or 80 watt (bare) light bulb for about 10 minutes after each feeding. The bulb should be 12 inches to 18 inches away from the body.[4]

Breast creams may increase soreness, because they act to hold in the moisture and may encourage infections. Some women use vitamin E oil but this may lead to higher-than-normal vitamin E levels in the baby.

If breasts continue to be very sore, or become painful, or bleed, a woman should contact her doctor immediately. If she seems more tired than usual, has a fever, and/or her breasts ache, she should also call her doctor immediately. This may be a sign of mastitis, or breast infection. Other symptoms include redness, localized soreness and tenderness, swelling, a painful lump in the affected breast, fever, and a general sick, tired, aching feeling.

A woman with a breast infection can, and usually should, continue nursing. The infection will not hurt the baby (often it actually is caused by him) and emptying the breast of milk can help keep the infection from becoming worse. The doctor may prescribe antibiotics that will not affect the baby. If only one breast is affected, that breast should be offered first at each nursing, to help keep it as empty as possible while it heals.

5. Supplementing with Formula

Whenever a woman begins to offer the infant a bottle in addition to breast milk, she has begun the weaning process. The easiest, most comfortable way to do this is to give one bottle a day as a replacement for one breast-feeding, and to continue doing this for 3 days to 5 days before introducing a second bottle at some other feeding. The bottles should be given at the same time each day. This helps the breast to begin producing less milk at that time. Leaking is less of a problem. Figure 14-5 gives a sample weaning schedule.

A woman who must suddenly stop all breast-feeding will find that her breasts will be very sore, full, and uncomfortable for several days. Expressing milk often relieves this, but may aggravate the problem, since it may stimulate the body to continue making milk. Cold packs, cold showers, and expressing only to relieve acute discomfort usually help in this situation.

The formula chosen for weaning should be a milk-based formula, not a soy formula (unless the doctor recommends soy). Milk-based formulas have a composition that is closer to breast milk than do soy formulas. Formulas will be discussed in more detail in Chapter 15.

A mother may be able to wean directly from

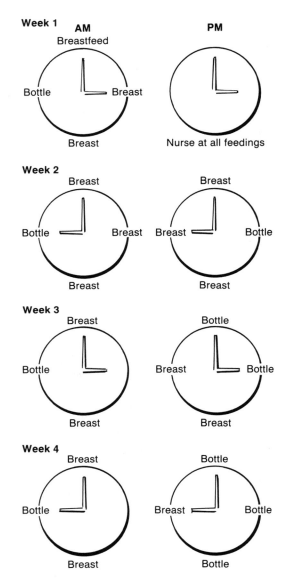

Figure 14-5
Sample weaning schedule.

the breast to a cup (a baby cup or a cup and straw) and never even offer a bottle, if the infant begins weaning at or after 8 months.

6. Do Breast-Fed Babies Need Vitamins?

Many pediatricians recommend that breast-fed babies receive vitamin supplements containing vitamin D, iron, and fluoride.[6] Vitamin D is not contained in breast milk, and some babies may not get enough sunlight to manufacture it themselves. This would put them at risk for rickets. Breast milk is very low in iron (most infants are born with a 4-month to 6-month store of iron), but the iron that is available is much more readily absorbed into the blood than the iron in any other food. Because of this, some pediatricians wait to prescribe supplemental iron until the infant is 4 months to 6 months old. Babies can become anemic if they do not get iron in some form by this age. Fluoride is important for a young baby's growing bones and teeth. Even though his teeth are not visible, they are forming. These three nutrients are the only ones that may be recommended for a breast-fed infant. The final decision is up to the pediatrician.

WHEN BREAST-FEEDING IS THE ONLY CHOICE

In the USA and in most developed nations, breast-feeding is not the only safe, healthy feeding choice for a new infant. Properly prepared, infant formulas can be a reasonable alternative for the woman who does not want to breast-feed. Where sanitation is good and formula can be made properly, the formula-fed baby will receive adequate nutrition for growth.

But in many parts of the world, bottle-feeding is still not a wise choice. These are places where

1. The water may not be clean, and is not always boiled before use
2. Refrigeration is unavailable, or unreliable
3. Containers are not washed regularly or thoroughly
4. People cannot always read their own language well enough to learn how to properly prepare formula

Formula is only sterile until it is opened. Then it can become contaminated very quickly. Bacteria may grow in any unwashed corner of a bottle, and make the infant very ill. Bacteria may also abound in the very water used for cleaning.

Formula is not the only nutrition problem for infants in these situations. In these communities (usually in underdeveloped countries), a mother who uses formula may mash up some other common food when the formula runs out. When cooked, many starchy roots that have been pounded and mixed with water look like formula. But they are of very poor nutritional quality for the infant, and he will not thrive, although he may survive.

Figure 14-6 graphically illustrates the effect this type of feeding may have on infants. Because of the high risk of death, breast-feeding is the *only safe* infant feeding choice unless the family has

1. Refrigeration for opened, unused formula

2. Clean, safe water

3. Enough equipment and fuel to boil all water and clean or sterilize all bottles

4. An understanding of why these are important

5. Knowledge of how to prepare formula

6. Enough funds to buy adequate formula for a growing infant

In many countries, few households possess all six of these requirements. This is why the World Health Organization strongly recommends breast-feeding and discourages formulas.[7] Under unsafe conditions formula, which would be an adequate choice for an infant in a developed country, becomes an unsafe choice. Until sanitation, equipment, and understanding can be improved, and funds are adequate to meet all the other needs of a poor household, breast-feeding will be the *only* wise choice.

STUDY QUESTIONS

1. What is one of the most important ingredients for successful breast-feeding? (Choose one)
   - The size of the woman's breasts
   - Her attitude
   - Her age
   - Whether or not she has breast-fed other children.

2. List and explain three advantages of breast-feeding for the woman and for the infant.

3. If a pregnant woman who came to you was a professional model, and worried that breast-feeding would "ruin" her figure, what would you tell her?

4. A woman who is totally breast-feeding her infant needs (a) more or (b) less calories than when she was pregnant?

5. What nutrients other than calories are important during lactation?

6. How much milk should a breast-feeding woman drink?

7. True or false: A woman who does not eat properly produces breast milk of poor quality.

8. What is the first fluid that the breasts produces called? What are its benefits?

9. True or False: If a baby does not seem to get enough milk from the breast in his first or

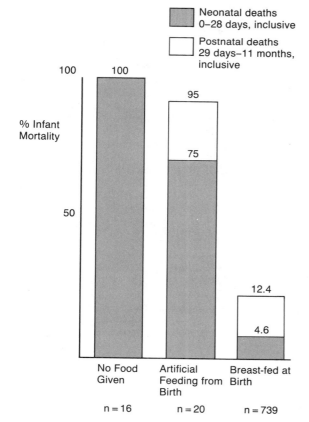

Figure 14-6
Infant death rates by method of feeding in seven Punjab villages, 1955–1959. (Adapted from Scrimshaw NS, Taylor DCE, Gordon JE: WHO Monograph No. 29, Geneva, 1968)

second day of life, the mother should give him some formula. Explain your answer.

10. When does the "full milk" come?

11. If a woman wants to breast-feed, but has to work full time, how can she still give breast milk to her infant? Describe at least two possibilities.

12. Is it true or false that a woman with a breast infection should stop nursing? Why or why not?

13. Should weaning to a bottle always be done suddenly? Why or why not?

14. Why might a breast-fed baby need vitamins or minerals?

RESOURCES

Community Organizations that Support or Encourage Breast-feeding (check your phone directory for local contacts)

Nursing Mothers Councils

La Leche League Chapters

Cooperative Extension Agencies

Women, Infants and Children's Program

Breast Shields (for inverted nipples) available from

La Leche League International
9616 Minneapolis Ave.
Franklin Park, IL 60131

Pamphlets, Speakers and Other Breast-Feeding Information Available from:

International Childbirth Education Association (ICEA)
P.O. Box 20048
Minneapolis, MN 55420

Health Education Associates Inc.
211 S. Easton Rd.
Glenside, PA 19038

Trainex Corp.
P.O. Box 116
Garden Grove, CA 92642

REFERENCES

1. Lawrence RA: Breastfeeding: A Guide for the Medical Profession, 2nd ed. St. Louis, CV Mosby, 1985
2. Worthington–Roberts BS, Vermeersch J, Williams SR: Nutrition in Pregnancy and Lactation, 3rd ed. St. Louis, Times Mirror/Mosby College, 1985
3. Kimball ER: Information Sheet No. 203, p 5. La Leche League International, 1964
4. Brewster DP: You Can Breastfeed Your Baby . . . Even in Special Situations, pp 91–92. Emmaus, PA, Rodale Press, 1979
5. Fomon SJ et al: Recommendations for feeding normal infants. Pediatrics 63: 52–59, 1970
6. Saarinen U: Need for iron supplementation in infants on prolonged breastfeeding. J Pediatr 93(2):177–180, 1978
7. World Health Organization: International code of marketing of breast milk substitutes. Nutrition Today 16:13, 1981

CHAPTER 15

Nutrition in Infancy

1. To explain changing nutrient and energy needs of the first 12 months
2. To discuss the supplemental nutrient needs of the breast-fed infant
3. To compare cow's milk and infant formulas: advantages, dangers, and recommendations for use
4. To provide practical, simple, and clear guidelines for introducing solids
5. To define several unwise or dangerous practices in infant feeding
6. To distinguish between practices that are unwise and those that are culturally distinctive

Infancy is the period extending from birth to the first birthday. During this period, an infant will usually double his birthweight by the age of 5 or 6 months, and triple it by one year.[1] He will never grow this fast again. Healthy growth depends on proper nutrition. And because changes happen so quickly during the first year of life, the type of foods infants can eat at different stages will also vary. This chapter will outline these changes in growth and in diet.

NUTRIENT NEEDS

An infant's growth is most rapid in the first 6 months. Then it slows down a little, so the Rec-

ommended Dietary Allowances for infant needs is divided into two groups, 0 to 6 months and 7 months to 12 months. During both of these periods, the most important nutrients are energy, protein, iron, vitamin D, and fluoride.

Energy

During an infant's first 6 months, he needs more energy, proportionate to his weight, than he will need during the rest of his life. The RDA for this period is 115 kilocalories per kilogram. So, a 10-pound infant (4.5 kg) needs about 525 Kcals each day.

Growth begins to slow down after 6 months, so the infant will need only an average of 105 Kcals per kilogram. His total needs may be more, however, because he will weigh more. A 20-pound infant (9 kg) who is 9 months old needs about 950 Kcals each day to continue growing.

Pediatricians can usually tell if an infant is acquiring enough energy by checking his weight gain. If a baby always fusses but is gaining the normal amount of weight for his age, he is getting enough food. Babies fuss and cry for many reasons other than hunger. Mothers who always feed a baby when he is fussy may be overfeeding him.

Protein

Babies from birth to 6 months need about 2.2 g of protein for every kilogram of body weight. After 6 months, the requirement drops to about

2.0 g/kg. This would mean that the protein in 1 liter (about 1 quart of formula or breast milk) is enough for a 10-lb (4.5 kg) infant. Until an infant reaches about 8 months of age, all the protein he needs can come from his mother's breast milk or from formula.

Iron

The need for dietary iron increases after the first 4–6 months. This is because most infants are born with a supply of iron "stored" in their bodies if their mothers were well nourished. If they do not get iron from their diet during the first few months, their bodies will draw needed iron from this supply until it runs out. Should this happen, an infant could become anemic by 6 months. Breast-fed infants get some iron from their mother's milk, although the amount that is absorbed may vary, and the baby's pediatrician may prescribe additional iron.[2] Infant formulas come with or without iron and the infant on iron-fortified formulas will probably get all the iron he needs from them.

Vitamin D

An infant who does not get a sufficient supply of vitamin D can develop rickets (see Chapter 6). Rickets can occur in infants who are completely breast-fed and who receive no vitamin supplement and little sunlight. Many pediatricians give breast-fed babies a supplement containing this vitamin. Infant formulas are fortified with vitamin D.

Fluoride

This is the third nutrient often recommended in a supplement for breast-fed infants. Fluoride is essential even before the infant has teeth, and breast-fed infants may not get enough, even when their mother drinks fluoridated water.

Formulas that are made with fluoridated water will contain enough fluoride, but formulas that are ready-to-feed or made with spring or distilled water may not.

FORMULA OR COW'S MILK?

What are the options, if a woman decides not to breast-feed? Can she give her infant fresh cow's milk or evaporated milk mixed with corn syrup, as her mother or grandmother did? Infant formulas are expensive, much more costly than evaporated milk, and many women who get most of their infant feeding advice from their older relatives believe cow's milk may be the best choice.

However, cow's milk is NOT a good choice for an infant, especially an infant under 6 months. Even though many were raised on it, and survived, it is not designed for infants and may prove to be an unnecessary stress on the baby's system. Table 14-1 illustrates how cow's milk differs from breast milk and formula. It contains a large quantity of sodium, much more than a baby needs. Its protein is harder to digest than the protein in breast milk. It contains almost no iron. Because the kidneys have to work harder to rid themselves of the extra sodium and protein, cow's milk places a greater stress on the infant's kidneys than does formula or breast milk. Finally, some children who can accept breast milk or formula seem to be allergic to cow's milk. These are some of the reasons evaporated milk formula is usually recommended only for the infant who cannot seem to tolerate any other formula, or when the mother simply refuses to breast-feed or feed the infant with another formula. Many pediatricians recommend vitamin plus iron supplements for infants on cow's milk.

When cow's milk is used in the first year, it should always be whole milk, never skim or low fat, even if the infant is overweight. Infants need the fat in whole milk.[3] They do not need the larger amounts of protein and sodium they would receive in a day's supply of low fat or skim milk.[4]

When evaporated milk is used, parents must understand how to mix it properly. Serious illness can result when a formula is not sufficiently diluted.[5]

Another possible danger that might be present with home-made formulas is food poisoning, especially *botulism*. Some corn syrup and honey have been found to carry the botulinum spore which causes this sometimes fatal poisoning.[6,7] Parents should avoid using these sweeteners when preparing infant formula. Table sugar is the most convenient and safest carbohydrate to use if a pediatrician recommends this type of formula.

Raw milk (milk that has not been pasteurized) may also be a serious health hazard for an infant on whole milk. If cow's milk must be used for infant feeding, it should always be pasteurized. Homogenization is not necessary.

INFANT FORMULA

There are two general types of infant formulas in common use: those based on (cow's) milk and those that use soy protein. Milk-based formulas have been commercially treated and fortified to make them the closest foods to breast milk available on the market.

Milk-based formulas with iron are the most appropriate food for the infant who is not breast-fed.[2] Infants should be on formula until they are between 9 months and 12 months old, and then should be switched to cow's milk. A child who is switching from one to the other may drink both cow's milk and formula during the same period. Properly prepared formula can even be mixed in the same cup with cow's milk. This may help an infant adjust to the different taste of the milk.

Formulas are not equal to breast milk. They do not contain the agents that, in breast milk, help protect an infant from infection and illness. They are not quite as digestible. Currently, no formula on the market is like colostrum, so the infant who is formula-fed from birth misses the benefits of that first food.

However, formulas *are* adequate, and most children on formulas grow well. A mother should never feel guilty about formula-feeding her infant, *if* he is growing well and *if* she is meeting his needs.

Soy formulas are quite different from breast milk, however. They *do* provide the infant with all the nutrient he needs, but soy protein is very different from the protein in human milk and in cow's milk. Usually soy formulas are given only to the infant who cannot tolerate a milk-based formula. There are still many questions concerning the adequancy of soy formulas, since some infants may have allergic reactions to them. All soy formulas are fortified with iron.

A soy *formula* is always better for an infant than is commercial soy *milk*. Soy milk often has little iron and little or no calcium. Fortified soy milk (which may contain these nutrients) may still have fewer vitamins and minerals than a growing infant needs. Vegan parents, who may feel strongly about avoiding dairy products, should be encouraged to use soy-based infant formula if the mother is not breast-feeding and will not feed her infant milk-based formulas.

Bacteria multiply quickly in *all* formula, so it should be used within 48 hours.

INTRODUCTION OF OTHER LIQUIDS AND SOLIDS

Water is usually given from birth, between feedings, and especially during the hot weather. Juices can be introduced by 3 months to 4 months. Tomato and citrus (orange, grapefruit) juices may be too acidic for the infant before he is 8 months to 10 months old.

Solids can be started between 4 months and 6 months. Table 15-1 outlines some guidelines for feeding the rapidly growing infant, month by month. Cereal is usually the first solid given, at about 4 months. Before formulas were iron-fortified, cereal was recommended earlier, as a source of iron. But infants cannot really digest it well before 4 months. The infant's mouth and tongue instinctively know how to suck, but they cannot move food from a spoon to the back of the mouth. It is not until the infant is about 4 months old that he is developmentally ready to do this. When a young infant is given a cereal-formula mixture, he will suck vigorously on it and consequently may choke.

Babies grow fast and often seem constantly hungry, even after drinking formula, so some parents still give cereal too early, often putting it in the bottle. Cereal fed in this form is not good for the infant. It is easy for the infant to get too much, and become overweight. A 4-month to 6-month-old infant needs less than a tablespoon

Table 15-1

Infant Feeding Guide

Foods	0–4 Mo	4–6 Mo	6–8 Mo	8–10 Mo	10–12 Mo
Breast Milk or Iron-Fortified Formula	5–10 Feedings 16–32 oz	4–7 Feedings 24–40 oz	3–4 Feedings 24–32 oz	3–4 Feedings 16–32 oz Whole milk can be introduced now.	3–4 Feedings 16–24 oz
Cereals & Breads	None	Boxed rice, oatmeal or barley (spoonfed) Mix 2–3 teaspoons with formula, water, or breast milk	All varieties of boxed infant cereal except Cera-meal or cereal with fruit or honey (Twice a day)	Infant cereals Cream of Wheat or other plain hot cereals Toast, bagel, or crackers	Infant or cooked cereals Unsweetened cereals Bread Rice Noodles & Spaghetti
Fruit Juices	None	Infant juice Adult apple juice, vitamin C-fortified (Avoid orange & tomato juice now) (2–4 oz a day)	Infant juice Adult apple juice vitamin C-fortified Try juice from a cup (4 oz)	All 100% juices Orange and tomato juice can be introduced now.	All 100% juices
Vegetables	None	None	Strained or mashed vegetables - dark yellow or orange (avoid corn) - dark green ($\frac{1}{2}$–1 jar or $\frac{1}{4}$–$\frac{1}{2}$ cup a day)	Cooked, mashed family vegetables Junior vegetables	Cooked vegetable pieces Some raw vegetables - carrots, tomatoes, cucumbers
Fruits	None	None	Fresh or cooked fruits - mashed bananas - applesauce Strained fruits (1 jar or $\frac{1}{2}$ cup per day)	Peeled, soft fruit wedges - bananas, peaches, pears, oranges, apples	All fresh fruits peeled and seeded Canned, packed in water
Protein Foods	None	None	Try *plain* yogurt	Lean meat, chicken and fish (strained, chopped or small tender pieces) Egg yolk, yogurt, mild cheese, peanut butter, cooked dried beans	Small tender pieces of meat, fish, or chicken Whole egg Cheese Yogurt Cooked dried beans Peanut butter

(From Massachusetts WIC Program)

of cereal each day. Formula can dissolve much more than this. It is more appropriate to offer milk (from the bottle) separate from cereal (mixed with milk and fed by spoon), and allow the infant to refuse one and accept the other. If an infant seems to be drinking far more formula than is recommended, his pediatrician should be informed.

Introduce one new food at a time. Wait at least 3 days to 4 days before introducing another new food. This way it is easy to determine which foods may cause allergies, or diarrhea, or other problems. An infant who develops a rash, begins vomiting, gets hives, or diarrhea may have a food allergy, or may have a virus. If the symptoms do not disappear quickly, again, the pediatrician should be informed.

An infant begins to eat "table food" (or foods that his family eats) between 8 months and 12 months. That is when he can begin to eat from the meat and protein group, and to try bits of tender meat or boned fish, cooked dry beans, peanut butter, and eggs. Cups begin to replace bottles. He can chew on soft vegetables and pick up and eat cut-up fruit and pieces of bread or toast. He now (usually) has teeth. Whole milk can be introduced, and he can try to eat with a spoon, although probably not successfully.

By 10 months to 12 months, these skills become more fine-tuned. The child may carry food to his mouth on a spoon. He uses his cup more successfully. Since growth begins to slow down, the infant is often more interested in playing with food than eating it. This is a normal part of learning how the world works. The infant who is still breast-fed should be drinking other beverages, including cow's milk, from a cup.

Listed on page 118 are further suggestions for parents who are introducing their infants to solids.

PROBLEMS WITH BOTTLES

While bottles are important and inevitable for the formula-fed infant, they can sometimes be used in dangerous ways. The most common of these practices include

1. Using animal-shaped bottles

2. Putting solids into the bottle

3. Allowing an infant to sleep with a bottle

4. Using the bottle to the exclusion of other feeding utensils

Animal-shaped bottles are hard to clean thoroughly. Milk is a rich food, and bacteria can grow very easily in it. If a bottle is not cleaned thoroughly after *every* use, residues accumulate in cracks and corners and bacteria begin to grow. Because these bottles are usually colored and opaque, it is often hard to tell if the bottle is completely clean. They are hard to clean with a bottle brush because of their unusual shapes. Such bottles should be used only for plain water.

It is not appropriate to put solids in a bottle. "Solids" includes cereal and baby food or table food in any form. If an infant is old enough to need solids, he is old enough to take them by spoon. Mothers sometimes put solids in the bottle to save time, but then neglect to spend the time the infant needs with her. It is important for an infant to learn to use a spoon, to smell different foods, to distinguish eating from drinking, to be able to see and handle different textures, and to learn to chew.

Infants and children who sleep with bottles of milk, juice, or sweetened water are in danger of *nursing bottle syndrome.* They may also be at a higher risk for ear infections. When he falls asleep, the infant will not continue swallowing. The liquid in his mouth will settle there until he awakens sufficiently to swallow it. During sleep, the inner passageway — the eustachian tube extending from ear to throat — is open. Liquid can flow up into the ears, where it can cause infections. In the mouth, as the liquid pools around the gums, the natural sugar it contains causes bacteria to make plaque. Cavities form. The longer the sugar source (milk and juice both contain natural sugars) is in the mouth, the more likely cavities will develop. When baby teeth are damaged by cavities, the forming permanent teeth may also be affected. So it is safest to offer infants a bottle when they are awake and can drink it readily. Parents who insist on offering a night bottle should fill it with nothing except plain (unsweetened) water.

The fourth problem occurs when a child who is able to drink from a cup and use a spoon does not do so, but continues to take only his bottle. Most children can take a cup by 12 months and

INTRODUCING SOLIDS

Avoid:

Salt. Infants get all they need in formula, breast milk and plain foods. Their taste buds are more sensitive than adults', and a "little" salt may be too much to them.

Sugar. It contains no vitamins or minerals and will only promote cavities. It should only be used as an energy source when evaporated milk formula is recommended.

Honey and Corn Syrup. These may contain botulinum spores, which can cause severe food poisoning. They also can cause cavities.

Opened, Stored Baby Food Should Be:

Covered.

Uncontaminated. Don't use the same bowl or spoon to feed the baby and to serve from the bottle or jar. The infant's germs can get into the food, on the spoon, from his saliva, and multiply in the refrigerator.

Used Promptly. Pureed meats should be used within one day, fruits and vegetables within 2 days.

Frozen, if it must be stored over a long period. Puréed food freezes well in ice cube trays. To thaw, put cubes in a dish (or baggie) in hot water.

Cereals Should Be:

Fed by spoon, not in a bottle.

Mixed to a soupy consistency with formula, milk, breast milk, or juice.

Iron-fortified, especially if the infant's formula is not, or if he is breast-fed.

Home-Made Baby Foods:

Can be *made ahead and frozen.*

Should be *made by* steaming, baking, or boiling the food thoroughly in a small amount of water, skins and seeds removed, and puréed in a strainer, baby food grinder, food mill, or blender.

Should *not be highly seasoned.*

Encourage Good Food Habits:

By setting a *good example.* The child will learn to eat what his parents enjoy. If they eat a wide variety of nutritious foods, so will he.

Give the infant *plenty of time.* If a child is excited or hurried, he will have trouble eating.

Use *child-size dishes.* Young children should not be expected to eat adult-size portions. If they want more, they will make this clear.

Allow him to *refuse food.* He may be tired, excited, or full.

Serve *foods that vary* in shape, color, texture, and taste.

Don't use sweets as *rewards* or treats. Reward with hugs, praise, and attention. Even "baby cookies" and "teething biscuits" have more sugar than a

(continued)

baby needs. Instead, snacks might be fresh fruit, cheese, or bread and peanut butter.

For Teething Infants:

Teething biscuits contain sugar. Instead, use crackers, chicken, or turkey bones, hard bread (*e.g.*, bagels, frozen fingers of toast), or clean, cold carrots.

Never give a teething infant (or any infant) items to chew on that are sharp or in small pieces that could make him choke.

Wash out his mouth daily, gently, with a cool cloth. This helps keep new teeth clean.

Adapted from US Department of Agriculture Program Aid No 1281, What Shall I Feed My Baby? A Month-by-Month Guide, pp. 28–35, 1981

give up the bottle completely by 18 months. If a child refuses even to try more than the softest table foods, he may be missing needed nutrients, and this may eventually affect his growth. In these situations, gradual weaning is ideal, but sometimes the only effective way to stop the bottle is to discard it, permanently and firmly, and to face — and consistently lovingly, say "no" to — an angry, upset child. The parent who says "no" and then later yields is actually encouraging the child to hold out for what he wants. The parent who lovingly but firmly enforces what is best will probably face several days of angry behavior. The child will give in when he realizes the parent will not. Cup and table food should be consistently offered but not forced. The new habits will be accepted gradually.

CULTURAL DIFFERENCES

Infant feeding practices vary widely according to culture. Cultures that do not use spoons will not teach infants how to use them. Some cultures use vegetables, rather than cereal, as the first solid. Others put strong-tasting foods into the infant's mouth, and then remove them, in order to introduce new tastes. Others may give no solids until the infant is 1 year old.

It is important for the health provider to distinguish between feeding practices that are culturally different and those that are unhealthy. Vegetables may be adequate as a first food, but

holding solids until one year is not. "Different" does not always mean unhealthy, but "different" should always be evaluated. Unwise practices may not cause an infant obvious harm. Dangerous practices, however, should be stopped whenever possible. Some examples of each include

Different, but healthful:

1. Introducing vegetables or fruits before cereals
2. Letting an infant taste a food he is not yet ready to eat, then removing it from his mouth
3. Breast-feeding an infant over 1 year old, (healthful only if the infant is eating a wide variety of table foods, as well as breast-feeding).

Unwise:

1. Feeding an infant every time he cries, because he must always be hungry, and believing fat babies are healthy babies
2. Feeding formula without iron, without first consulting the pediatrician
3. Feeding evaporated milk formula before an infant is 6 months old
4. Putting sugar in water
5. Giving low fat or skim milk when a child is between 12 months and 18 months (if the pediatrician has not specifically recommended it.)

Dangerous:

1. Giving low fat or skim milk to an infant under 12 months[4]
2. Giving an infant undiluted formula or evaporated milk[5]
3. Allowing an infant to sleep with a bottle
4. Exclusive breast-feeding beyond 7 months or 8 months, without introducing solids
5. Withholding water, especially if a child has diarrhea

The final authority on the best feeding for an individual infant is the pediatrician. He should be seen regularly for immunizations and checkups and called when there is a question. How well the infant is growing, and whether or not he needs vitamins, should be determined by his physician.

STUDY QUESTIONS

1. How many calories does a 4-month-old infant need? How does this compare to his needs at 9 months?
2. How does a 3-month-old obtain (a) the protein and (b) the iron he needs?
3. What vitamins and minerals are often prescribed for breast-fed infants?
4. List and discuss the pro's and con's of feeding an infant cow's milk rather than infant formula.
5. Is honey better than table sugar for an infant? Why or why not?
6. If a baby is not breast-fed, how long should he be fed infant formula? When can he try cow's milk?
7. What are the two major groups of infant formulas? What source of protein is used for each? Which is most like breast milk?
8. Should an infant be fed formula with or without iron? Why?
9. When should solids be started? What kinds usually are introduced first?
10. When should an infant begin
    a. to eat from a spoon?
    b. to drink from a cup?
11. Jeannie is 11 months old and tries to feed herself. Her mother works fulltime and often tries to feed Jeannie in the 15 minutes before she leaves for work, and the 15 minutes before her husband gets home at night. When Jeannie feeds herself, she takes a long time, and gets food all over the floor. But when her mother insists on feeding her, she cries and sometimes refuses to eat. Her growth is good, but both Jeannie and her mother are very frustrated at mealtimes. What would you discuss with Jeannie's mother?
12. True or false:
    - Infants have poorly developed taste buds, so baby foods should be highly seasoned.
    - Cereals fed by spoon should be of a soupy consistency.
    - Infants who refuse to eat are being stubborn.
    - Bottles with unusual shapes are hard to clean. Bacteria may grow in them, making infants sick.
    - An infant who sleeps and sucks on a bottle of sugar water will probably sleep through the night and be more content and healthy.
    - An infant who sleeps with a bottle of milk may develop cavities.
    - Cooked rice and cornmeal are high in iron and are recommended for infants beginning to eat solids.

REFERENCES

1. National Center for Health Statistics: Physical growth chart: Birth to 36 months (in percentiles). Am J Clin Nutr 32:607–629, 1979
2. Fomon SJ et al: Recommendations for feeding normal infants. Pediatrics 63:52–59, 1979
3. Massachusetts Department of Public Health: Maternal and Child Health, Infant Feeding Policy, 1983 ed, p 12
4. Fomon SJ et al: Skim milk in infant feeding. Acta Pediatr Scand 66:17, 1977
5. Abrams CAL et al: Hazards of overconcentrated milk formula, JAMA 232(11):1136–1140, 1975
6. Community Nutrition Institute: Nutrition Week, February 24, 1983
7. Arnon SS: Honey, infant botulism and the sudden infant death syndrome. West J Med 132(1):58–59, 1980

CHAPTER 16

Nutrition in Childhood

OBJECTIVES

1. To define the changing energy and food needs of childhood

2. To provide specific guidelines for meal planning for children in the age groups of 1–3 years, 4–6 years, and 7–10 years

3. To discuss
   a. Different nutrient needs of each of these three groups
   b. Eating-related developmental maturity
   c. Unique, food-related characteristics

4. To list, describe, and discuss seven common nutrition-related childhood problems, and provide general guidelines for initiating solutions

An infant is considered a child after his first birthday. At that time, the phenomenal growth of infancy slows down. Needs — and appetite — begin to decrease. Growth during childhood is steady, and a child will usually gain about 2 kg (4½ lbs to 5 lbs) each year until he enters adolescence.

Even though growth is steady in childhood, food needs are not the same for all ages. Less food is needed to help the 2-year-old grow than is needed for the 7-year-old, because the younger child's body is smaller, and his basic needs are different. A 2-year-old may need 1100 kilocalories (Kcals) to continue growing while a 7-year-old, with a larger body to support, may need around 1600 Kcals.* Because needs vary in

childhood according to age, the Recommended Dietary Allowances are divided into three groups: ages 1 to 3, 4 to 6 and 7 to 10. Table 16-1 illustrates this difference with a sample menu modified to meet the RDA for each of the three groups.

The easiest way to plan menus for children is by using the four food groups as a guide. This is a practical guideline, because all children need the same number of servings from each group, although the serving *size* each needs may vary. This is illustrated in Table 16-2. One serving of meat measures one ounce for the 2-year-old and two ounces for the 8-year-old. This variation in portion size applies to all four food groups. Still, each child is different, so the four food groups is intended only as a guideline to assist in meal planning and to educate parents on standard portion sizes. Individual children may require more or less.

While mealtime for children is usually a family event, involving children of different ages (see Fig. 16-1), needs do differ according to age, so it is helpful to consider each category as a separate unit.

AGES 1 TO 3

During the three pre-school years, a child is totally involved in learning about his world and what he is able to do with it. He will gain 2 kg to

*This average can easily be calculated for any age child by allowing 1000 Kcals for the first year and 100 for every year after age one.

Table 16-1

Sample One-Day Menu for Children

Meal	Ages 1–3	Ages 4–6	Ages 7–10
Breakfast	Cereal: ½ cup Instant oatmeal ¼ cup Milk ½ cup Orange juice	½ cup Instant oatmeal ¼ cup Milk ½ cup Orange juice ¾ cup (6 oz) Milk	½ cup Instant oatmeal ¼ cup Milk ½ cup Orange juice ¾ cup Milk 1 slice Toast
Lunch	1 slice Whole wheat bread 1 oz Chicken salad ¾ cup Milk ½ Banana	2 slices Whole wheat bread 2 oz Chicken salad 1 cup Milk	2 slices Whole wheat bread 2 oz Chicken salad (with mayo) 1 cup Milk
Snack	6 Saltine crackers 1 tbsp Peanut butter small Orange, peeled and cut up ¾ cup Milk	1 Banana ¼ cup Mixed peanuts & raisins ½ cup Milk	2 slice Bread with: peanut butter and 1 banana ½ cup Milk
Dinner	Chili with: 2 oz Hamburger ¼ cup Kidney beans ¼ cup Spinach ½ cup Milk	3 oz Hamburger ¼ cup Kidney beans ¼ cup Spinach salad ½ cup Orange juice	3 oz Hamburger ¼ cup Kidney beans 1 Baked potato ¼ cup Spinach salad ½ cup Orange juice
Snack	¼ cup Milk	½ cup Milk	½ cup Milk 1 slice Raisin toast

2.5 kg (4½ lb to 5½ lb) each year and grow 7 cm to 12 cm (3 in to 5 in) each year. His muscle control becomes more fine-tuned, and he will want to use every new ability to gain self control and to learn to make choices. Mealtimes are often messy, and he may want to wander around the house with food. He has a very short attention span, and may become frustrated with his own clumsy use of utensils. Meals should be short, yet unhurried, with little to distract him. Sometime between ages one and three, his molars will erupt, and help him to chew more easily.

Preschoolers are struggling to gain control of themselves and their environment. So they often say "no" to foods. Their health may suffer if they continually refuse essential foods, but this is usually not a problem. Parents can avoid this struggle by offering the child a choice between two nutritious foods.

Food jags are common. A *food jag* develops when a child wants only one or a few of the same foods every day, for several days. These jags are normal and usually harmless. After several days or a week, the child should begin to choose some of the other foods that are regularly offered to him. During food jags, parents may

1. Meet the child's demands, as long as they are reasonable
2. Refuse to pay much attention to the child's monotonous diet
3. Continue to offer him other foods, allowing him to refuse

Parents may want to intervene if a food jag lasts more than a week. Most children grow out of these jags and remain healthy.

During the first 3 years, the child is exposed to most of the foods of his culture; he develops preferences. Each introduction to a new food

Table 16-2

Child's Feeding Guide

Food Group	Major Nutrients	Servings/Day	Serving Size By Age (in years)		
			1–3	4–6	7–10
Milk & Milk Products	Calcium Protein	3	¾ to 1 cup Milk ¾ cup Milk = 1 oz Cheese = 1¼ cup Ice cream = ¾ cup Pudding = ¾ cup Plain yogurt = 1½ cup Cottage cheese	1 cup Milk 1 oz Cheese =	1 cup Milk = 1½ oz Cheese 1 cup Pudding 1¾ cup Ice cream 2 cups Cottage cheese
Meat or Protein Equivalent	Protein Iron	2	1 oz Meat, fish, poultry = ½ cup Dry, Cooked peas, beans, tofu = 2 tbsp Peanut butter = 1 Egg	1½ oz Meat = ¾ cup Peas, beans = 3 tbsp Peanut butter = 1 Egg	2 oz Meat, fish, poultry = 1 cup Beans = 4 tbsp Peanut butter = 2 Eggs
Fruits & Vegetables	vitamin A vitamin C Fiber	4	2–4 tbsp (up to ¼ cup) ½ cup or small piece ¼ cup or 1 small piece		½ cup ½ cup or medium piece ½ cup or medium piece
Breads & Cereals	B vitamins Iron, if product is enriched or fortified	4	½ slice Bread ¼ cup Rice, macaroni, dry cereal 1–2 tbsp Hot cereal	1 slice Bread ½ cup Rice, macaroni, dry cereal 3–5 tbsp Hot cereal	1 slice Bread ½ cup Rice or macaroni 1 cup Dry cereal ½ cup Hot cereal

Adapted from Massachusetts WIC program, WIC Form #51: Preschool Feeding Guide, October 1983, and National Dairy Council Guide to Good Eating, 4th ed, 1982

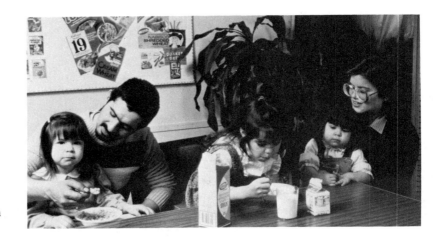

Figure 16-1
Nutritious eating in childhood involves the whole family. (Photo courtesy Massachusetts Department of Public Health. Used with permission.)

involves many decisions. Figure 16-2 illustrates some of the things that may influence a child's decision to taste or refuse a new food. However, tastes will continue to change during childhood. A child who refuses certain vegetables at age 2 may try them at a later date, or in a different form, and enjoy them.

Preschools and Headstart programs also help introduce the young child to a variety of foods, in a setting where he sees other children eating them. These social situations may also influence preferences for foods during preschool years.

AGES 4 TO 6
Children between 4 and 6 will gain about 3½ lb to 5 lb and 2¼ in to 3 in each year. They may appear to "thin out" and this is normal. They are usually full of energy, and eager to learn how to do things by themselves. They may prefer to talk rather than eat, and have trouble remaining seated throughout an entire meal. Since they are learning how to use objects for their own convenience, they may try to use food and food behaviors (such as refusing foods or insisting on a particular snack) to have their own way, if they can. During this time, they enjoy eating with their fingers, although they can learn to use a knife safely. They enjoy snacks and have strong likes and dislikes. The 4- to 6-year-olds may "hate" mixed dishes, such as casseroles, and prefer to taste each food separately.

They need about 80 Kcals for each kilogram of weight. They are still growing steadily, and should not lose weight, even if they are overweight. If overweight is a problem, controlled portion sizes and limits of foods to help slow down their rate of gain are more appropriate.

Occasionally, a child of this age may have a small appetite, and get most of his energy from beverages. Milk and juices have many nutrients, but little or no iron, so anemia may be a problem. Other nutrients are usually missing as well, and the child's pediatrician should know if the child refuses to eat over an extended period of time.

AGES 7 TO 10
Between 7 and 10, the child's body begins to prepare for adolescence. Both weight and height begin to increase more quickly than during the previous 6-year to 9-year period. This increase is less predictable than other such periods of growth increase. It may begin at any time. Girls usually begin their growth spurt before their tenth birthday, boys afterwards.

The 7-to-10 year-old knows what foods he prefers. He usually has enough self-control to eat a meal in one sitting, and is comfortable using utensils. He may want to help prepare food, and to socialize with peers at meal times. He can learn why nutrition is important, and is often very interested in learning how and why

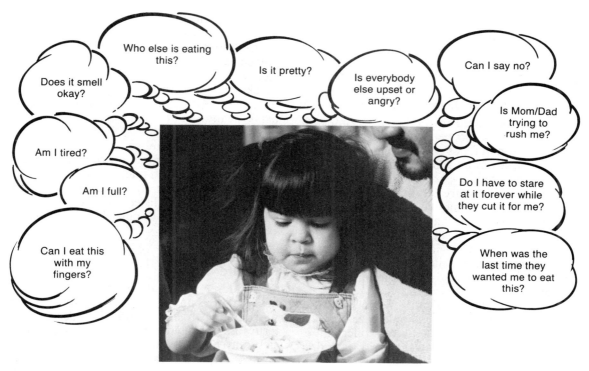

Figure 16-2
The success of new foods may depend on many of the above factors. (Photo courtesy of Massachusetts Department of Public Health. Used with permission.)

things work. Nutrition is often built into many school curricula for this age group. Some suggested reading material pertaining to nutrition education for children is found at the end of this chapter.

The school child may have one or even two meals at school. The National School Lunch Program, which began in 1946, insures that a child will be offered a selection of foods that can meet one third of his daily nutrient needs. This type of lunch is called the "Type A" lunch, and includes

1 cup milk

2 oz protein in a main dish

¾ cups vegetable and/or fruit

1 slice bread

1 tsp margarine

The child is offered these foods but he is not required to eat them. He may not eat foods that he needs unless he has learned to enjoy them.

Some children may have a school breakfast as well as a school lunch. Where it is offered the school breakfast program (begun in 1966), provides:

1 cup milk

½ cup fruit or full strength (100%) fruit juice

1 serving bread or cereal

The school breakfast does not provide one third of the the RDA. It is also low in protein. But sometimes it is the only breakfast a child may have, and children are usually able to study better after having had breakfast than on an empty stomach.[2]

NUTRITION PROBLEMS

Many eating problems may occur during the childhood years. Some of the most common are discussed below.

Anemia Due To Low Iron

Iron must be stored in the body, in order to prevent anemia. To be stored, there must be sufficient iron in foods eaten to meet the child's immediate needs and to put some iron in reserve. If there has never been quite enough iron in the diet, a child can easily use up his marginal stores and become anemic. As mentioned earlier, this sometimes happens when children drink too much milk, suppressing their appetite for other foods, higher in iron. Iron-deficiency anemia may affect a child's energy and interest in learning. It may also put an urban child at greater risk for lead poisoning.

If a child becomes anemic, his doctor must decide whether or not he should take supplements. However, the parent can offer more high-iron foods, such as raisins, red meats, dry cooked beans or peas, fortified cereals, and (if it is acceptable to the child) liver. Water or 100% fruit juices can replace any excess milk intake. Juices high in vitamin C (orange, grapefruit, and fortified apple, or grape juice) do not contain iron, but can help the body use the iron it may get from other sources.

Cavities

Children like to eat frequently. This can lead to tooth decay if the foods they eat are sticky or contain large amounts of sugar. Cavities in baby teeth are not harmless. They may result from habits that can later cause decay in the adult teeth. They may attack the permanent teeth before the new teeth come fully through the gum. They may interfere with a child's ability to try new foods.

Some foods that lead most easily to cavities include potato chips, regular gum, creme-filled cookies, hard candy, chewy candy, cakes, pies, and sweetened beverages. Even too many raisins or other dried fruits can cause cavities, if they are eaten regularly.

Brushing teeth with a fluoride toothpaste helps prevent cavities. Fluoridated water gives the teeth strength to resist decay. The best way to prevent cavities by diet is to avoid frequent contacts with very sticky or sugary foods. Healthy snacks such as fresh fruit, vegetables (raw carrots, celery, broccoli, green or sweet red peppers), peanut butter, crackers, and nuts and seeds are lower-cavity risks. Fruit juices may not be less cariogenic than fruit punches and sweet drinks, but they are more nutritious. Popsicles can be made with fruit juices frozen on sticks in ice cube trays. Some other snacks that do not promote cavities are listed on page 127.

Dental care will be discussed in more detail in Chapter 41.

Chronic Illness

Sick children often have poor appetites. An illness that does not, in itself, threaten the child's nutrition may retard growth if it leads to a long-term loss of appetite. Children who are often sick may also have a smaller appetite simply because they are not as active as other children.

Large meals and certain foods often overwhelm or nauseate a child who is ill. To entice a child to eat a balanced meal during a long sickness, the four food groups must be used creatively. Very small meals, prepared attractively with a little food from each group can sometimes perk up an appetite. Mixed milk drinks, such as eggnog, or milk with fruit, peanut butter, ice cream, or juices, may appeal. Raw, cool vegetables may be more attractive than cooked ones. Tuna salads or egg salads may be preferred over hot dishes.

Good nutrition is vital when a child is sick, but it should never take the place of good medical care.

Overweight

A child is considered overweight when his weight compared to his height is *at* or *over* the 95th percentile. This means that 95% of the children of his height weigh less than he does. The overweight child may be teased by other children. He may not be able to do everthing his

SNACKS FOR HEALTHY TEETH

Instead of:	Try:
Candy	Fresh Fruit
Cookies	Popcorn
Lifesavers	Peanuts
Caramels	Pretzels
Raisins*	Cheese
Pie	Yogurt
Cake	Crackers with peanut butter
Tonic	Fruit & vegetable juice
Caramel popcorn	Fresh vegetables
Chewing gum	Sugarfree gum
Sugar-coated cereals	Low – sugar, unsweetened cereals
Lollipops	Pickles

*Raisins have many vitamins and minerals that make them nutritious snacks. But they are high in natural sugars, so should be used moderately.

peers do, may become less active, and then gain even more weight. Unless overweight is controlled in childhood, an overweight child can become an overweight adult. He can develop the weight-related health hazards of overweight: heart disease, hypertension, diabetes.

Children become overweight for the same reasons adults become overweight: their energy input is greater than their energy output. Perhaps a child is always served (and eats) adult-size portions of food. Perhaps he has high-fat, high-sugar snacks and desserts as rewards. He may be overweight because he eats too much of one particular food (or beverage), or even because he does not exercise enough.

Unlike adults, overweight children in general should not lose weight. If they lose weight, they may also lose nutrients needed for growth. Instead, they should stop gaining, or gain very slowly, until their height, proportionately, catches up with their weight. As they become taller, their weight will usually become more appropriate to their height; they "thin out." Slowing weight gain does involve eating less and (often) exercising more. The whole family is often involved in successful weight control for a child. If overweight is a problem for the family

members, diet and exercise may be essential for everyone.

Pica

Pica is the practice of eating clay, dirt, ice, laundry starch, or other nonfood substances. It is more common in some places than others and seems prevalent among poorer sections of the southern USA. Some researchers believe there may be a relationship between pica and nutrient deficiencies.[2] Others disagree, suggesting pica may be a result of emotional deprivation.[3]

Pica is *not usually* a life-threatening practice. It *can be* life-threatening to the child, however, if it involves eating something toxic, such as paint chips containing lead. Lead poisoning can lead to mental retardation if it is not detected and treated in time. Pica may also threaten a child's health if it results in a loss of appetite by filling the stomach. If pica is a regular practice, medical providers should be aware of it and be ready for intervention.

Toddlers often put anything in their mouths, and try to eat nonfood items. This should not be confused with pica; it is a normal phase of development. The toddler uses his mouth to learn about his world. He needs close supervision but, unless he persistently eats the same substance, this behavior is usually unrelated to pica.

Television

TV appeals to children because of its bright colors and catchy tunes and messages. Children memorize and accept what they are told on TV. They cannot critically evaluate what they see and hear. As a result, they may be convinced that candy, potato chips, and other advertised *junk food* goodies are really good for them. They come to want what the ads promote without knowing why they want the junk food.

Consequently, television ads can lead to a common childhood feeding problem. Healthy snacks are rarely advertised, and are usually surrounded by ads for other snacks with little more than energy, fat, and artificial flavors. Some organizations are fighting for change in children's TV, but changes are slow and meanwhile, parents must make choices. Some choices include

Limiting or decreasing TV time or the stations a child may watch

Using public television and radio, since they have no advertising for products

Doing aggressive teaching at home about the false claims of TV ads, and providing fun, nutritious snacks.

Underweight

A child whose weight for his height is less than the 5th percentile of his growth chart is considered underweight. Pediatricians may also become concerned if a child drops from one percentile (*e.g.,* the 50th) to a lower percentile (*e.g.,* the 10th) or simply does not gain weight between check-ups. Underweight in a growing child can be a serious problem. It may reflect poor eating habits. A diet that is not adequate in the major nutrients can stunt height as well as weight, if it is continued. The underweight child may develop diseases, flu, or infections more easily than a heavier, better nourished child. Frequent illness can make underweight even more severe, creating a harmful cycle.

As with overweight, the best way to begin treating an underweight child is to find the causes for the low weight and do whatever is possible to resolve them. Is the child eating or drinking foods that regularly cause him to vomit or to have diarrhea? Is there always enough food in the home? Is the child missing breakfast or other meals? Is he filling up on low-calorie or low-nutrient-dense foods? Is he on what seems to be an extended food jag? Does he get enough sleep? Does he have a chance to watch others eat and imitate them? Are mealtimes full of tension? Any of these could lead to underweight, and weight gain will begin when the problem can be resolved.

Vitamins alone cannot help a child gain weight. They contain no energy. Energy for weight gain must come from foods, sometimes foods *dense* in energy. Nonfat dry milk mixed in whole milk adds calories and protein. Peanut butter, margarine, mayonnaise, instant breakfast drinks, and sugars are other foods to add for extra calories. It is up to the physician, dietitian, and related health care providers working with the parents to decide which changes are most appropriate for the child.

Good nutrition in childhood helps lay the foundation for lifelong health. Children who learn that nutritious meals and snacks can be fun may begin healthful habits that will continue into adolescence and adulthood.

STUDY QUESTIONS

1. Approximately how many calories does an average 2-year-old need each day? An average 6-year old?

2. Into what three age groups do the RDAs for children fall? Why?

3. Why are most 18-month-old toddlers messy eaters?

4. What is a food jag? Is it harmful?

5. True or false: (Explain your answer)
   - Lifelong taste preferences are formed by age 2.
   - Headstart and preschool programs may help a child learn to like more and different foods.

- A 5-year-old needs about 100 kilocalories per kilogram of body weight.
- Most children become heavier when they reach age 4 or 5.
- The school breakfast guidelines are low in protein.
- Most children can learn more readily after eating breakfast than they can on an empty stomach.

6. When a toddler is introduced to a new food, what might influence whether or not he likes it?

7. What snacks are better than gum and candy for healthy teeth? Why are these snacks more healthful?

REFERENCES

1. National School Lunch Act, Public Law 396, 79th Congress, June 4, 1946, and the Child Nutrition Act of 1966

2. Coltman CA Jr: Pagophagia and iron lack. JAMA 205:513, 1969

3. Goodhart RS, Shils ME: Modern Nutrition in Health and Disease, 6th ed, p 773. Philadelphia, Lea & Febiger, 1980

SUGGESTED READING

Some sources for nutrition education materials for children include:

The National Dairy Council, Rosemont, IL 60018-4233

Creative Food Experiences for Children, by Mary Goodwin and Gerry Pollen, available from the Center for Science in the Public Interest (CSPI), 1755 S St NW, Washington, DC 20009

Learning for Life (two curricula for 6–8 and 9–13 year-olds), Dept. A, Management Sciences for Health, 165 Allandale Rd., Boston, MA 02130

Nutrition in Adolescence and Adulthood

Adolescence is the period in which a person develops from a child into an adult. It is a period of rapid change — physical, emotional, mental, and spiritual. It marks the end of childhood and the beginning of a different kind of maturation process, a maturing that will continue into adulthood and old age. Because the lifespan is a continuum, these three growth periods — adolescence, adulthood, and the older adult years — will all be considered in this chapter. Some of the nutrition questions and issues that overlap these age groups will also be discussed.

ADOLESCENCE

Adolescence is often a series of unpredictable changes. The adolescent is frequently confused and troubled about his body, even when he understands its physical and emotional changes. The physical changes, together with peer pressure, often have a strong influence on the way the teenager eats. What he needs may not always be what he chooses. But what does he need?

Energy

Chapter 2 discussed the many factors that determine how much energy (and other nutrients) a person needs. Of these factors, growth, sexual differences, and activity levels have the greatest influence on energy needs during the teen years. Growth in adolescence may be more rapid than during any other period of life (except infancy). Children (of yesterday) overnight seem to reach their adult height and to mature sexually.

Usually the growth in height comes before sexual maturation; the time of fastest growth is called the *peak height velocity.* Girls usually reach this period 2 or 3 years before boys, and before their menarche (or first menstrual period).[1] This time of peak height velocity is when nutrient needs (especially energy needs) are the greatest.

However, each adolescent is separate and distinct. Sexual maturity may begin at 9 years or at 16 years of age. Rates of growth may vary. Even during the "growth spurt," growth may be faster at some times than at others. Some adolescents grow more than do others. There are wide variations between the sexes, among cultures, and even within families. Some teens may be more deeply involved in athletics than others. This enormous variation in growth, activity, and sexual maturity makes it extremely difficult to discuss specifically just what an individual adolescent should be eating. It is possible, though, to make some generalizations.

Adolescents need more energy than they did as children. They also need more energy than they will as adults. Some nutrients are also *especially important* during this period. For example, rapid bone growth increases the need for vitamin D and calcium. Figure 17-1 illustrates the Recommended Dietary Allowances for six

of the most important nutrients. The RDAs are not as accurate a predictor of needs during this period as they are during other, more predictable, growth periods, but they are the most comprehensive and well-researched public guidelines available. The RDAs divide adolescence into three segments: ages 11 to 14, 15 to 18, and 19 to 22, and divide adolescence by sex as well. Teens have usually completed most of their growth by age 19, so that age may mark the beginning of early adulthood.

An adolescent who plans meals around the RDA or the four food groups should use these guidelines as a skeleton structure. As long as the skeleton (the basic amounts of various foods) is present, the teen will probably not be malnourished, but he should also eat more, if necessary, to satisfy hunger. Besides energy and protein, adolescent needs for vitamin D, iron, and calcium are at an all-time high and these needs may be hard to meet without planning. For example, a teen needs to make the same choices from the four food groups as does a breast-feeding woman. (A pregnant teen needs even more!) Illustrated on page 132 are sample menus for teenagers based on the four food groups, showing how an adolescent boy or girl might meet their requirements on a typical day.

During this time, when nutrient needs are the highest, powerful social influences often make good nutrition an adolescent's lowest priority. Teens want to make their own decisions, and peers may influence these decisions much more strongly than would a sense of physical responsi-

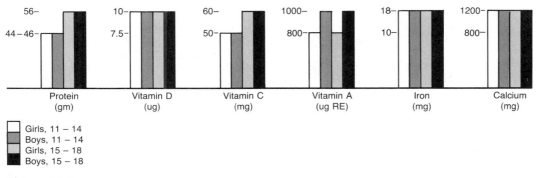

Figure 17-1
Key nutrient needs for adolescents, as compared to adult needs.

THE FOUR FOOD GROUPS: SAMPLE MENUS FOR ADOLESCENTS

	Girls	Boys
Breakfast:	1 cup low fat milk	1 cup low fat milk
	1 piece fruit	2 scrambled eggs
		2 pieces toast
Lunch:	1 cup yogurt	Submarine sandwich with lean
	Tuna salad sandwich	meat, lettuce and tomatoes
	(2 ounces tuna)	Fruit juice or fruit
	Banana or juice	1 cup low fat milk
Afternoon:	1 orange	1 cup low fat milk or ice cream
		1 banana
Dinner:	Cheeseburger (4 oz meat)	Cheeseburger (4 oz meat)
	Salad or green vegetable	Salad or green vegetable
	Beverage	Beverage

bility. An adolescent may not believe that what he does affects his body, and his health. Long term benefits are not good motivators for teenagers. Other, more immediate concerns simply seem much more important. This is a perpetual situation for anyone who works with teens. Effective work with adolescents involves relevant education and respect for the teen and his decisions.

Social Concerns

The strongest influences on a teenager's eating habits relate to self-image and include the following:

How their Peers Eat. Peer approval is the strongest approval a teen may feel, and value. A teen may accept himself only when his peers accept him. He may feel that, if he chooses differently than his peers, they will reject him. He will probably not order milk if his peers order Coke or order spinach if they order french fries.

Weight and Body Image. Boys often want to eat food that will help develop muscle. But they may not know what foods help to do this. Girls want to avoid foods that seem to add fat. They may be on perpetual diets, or try crash diets. Overweight teens may establish what becomes a lifelong habit of filling empty or lonely times with food. Lifelong eating habits can develop

from adolescent weight concerns. These concerns often make teens very open and interested in nutrition and willing to try anything that promises to improve weight and body image.

Advice from Heroes. Teens often look to nonparent role models for advice and guidance. They choose heroes and try to conform their lives to theirs. However, heroes, such as athletes (and coaches), models, and other "celebrities" offer a lot of advice, but actually may know very little about nutrition.

Exploring Various Lifestyles. Adolescence is often a time for discovering and thinking through individual beliefs. This is an important part of adolescent development, and may include trying new foods or eating patterns.

Some of these influences may lead to potentially dangerous eating habits. For example, a teen exploring various religions or philosophies may try diets that are deficient in certain nutrients. Overweight teens may try crash diets that do leave them thinner, but also weaker. In a long-term crash diet, an adolescent may lose muscle and become more susceptible to illness and infection. Inadequate calories in a growing child or teen may also affect bone growth and adult height. Adolescent dieting that becomes extremely stringent may (in rare cases) develop into *anorexia nervosa,* an extremely dangerous syndrome of self-starvation which will be discussed in more detail in Chapter 37. Or a teen may develop *bulimia,* that is, the person may eat large amount of foods, then immediately purge with laxatives and/or induce vomiting so as not to retain the food and thus to avoid gaining weight. Bulimia, which is much more common than anorexia nervosa, is also dangerous and can severely damage the digestive tract and destroy the enamel on the teeth.

Working with Adolescent Food Problems

Iron Deficiency Anemia

This condition is common, especially in teenage girls.[2] A girl, who requires a good deal of iron, may not be eating enough foods with iron. Physicians may recommend iron supplements to help meet the RDA of 18 mg. See Chapters 8 and 27 for lists and information about high-iron foods.

Overweight

A teen's self image is an extremely fragile thing, and overweight teens are often upset by their extra weight, to a far greater degree than are overweight adults. Often, the overweight teen may not eat more then his normal-weight peer, but he may not be sufficiently active to burn off the food he does eat.[3]

The adolescent years are a good time to resolve weight problems. Most teens are often highly motivated to lose weight. A teenager, particularly a girl, may not have a long history of diets that failed, so she may be optimistic and faithful to a diet. With fast growth occurring, the weight may come off far more quickly than at other times in life. And there are usually many opportunities for activity, one of the key ingredients in all weight loss. Track, swimming, dancing, and gymnastics are accessible to most teens, in school or in the community.

Underweight

Some teens, especially boys, feel underweight as acutely as others feel overweight. They may be growing so fast that their huge appetites seem to add no flesh to their bodies.

Underweight can be more difficult to correct than overweight. Both require the same atten-

tion to activity, enough sleep, and a sensible, nutritious eating pattern. Activity helps to build muscles. In some sports, a thin, muscular body is more effective than a heavier one. The adolescent who does not get enough sleep may need more energy, yet eat less than one who does get enough sleep. Nutritious foods help ensure good health for both weight extremes. A thin teen may be quite healthy if he is eating according to the recommended guidelines. If he is not eating correctly, and becomes ill frequently, a balanced diet may help improve his health (by giving him nutrients he is missing, and protein and energy to fight infection). However, his weight may not be affected. Sometimes the only solution to an underweight problem is time: time for the growth spurt to slow down (though during this time the adolescent should certainly eat as much as he can).

Unusual Preferences

The teen who decides to become a vegetarian, for example, may refuse much of the food offered at family meals. He may not know what nutrients need be replaced, or even know how to begin to do so. The teen may only know what he will *not* eat. However, a "different" eating pattern may not necessarily be a "bad" habit. Cultures around the world eat "different" foods and yet acquire all the nutrients they need. (Cultural eating habits will be discussed in Chapter 18.) A teen who adopts an unusual food preference, even for a short time, should learn as much as possible about making it nutritionally balanced. A registered dietitian in the community should be able to help the teen plan a diet or recommend books, organizations, or other reputable resources.

Food Fads

Fads and diets are sometimes the teen's motivation for unusual preferences. These fads may be dangerous, especially if they are strictly adopted (or if one fad quickly follows another) over a long period of time. Just like an adult, a teen may begin to rely on fad diets to lose weight quickly, and often. A healthier lifelong pattern of slow weight loss and remaining at an ideal weight level may never be learned.

A teen has the right to know all about a fad

diet and why it may not be adequate or wise. Physicians, local dietitians, and home economics teachers are resource persons with whom the adolescents could discuss questions relating to diet.

Pregnancy

A pregnant teen requires a lot of food. She should have at least 5 cups of milk, 3 servings of meat, 4 servings of fruits and vegetables, and 4 servings of breads and cereals each day (or come as close as possible to these recommendations). But she also often needs a good deal of support for many social concerns and problems, and it may be very hard for her to eat properly. Some of her problems might include nausea and vomiting, anxiety, depression, family conflicts that make mealtimes unpleasant, lack of knowledge, or lack of resources if she leaves home. She may deny her pregnancy and try to lose weight to "hide" it. She may have a naive belief that "if I don't eat, maybe it will go away."

Communities vary widely in the resources available to the teenager in a crisis pregnancy. Some have pregnancy centers that offer support to the teen so that she can make the decisions necessary to carry her pregnancy to term. Hospitals may have special programs. Some national organizations have set up hotlines to help a pregnant teen locate support agencies in her area. But to begin this process, a teen must first admit she is pregnant. If good eating habits have become a lifestyle for her *before* her pregnancy, she is more likely to have a healthy pregnancy, even during this crisis period.

In some cultures, adolescence is the normal time to begin having children. For these women, pregnancy is not a crisis, but a normal part of life for their age. The available evidence seems to indicate that pregnancy to a teenager in such a culture is no greater a health risk than is pregnancy in early adulthood. It is the social situation that makes the difference.

About Breakfast

Teens often skip meals, and eat snacks later. Breakfast is often skipped. But breakfast is just as important in adolescence as in childhood. Skipping breakfast, a teen (or adult) may then snack several hours later on something high in sugar and calories and low in other nutrients. Candy bars, sweet rolls, or donuts may have just as many calories as a bowl of cereal and an egg, but have few of the other nutrients. And there is some indication that a breakfast high in protein may lower a person's intake of high sugar foods by satisfying hunger.[4] It would mean that breakfasts of cereal and milk, an English muffin with cheese, peanut butter, eggs, meat, or even leftover pizza may actually help weight control in the long-run.

Breakfast need not be the traditional cereal, eggs, and bacon to be nutritious. A teen who warms up a bowl of chili, fixes a salad with cheese, eggs, and cold meat, or has a peanut butter or tuna sandwich, or yogurt and some fresh fruit will be just as well nourished as one who has the "traditional" breakfast. And all of these "nontraditional" breakfasts can be prepared quickly.

So, adolescence is both the end of being a child and the beginning of adulthood. It can be a hard time, physically, emotionally, and nutritionally. The choices an adolescent is learning to make will help prepare him for adult decisions. A basic knowledge of how to choose nutritious meals will lay the groundwork for a lifetime of healthful eating habits.

ADULTHOOD

The RDAs for the adult years are divided into three age groups: 19 years to 22 years, 23 years to 50 years, and the over 50 group. The major difference in the human body within these three age groups is the varying need for growth and maintenance.

Both men and women complete their growth between the ages of 19 and 22. Bone length and strength reach their maximum. Sexual maturation is completed. But some growth *does* continue, so needs are still slightly higher than later on in adulthood. For example, the RDA for both men and women between 19 years and 22 years suggests that they need as much vitamin D daily as is provided by 3 cups of milk. After age 23, this need can be met by 2 cups of milk each day. Energy needs also are higher. Most women should get 1700 Kcals to 2500 Kcals each day and most men, 2500 Kcals to 3300 Kcals.

By age 23, most growth has ended. Only the severely underweight will need to gain. Basic energy needs (to maintain the health of all the tissues in the body) begin to decrease about 2% every 10 years after age 23.[4] Depending on activity, a woman between 23 years and 50 years of age might need 1600 Kcals to 2400 Kcals per day and a man, 2300 Kcals to 3100 Kcals.[4]

Nutrient needs in the years after 50 will be discussed later. Nutrition needs in pregnancy and lactation are discussed in Chapters 13 and 14.

Meal Planning

The four food groups guideline discussed in Chapter 12 is as useful when planning meals for adults as for children. Since fats, oils, and sweets are not included in this guideline, these basic needs can be met with an intake of about 1200 Kcals. A person could meet his basic needs and still lose weight (since almost all adults need more than 1200 kcals to maintain weight). This low level also allows some extra energy in the form of sweets and oils, if desired, or more portions from each of the four food groups. A diet providing less than 1200 Kcals may not furnish all the nutrients the body needs, and thus the body may use those nutrients it *does* get for basic functioning, rather than for health and maintenance.

Another, more general set of guidelines for meal planning is the dietary guidelines described in Chapter 12. Table 17-1 illustrates a typical daily menu and how it can be adapted to meet the basic four and the dietary guidelines. Consult the RDA in Appendix One for other specific nutrient needs in adulthood.

Nutrition, The Athlete, and Exercise

Athletes do not have any special needs for vitamins, protein, fats, or most minerals. However, they have higher than average needs for two nutrients: energy and water. A person needs to eat more, if he is in training as an athlete, than he

did during nonathletic periods of his life. Because it is energy (calories) and not protein or fat that is needed, the easiest (and cheapest) way to get these extra calories is with carbohydrate foods, such as breads, whole grains, fruits, and sugars. To plan meals for an athlete, the four food groups are still an appropriate general guide, but portions of breads and cereals, fruits, and vegetables should be increased.

Athletes also need more water than nonathletes (see Chapter 9), because water is lost in perspiration. Some believe that athletes also need more salt, but this is not true. The average diet contains more salt than any body absolutely needs, and thus there is more than enough in reserve for the needs of most athletes. An athlete who consumes extra salt is forcing his kidneys to work overtime excreting what is not needed. The kidneys use water to flush out the body's extra substances. So too much salt may actually rob the athlete's body of needed water. Highly concentrated, sweetened drinks may have the same effect, and may actually make the athlete thirstier. The average diet contains far more than enough salt for most athletes. Several references are listed at the end of this chapter, for those interested in a deeper discussion of nutrition and the athlete.

An athlete does not use his food any differently than does a nonathlete. However, he may use it *more effectively.* This is true for any person involved in regular, strenuous, prolonged exercise, such as walking, jogging, swimming, aerobic classes, rowing, and so forth. The heart is a muscle and these types of exercises help to "tone up the heart." When it is working well, blood can flow and "feed" the body effectively. Cells acquire the oxygen they need to complete all their functions. Body fat is "burned" and muscle "built." As the body improves overall, it becomes more and more finely tuned in the way it uses food to make energy.

For this fine tuning to be most effective, these "aerobic exercises" (that make the heart work harder and take in large amounts of oxygen) or sports should become part of a person's lifestyle. Listed on page 137 are exercises that do, can, or do not help condition the heart. Government publications and other information devoted to

Table 17-1

Sample "Typical" Menu Revised To Meet Dietary Guidelines

	Instead of:	(Problem) ↑ = High ↓ = Low	A better choice might be:
Breakfast	Sugar-coated cereal with whole milk	↑ Sugar ↓ Fiber ↑ Saturated fat	Instant hot oatmeal Low fat or skim milk
	2 slices white toast with butter	↓ Fiber ↑ Saturated fat ↑ Cholesterol	2 slices whole wheat toast with peanut butter or corn-oil margarine
	Coffee	No nutrients stimulant	Orange Juice
Lunch	Ham and cheese sandwich	↑ Sodium ↑ Cholesterol ↑ Saturated fat	Water-packed tuna sandwich
	On white bread, bag potato chips	↓ Fiber ↑ Sodium, "Empty" calories	On whole grain bread, fresh fruit
	Soda	↑ Sugar, few nutrients	Low fat milk
Snack	Small candy bar	↑ Sugar ↑ Fat "Empty" calories	Low fat yogurt
Dinner	Cheeseburger with pickles, ketchup	↑ Fat ↑ Cholesterol ↑ Sodium	Baked fish with lemon, onions, parsley
	Salad drenched in salad dressing	↑ Fat, ↑ Sodium	Salad with lemon juice, spoonful oil/vinegar
	French fries	↑ Fat, few nutrients	Baked potato with melted cheese
	Soda	↑ Sugar	Juice or tea with milk
	Ice cream cone	↑ Fat ↑ Sugar	Fresh fruit cocktail
Evening	Cheese Curls	↑ Fat "Empty" calories	Air-popped popcorn
	Several alcoholic beverages	↑ Calories, ↑ Alcohol intake Few nutrients	Chilled juice or soda or 1 small alcoholic beverage

physical fitness, designed for the average person not interested in becoming a professional athlete, are usually available from health centers, libraries, and even insurance companies. Many local programs are available to help persons start a beneficial exercise routine. It is important to check first with a physician if these routines will involve more exercises, or more *strenuous* exercises than an individual is used to doing.

Contrary to some beliefs, there is little evidence that regular exercise will lead to a substantially *longer* life. But, combined with good nutrition and other health practices, it may lead to a more *healthful* life.

Premenstrual Syndrome (PMS) and Nutrition

In the 7 to 14 days before menstruation, many women complain of mood swings, fluid retention, food cravings, acne, and/or headaches. These classic premenstrual symptoms have come to be called "premenstrual syndrome" or PMS.

EXERCISES TO CONDITION HEART AND LUNGS. WHICH ONES HELP?

A *Do Condition* *Heart and Lungs*	B *Can Condition*	C *Do Not Condition*
Cross-country skiing	Bicycling	Baseball
Hiking *(uphill)*	Downhill skiing	Bowling
Ice hockey	Basketball	Football
Jogging	Calisthenics	Golf *(on foot or by cart)*
Jumping rope	Field hockey	Softball
Rowing	Handball	Volleyball
Running in place	Racquetball	
Stationary cycling	Soccer	
	Squash	
	Swimming	
	Tennis *(singles)*	
	Walking	

(Exercise and Your Heart. US Department of Health and Human Services, NIH Publ. No. 81–1677, p 21, May 1981)

Because PMS involves subjective and/or emotional changes rather than clearly measured physical change, it is difficult to predict, to diagnose, and to identify a rationale for treatment. Not every woman experiences the symptoms. Women who do may have quite different complaints from one another and even from month to month. Aside from prescribing tranquilizers, little has been done to help women cope with the symptoms of this often doubted syndrome.

Hormone levels do change considerably in the 14 days each month between ovulation and menses. Potentially, hormone balance can influence water retention, electrolyte balance, appetite, glucose tolerance, and mood. But it is not clear why some women experience these changes more than others.

The popular press often advises dietary change as part of treating PMS. Women are told to cut down on caffeine, salt, and simple sugars, to eat more protein or calcium, and to take vitamin or mineral supplements, particualrly pyridoxine (vitamin B_6). Theoretically a low-sodium diet minimizes water retention. And though caffeine is a mild diuretic, there is some evidence that high caffeine intake makes the emotional symptoms even worse.[5] Beyond this, however, there is no evidence that the therapies have reproducible benefits, though decreasing caffeine, salt, and sugar and increasing protein and calcium foods is not harmful.[6] However, supplements may be dangerous and should not be used unless specifically recommended by a physician who can monitor their effects. B_6 has not been shown to have any reliable effect on PMS and megadoses, like megadoses of anything else, may have serious side effects.[7]

Nutrition After 50

It is true that the body begins to age as soon as it begins to grow. Cells are sloughed off constantly and replaced with new cells. But after a person reaches physical maturity in the early 20s, growth slows. Changes begin that will eventually lead to the noticeable signs of "aging," such as wrinkles, dry skin, deteriorating eyesight, hearing, and endurance. By age 50, most of these changes are evident. It take more effort to keep the body in shape than it did at age 25. Nutrient needs and considerations are different.

The body's fat-to-muscle proportions are different. And the diet may be different as well, as a result of taste changes, financial limitations, or dental problems.

In the years after age 50, changes become more and more noticeable. Individuals may not be able to be as active as they formerly were, so they need fewer calories. The body does not make secretions (such as saliva and digestive fluids) as well as it used to make them. Muscles, including the walls of the digestive tract, are weaker. This makes indigestion and constipation more likely. Taste and smell may change or weaken due to minute changes in the nervous system.

Lifestyle may also affect changes. After retirement, there may not be enough money to buy the same nutritious foods as there was before retirement. Many persons are afraid of aging. Older adults often have some chronic complaint, some point at which their body is weaker than it has been. They may develop strong interests in "health fads," unproved or plainly false claims that promise health or longer life through pills or a special diet. Trying these gimmicks, including large doses of vitamins or the regular use of some acclaimed powder or other substance, may be the ways these older adults try to regain lost health or retain what health they have.

Chapter 20 will discuss these fads in more detail. If the substances are not dangerous, the only problem may be a financial one. Usually such products are extremely expensive. When funds are limited, a person may need to choose between buying foods that are obviously nutritious, and these other substances that provide few calories, poor nutrient balance, and questionable benefits.

The adult over 50 still needs all the nutrients he needed at age 30, *except* energy. This situation is the opposite of the athlete. Because the older person's needs are less, it is easy to gain weight, even on the same diet that maintained weight for many years. The four food groups, and the prudent diet (based on the dietary guidelines) are still recommended for meal planning. However, there is less leeway than before for "extras" and sweets. Planning meals for the older person's specific mechanical or neurological problems, when they affect eating, will be discussed in later chapters.

STUDY QUESTIONS

1. What makes it difficult to determine how much of a nutrient a teenager needs?

2. Define "peak height velocity." When does it occur in adolescents?

3. Which age group, from 11 years to 14 years, or 15 years to 18 years, needs more of the nutrients listed below? Explain your answer.
   - Calcium
   - Energy
   - Iron

4. How many choices should a teen pick daily from each of the four food groups?

5. List three social concerns of adolescence. Describe how each concern may influence a teenager's food choices.

6. List and discuss some of the problems an adolescent may face in a crisis pregnancy. How might each problem affect her eating habits? What can be done about each, assuming she plans to carry the baby to term?

7. Is breakfast important for adolescents and adults? Why or why not?

8. Why do adults who have stopped growing still need nutrients?

9. Why might a 21-year-old college student need more calcium than his 25-year-old brother?

10. Approximately how much energy do adults between ages of 23 and 50 need each day?

11. List three aerobic exercises.

12. How do nutrient needs change after age 50? What might be some concerns of an elderly person about his nutrition?

13. The older body produces less _____, which makes digestion more difficult and constipation more frequent.

14. True or false. Explain your answer:
   - Anemia is rare in adolescence. High levels of iron are not needed until the end of puberty.

- Adolescence is an optimal time for an overweight teen to diet successfully.
- Underweight teens are healthier because they are not carrying a lot of excess fat.
- Unusual eating habits are common in the teen years and may not be harmful.
- An underweight teenage girl usually has anorexia nervosa.
- Teens need to eat about as much as breast-feeding women.
- Athletes should take salt tablets regularly while they are in training.
- Sweetened beverages are healthier for a runner than plain water.
- Regular aerobic exercises help tone the heart muscle.
- Adults over 50 years of age should eat less candy than their 30 year old children.
- A 17 year old teenage girl needs more protein than her mother.

REFERENCES

1. Shuttleworth FK: The physical and mental growth of girls and boys age six to nineteen in relation to age at maximum growth. Monograph No. 4 of the Society for Research in Child Development, Serial No. 22:16, 1939

2. National Academy of Science: Iron Nutrition in Adolescence, Publication No. (HSA) 77-5100. US Department of Health, Education, and Welfare, 1976

3. Bullen BA, Reed RR, Mayer J: Physical activity of obese and nonobese girls as appraised by motion picture sampling. Am J Clin Nutr 14:211–223, 1964

4. Food and Nutrition Board, National Academy of Science: Recommended Dietary Guidelines, 9th ed, pp 22–23. Washington, National Research Council, 1980

5. Rossignol AM: Caffeine containing beverages and premenstrual syndrome in young women. Am. J. Public Health 75:1335, November 1985

6. Jones DY, Kumtiyika SK: Premenstrual syndrome: A review of possible dietary influences. J Canadian Diet Assoc 44:194, July 1983

7. Vitamin B_6 toxicity: A new megavitamin syndrome. Nutr Rev 42:44, February 1984

SUGGESTED READING

Suggested references for nutrition and the athlete:
Clark N: The Athlete's Kitchen. Bantam, 1981
Smith NJ: Food for Sport. Palo Alto, Bull Publishing Co., 1976
McArdle WD: Exercise Physiology. Philadelphia, Lea & Febiger, 1981

CHAPTER 18

Cultural Food Patterns

OBJECTIVES

1. To discuss briefly the historical effects of foreign culture on "American" food patterns

2. To discuss the effect "American" food habits may have on the cultural food habits of immigrants

3. To list some common factors in the practice of culturally different food patterns

4. To equip the student to counsel in a sensitive manner those clients who eat in a culturally different way than Americans, by discussing basic principles for sensitive, cross-cultural communication and by suggesting ways of communicating across language barriers

5. To discuss the general food patterns, beliefs, and preferences of the following predominant food cultures in America:
   a. Chinese
   b. Hispanic (Mexican and Puerto Rican)
   c. Italian
   d. Kosher
   e. Southeast Asian
   f. Southern (USA)
   g. Vegetarian

Within the USA, there are many different Americas. Except for the native Indians, all Americans have family roots in other nations, even though these roots may be decades or generations in the past. Each nation had its own food patterns. Each nation was located in a specific climate, with a certain range of available foods. Each nation had its own problems with storing foods, and its own beliefs about the values and dangers of certain foods. When the immigrants came to America, they brought their beliefs and practices with them.

Through the generations, some of these foods became more "Americanized" than others. Foods such as spaghetti, roast beef, coffee, milk, and pies have become "American" although they originated in other cultures. Many other new foods, such as hamburgers, potato chips, and carbonated beverages today seem more American than the fish, pumpkin, and wild game that had been staple foods for centuries in America. Most immigrants and even the Indians today have made major changes in their diet to reflect the current "American" diet.

But some have not. There are many persons in the USA and Canada who still eat according to their native culture. When hospitalized, they may refuse to eat or to comply with a special diet because it goes against their cultural preferences and/or beliefs. These persons will be the focus of this chapter. The individual who can best help them eat properly is the individual who understands their cultural food patterns.

Those who resist widespread Americanization in their eating habits share certain similar characteristics. Often they still have relatives and friends in the homeland. They may visit the homeland regularly. They may live in a community surrounded by others of the same native culture. They may speak one or more languages, other than English. They may be married to someone from the same culture. They may belong to a very close-knit family unit. And anyone who works with them must also be willing to work with the entire family and its social system.

EFFECTIVE CROSS-CULTURAL COMMUNICATION

Genuine respect is crucial in order to work effectively with people from other cultures. Their "unusual" habits should never be mocked. Preferences should be met, whenever possible. The counseling atmosphere should enable the individual to feel free to talk about his dietary patterns with a counselor who is eager to understand.

Respect also means that the client will not be stereotyped. Not everyone will eat exactly the same way, even within a culture. For example, some persons will like boiled chitterlings (pig's intestines) or boiled plantains, while some will not. Some will accept more "American" foods than others. Each culture is simply a framework of food patterns. The framework may overlap with other frameworks; each is surrounded by the "American" framework. Within each, and overlapping to different degrees, is the individual. Other essentials for good communication with people from another culture include

- Warmth, friendliness
- Patience; the client may have as much trouble with understanding as does the counselor
- Respect for privacy
- Respect for differences
- A professional (but not distant or cold) manner

OVERCOMING LANGUAGE BARRIERS

While culture or background alone can sometimes be a "language barrier," communication is even more difficult when the individual client knows little English. If this is the case, the following guidelines may help improve communication:

1. Use simple words that are easily understood. If a concept is extremely important, find out if someone at home speaks or reads English. Write down the most important suggestions. If pamphlets are available in the native language, get them and use them.

2. Speak slowly and clearly, but no louder than normal.

3. Use pictures and gestures as much as possible.

4. Above all, use an interpreter if one is available. Find out and keep in mind:
   a. How well the interpreter knows both languages
   b. How well he knows the subject
   c. The national background of the interpreter. Is he a stranger to the client? Is the interpreter from a nation against which the client may have a strong bias? Are there other possible barriers that might bias information?
   d. The possibility of both parties misunderstanding the message. Clarify. Ask questions.
   e. The client. Maintain good eye contact. It is the client, not the interpreter, who is the focus of the conversation. It is the client's concerns that matter most.

5. Never assume all clients of a certain culture eat the same amounts or varieties of the cultural foods. Never assume that all will refuse the same "American" foods. Never assume.

6. Use the general practices that do seem to recur with clients to develop practical, relevant suggestions for future clients. Use available translators to put these suggestions in writing.

The following pages will discuss the general food patterns and beliefs of seven different cultural groups common in America. These outlines cannot be comprehensive. But they do cover general information that can be helpful in trying to influence the food choices of persons from these groups.

CHINESE

Highlights

Chinese-Americans may come from Hong Kong, Taiwan, and occasionally mainland China. Language may be a problem for the health care provider, though family members are usually available to translate. The Chinese family is usually a very strong, supportive, cohesive unit.

Many Chinese, as well as other Asian groups, reject much of Western medicine in favor of their own cultural remedies and beliefs. This may result in conflict when they are forced into medical care. The value of foods is often a major part of these beliefs and the *Yin – Yang* or *Hot – Cold* theory, described on page 143, is a commonly used interpretation of the role of food in health and in disease.

The Four Food Groups

Dairy. The Chinese do not eat many dairy products. They may drink milk occasionally, and enjoy ice cream, but the use of cheese is rare. Most of the calcium in the diet comes from fish, some green vegetables, and tofu (bean curd cakes). Some Chinese may not be able to tolerate milk, and develop diarrhea as a result. These persons may be willing to eat yogurt or custards, instead, and tolerate them.

Protein. Most meats and poultry are found in the Chinese diet. However, shellfish, canned, and fresh fish may be more popular than meat. *Tofu,* a white, cheeselike cake made from soybeans, is also common. These protein sources are chopped in tiny pieces and cooked with rice, vegetables, and seasonings. Chinese rarely eat meat as a separate dish.

Fruits/Vegetables. These are used daily. Some common fruits and vegetables (where available) include figs, kumquats, mango, persimmon, bamboo shoots, cabbage, celery, Chinese cabbage, greens, leeks, snow peas, taro, white radish, water chestnuts, white turnip, and winter melon.

Grains and Cereals. Rice is the staple food. Noodles, barley, millet, and some bread may also be used. Chinese rice may not be enriched with iron or B-vitamins, and usually has a different texture than American "instant" or "converted" rice.

Seasonings

The most popular seasonings are soy sauce and monosodium glutamate (MSG). Other common seasonings include sweet and sour sauces, mustard sauce, ginger, red bean paste, black bean sauce, oyster sauce, and sweet vinegar.

Beverages

Tea is served with every meal. It is usually plain, without milk, cream, or sweeteners. Very little milk is used, except by young children. It may be considered a luxury. Some Chinese drink coffee. Sugar cane drinks or sweetened soy milk may be common snack beverages, where they are available. Alcoholic beverages are a part of the Chinese diet for celebrations and holidays.

Meal Patterns

The Chinese-American diet fits many of the dietary guidelines (see page 86). It is low in fat and cholesterol, since little meat or saturated fat is used. Fresh fruits and vegetables contribute fiber. The Chinese *do* make rich, heavy desserts, but they are not a daily part of the diet.

All Chinese meals are based on rice (or noodles). Even the question, "Have you eaten today?" means "Have you had rice today?"* Many Chinese in America have adopted American breakfast foods, but still serve rice at other meals.

Meats, fish, vegetables, and seasonings are often fried in oil, after being cut up finely. Food may be well seasoned with sauces and spices.

Rice congee, a souplike mixture of cooked rice and water, is often used when an individual is ill. The Chinese believe it is very healthful and easily digested.

---

* Personal communication. Chinese nutritionists, South Cove Community Health Center, Boston, MA

Infant Feeding Practices

Bottle-feeding is more common than breast-feeding. Mothers may return to work quickly, so fathers and other relatives may share infant care and feeding.

Some may believe that a child should have only milk and rice congee until he is 18 months to 24 months old. Children who wait this long before starting on meat, fruits, vegetables, and other cereals may become anemic. Milk (or infant formula) and rice do not sufficiently meet the nutrient requirements of a child over 6 or 8 months old. Even when solids are offered, meat and fish are sometimes given in very small quantities. Or the child may be fed the broth, with the meat discarded after cooking. However, most parents are willing to feed the small child eggs. These may be the best protein source available until the parent is willing to give the child more meat and fish.

Sometimes a child's first solid foods include candy, potato chips, or soda. He may demand these foods only, and be full enough from eating them to refuse necessary vegetables, fruit, and meats, when they are offered. The infant's teeth may suffer as a result.

Common Nutrition Problems

The Chinese diet is high in sodium. Most of the sodium is found in the sauces and MSG, the white powder used to enhance flavor. In some communities "reduced sodium soy sauce" is available, but it may not be well accepted.

The low calcium content of the Chinese diet may be improved by increasing green leafy vegetables, small boney or pickled fish, and tofu, which has been made with some form of calcium.

The "Hot–Cold" Theory

As mentioned above, this theory often influences the food choices an Asian person might make under certain conditions. It is based on the eastern religious belief that there are two equal but opposing forces in the universe, the *Yin* and the *Yang* or, in food, "Hot" and "Cold" forces. Health is believed to occur when the two forces are in a proper balance in the body. Sickness occurs when there is imbalance of the two forces in the body.

Persons who believe this theory try to help cure sickness by bringing the body back into proper balance through diet and other practices. They believe certain foods are either hot, cold, or neutral in their properties. "Hot" or "cold" qualities have nothing to do with temperature, spice, or taste. They refer to the forces that are believed to be contained in the foods.

This system is "both individual and arbitrary.[1] That is, not all cultures see the same foods in the same way. To the Chinese, fruits and vegetables are "cold" and meats, condiments, alcohol, and fatty foods are "hot." This might differ in another culture. People from Southeast Asia, Haiti, the West Indies, and many other groups also practice some form of this system.

Sickness is not the only condition where the body is "out of balance." Pregnancy is also seen as a time when the body forces change. Some parts of pregnancy may be "cold" periods when "hot" food is needed for balance (and "cold" foods avoided). Other periods are "hot," when "cold" foods are needed (and "hot" foods avoided). Menstruation and the postpartum period are also times when women often eat according to a prescribed pattern based on "hot" and "cold."

For the Chinese, the postpartum period is "cold." The body has lost heat, and needs to have it restored. As a result, women are expected to eat rice with "hot" foods such as sweet vinegar, ginger, and meat for one month postpartum.* Milk may be allowed, if it is "neutral," but the "cold" foods, such as fruits and vegetables, are not permitted.

Other beliefs often accompany this system in various cultures. Some foods are believed to increase or decrease the blood supply. Some foods are thought to cause disease directly and others to have "magical" properties (for example, some cultures forbid double-yolked eggs in pregnancy, since they may "cause" twins).[2]

---

* Personal communication. Chinese nutritionists, South Cove Community Health Center, Boston, MA

Even vitamin and mineral supplements may be "hot" or "cold" and taken or avoided, accordingly.

When a health provider works with people who practice this system, the beliefs must be respected. It is unlikely—and usually unnecessary—that the beliefs can be challenged. The client may not understand—or agree with—the system, but may follow it because it is such a strong cultural norm. He does not need to understand digestion and metabolism in order to eat as well as possible within this belief system.

The most effective response is one that works within the perceived beliefs. Respect the person and accept his beliefs, even if it is not possible to agree with them. If a hospitalized person, for example, refuses orange juice (because it is "cold" and the body needs "hot" foods), determine what beverages—and high vitamin C foods—are acceptable. Find out if the family can bring foods from home. Make sure the dietitian and physician are aware of the problem.

If the proscription is a temporary one, as in the postpartum period, it is not likely that a nutrient deficiency will have time to develop, as long as the client returns to a complete diet in a short time.

HISPANIC

Highlights

Hispanic-Americans usually come from Mexico, Puerto Rico, Cuba, Central or South America. The diet in each of these cultures is a bit different. Moreover, the American culture may influence each diet and each culture differently. Only those of Mexico and Puerto Rico will be discussed here, since they are usually the most common.

Mexican-Americans may be very poor, especially if they have recently arrived in the USA. Some may be unable to read or write either Spanish or English. They may buy food only if it is cheap, or if they recognize the packaging. They may have no desire to return to Mexico.

In contrast, Puerto Ricans may travel back to their native land frequently, since Puerto Rico is part of the United States. The conditions there are frequently better for the average person than those in Mexico, and literacy is not usually a problem, although Puerto Ricans may read and speak only Spanish.

• Mexican

The Four Food Groups

Dairy. Fresh, evaporated, flavored, and condensed milk are all accepted but used in small quantities. Ice cream is used. American, hoop, and Monterey Jack cheese are the most common cheeses found in the Mexican diet.

Protein. Pork may be more common in the diet than beef. Chorizo, a spiced sausage, is used frequently. Dried, cooked beans are the mainstay of most diets, and are eaten daily.

Fruits/Vegetables. These may be "too expensive." Some that are preferred include avocado, chilies, guava, mango, corn, green beans, lettuce, prickly pear, cactus leaf and fruit, sapote, tomato, sweet potatoes, and zucchini.

Grains and Cereals. Most meals include corn or flour tortillas, rather than bread. Sweetened cereals are often chosen, instead of plain cereal. Noodles, spaghetti, and sweet bread are common, and white bread, though it contains fewer nutrients than whole grain bread, may be regarded as a status symbol.

Seasonings

Chili sauce, guacamole (avocado and tomato, mashed together with oil and seasonings), pork cracklings, lime, and salsa (a tomato-pepper-onion relish) are the chief seasonings. Lard is usually used as the fat source in cooking.

Beverages

Mexican-Americans drink coffee and tea, often with sugar and canned or sweetened condensed milk. Hot chocolate may be accepted but is not common. Soft drinks and fruit drinks are the most common beverages for many. All of these contain a good deal of sugar and few, if any, necessary nutrients, other than energy.

Local beers are often brewed; alcohol may be

a regular part of life for many, and sometimes serves as a temporary escape from the chronic problems of poverty.

Meal Patterns

Breakfast frequently consists only of bread or sweet cereal and sweet coffee or tea. Lunch usually includes beans and tortillas, fried potatoes, and/or fried macaroni. Tomatoes and chilies are included in most meals.

Infant Feeding Practices

Used for generations, canned milk is sometimes preferred over infant formula. This may be only because it is cheaper. Parents who cannot afford infant formula, and do not choose to breastfeed, should be referred to the Women, Infants and Children's (WIC) program for help and for supplemental formula.

As a result of this high use of canned milk without supplementation, of cereal added to baby bottles, and of early feeding of candy and soda instead of fruits, vegetables, and pure fruit juices, obesity and poor nutrition may begin in infancy.

Common Nutrition Problems

Obesity, with its many related problems (such as diabetes, hypertension, and heart disease), is one of the most common nutrition-related health problems among Mexican-Americans. This is largely due to a diet high in sugar and low in fresh fruits and vegetables, foods frequently fried in animal fats, and large quantities of starchy foods low in fiber.

• Puerto Rican

Four Food Groups

Dairy. Except for children, Puerto Ricans rarely drink cold milk. The adults, however, may use it in their coffee, and coffee may be as much as half milk. Cheese is well accepted.

Protein. Chicken is most commonly used, although fish, beef, pork, and eggs are also a regular part of the diet. Dried, cooked beans are boiled with spices and sauces, and usually served daily with rice.

Fruits/Vegetables. All fruits are well accepted. Papaya, mangoes, oranges, bananas, and nectars of peach, apricot, and pear are common. Tuberous roots and other starchy vegetables are called *viandas* and are as common as rice and beans. Viandas may be boiled or fried, and the most common are plantains (green bananas), batata, namé, yautio, malanga, and apio. Other accepted vegetables include pumpkin, carrots, tomatoes, sweet potatoes, lettuce, onions, cabbage, and green peppers.

Grains and Cereals. Rice with beans is served daily in many Puerto Rican households. Sometimes cooked plantain may be considered a bread. Crackers, white bread and rolls, and cereals are well accepted.

Seasonings

A sauce called *sofrito* is commonly prepared and cooked with rice and beans. It is made from onions, peppers, garlic, tomatoes, lard, spices, and annatto seed. It is commercially available, but most housewives will make it from scratch. Other common seasonings include bay leaves, *achiote* (annatto), *cilantro* (coriander leaves) vinegar, oregano, and tomato products.

Beverages

The most popular beverage is coffee with milk. Soft drinks, fruit drinks, fruit nectars, and *malta* are also common. Malta is a sweet, nonalcoholic drink made from malt extract, sugar, and caramel. Many Puerto Ricans believe it is healthful, although it actually contains a good deal of sugar and very few nutrients.

Alcoholic beverages are common, although women rarely drink them.

Meal Patterns

Breakfast usually consists of French bread or plantains, sometimes cereal and/or eggs, coffee with milk, and perhaps, cheese. Lunch may be canned American soups, sandwiches, hamburgers, or pasta products, or it may be rice, beans, and meat with a salad. Supper is usually the main meal of the day and includes rice and beans with meat, salad, viandas, a beverage, and maybe dessert. Custard, fruit, or ice cream are common desserts.

Infant Feeding Practices

Few Puerto Rican women breast-feed, although some may be willing to give it a try, if encouraged by husband, mother-in-law, or mother. Early marriage may be common, and these other relatives often strongly influence a young mother's feeding decisions. Formula is well accepted, and widely used. Cereal is often added to the formula in the bottle, sometimes by the second month. This practice may continue long after the infant is able to eat cereal with a spoon.

Common Nutrition Problems

The Puerto Rican diet has very few built-in problems. It may be low in calcium, because of poor milk and cheese intake, but is usually adequate in other major nutrients. The problems that may occur include

Eating too little. Some women eat very little and are chronically underweight. As a result, they may have poor resistance to disease and few reserves to carry into pregnancy.

Too much junk food or sugar, especially for children. Teenagers, as well, may reject the cultural meals and depend on fast foods and soft drinks to satisfy hunger.

Puerto Ricans who must limit sodium should avoid sofrito and other popular sauces for rice, since they are high in sodium.

ITALIAN

Highlights

Food is a very important part of the Italian-American culture. To serve food is to show love. To reject food is to reject love, and may be an insult to many cooks. Guests are always offered food in large quantities, and, as a result, the overweight figure is common, and acceptable within this culture.

The Four Food Groups

Dairy. Milk is used by adults only in coffee. Cheeses, however, are quite popular. Common Italian cheeses include mozzarella, ricotta, parmesan, romano, provolone, and imported cheeses that are usually high in sodium.

Protein. All meats, fish, and poultry are used. Many varieties of cold cuts (also high in sodium, as well as fat) are prevalent. Meat is often fried, while nuts make a popular condiment and snack.

Fruits/Vegetables. Italian-Americans eat large quantities of fresh fruit. Most meals include vegetables, although they may be cooked (or covered) with oil. Olives, high in natural olive oil, are also used as a condiment.

Grains and Cereals. Pasta and/or bread is served with every meal. Rice and *polenta* (cornmeal) are also common.

Seasonings

Many herbs and spices are used, with butter and olive oil the preferred fats used in cooking.

Beverages

Expresso coffee is usually a part of breakfast and is served after supper. Wine is frequently drunk at lunch and supper. Many older Italians drink mineral water and imported fruit drinks, while anisette is occasionally added to coffee.

Meal Patterns

Traditionally, the heaviest meal is the noon meal, consisting of soup, pasta, meat, salad, vegetables, and bread. Cheese and fruit are served at the end of every meal. Sweet desserts are common and usually abundant on religious holidays and festivals. The diet may be more or less Americanized, depending on the individual family.

Infant Feeding Practices

Because Italians have been part of the American culture for a longer time than have the preceding groups, their infant feeding practices vary according to individuals and the American influence. Overfeeding may be a problem, beginning with infancy.

Common Nutrition Problems

The common diseases that may result from overeating and overweight are the key problems of this culture's diet. Much of the food is high in sodium, and may also be high in cholesterol content and saturated fats, from meat, cheeses, and butter.

KOSHER

Highlights

The *kosher* diet, which is followed by many (especially Orthodox) Jews, is based on interpretations of dietary restrictions in the Hebrew Scriptures. First, a kosher diet forbids all foods that are clearly forbidden in the Mosaic Law. Second, milk and meat products are bought, stored, prepared, and eaten separately, out of obedience to the Jewish interpretation of the Bible verse, "You shall not boil a kid in its mother's milk".[3] Milk and meat must never be consumed at the same meal or with the same utensils if at all possible. Sometimes utensils may be used for both milk and meat if they are thoroughly cleaned between uses. Some families have two sets of dishes, eating utensils, pots, and even refrigerators. One set is used for meat products and the other, for milk. "Keeping kosher" is a lifestyle, not merely a way of eating.

The Four Food Groups

Since Jewish people are part of the American culture, the four food groups differs little from the usual American diet. All dairy products are accepted at milk meals. Meats must be kosher, that is, they must be slaughtered by a kosher butcher in a way that properly drains the blood from the animal. This process involves salting the meat, so kosher meat is slightly higher in sodium than its unsalted counterparts. Soaking meat in water before cooking may help rinse out

some of this salt. Meats that are forbidden include pork, shellfish, and scavenger fish. Other fish, as well as eggs, are not considered "meat." They are regarded as *pareve* or neutral. Foods that are pareve can be served with dairy products, or with meat. All fruits and vegetables are acceptable, and all grain products are used. However, bread made with milk or milk solids could not be served at a meat meal. Leavened, or raised, breads are forbidden during Passover, in accordance with the Mosaic Law.

Butter may be preferred over margarine. Any margarine that has been marked with a "U" on the package is kosher. This means that no milk (or whey) solids have been added to it. Consequently, it can be used with either milk or meat meals. Margarines should be encouraged by the health provider in place of butter, particularly if a client is at risk for heart disease, since margarines are usually much lower in saturated fat, and contain no cholesterol.

Beverages

Since milk cannot be served with meat meals, soft drinks, juices, and wines are common. Coffee and tea are both acceptable, with nondairy creamer used as a milk substitute at meat meals.

Meal Patterns

Meals are either "milk" (sometimes called *Milchig*) or "meat" (*Fleischig*) meals. Individuals must wait 30 minutes after drinking milk to eat a meat meal, and 6 hours after a meat meal before having any milk.

This means such common foods as ham and cheese sandwiches, cheeseburgers, spaghetti with melted cheese and meat sauce, pizza with sausage, or a chef's salad with a milk-based salad dressing would never be a part of the diet, or even brought into the home of a person "keeping kosher."

Infant Feeding Practices

This depends both on the culture and the individual family. There is no part of the kosher diet that would be a nutritional problem for an infant.

Common Nutrition Problems

Whenever someone who "keeps kosher" is told to lower his sodium and cholesterol levels, the diet is a potential problem. This is because of the high fat and sodium levels in many preferred foods. Low fat cheese (such as farmer's or pot cheese) can be substituted for high fat cheeses (such as cream cheese). Commercial low cholesterol egg substitutes (which come in powder or frozen liquid form) can be substituted for eggs in challah (egg bread) or other recipes. Margarines made from polyunsaturated vegetable oils can substitute for butter. All added salt (that is, the salt added at the table and in cooking) can be controlled, with herbs and spices used for flavor. None of these changes affect the kosher dietary restrictions.

SOUTHEAST ASIAN

Highlights

Even though the Southeast Asian "boat people" will be discussed together, as a group, in this section, they are not all alike. They may come from Vietnam, Laos, or Cambodia, three separate nations. They may come from the city or from a hill tribe. They may have strong feelings against "boat people" from another nation. They may read and write one, two, or three (or more) languages. They may have lived in a Western-type culture in Asia, or in a very simple manner. They may have been very rich or very poor in Asia. Since the Southeast Asian group includes persons who were enemies in war, it is very important to be sensitive to these differences.

However, some generalizations can be made. Southeast Asians (SEA's) are usually very polite and private people. They rarely express hostility, feeling that it is more polite to say "yes" than to admit they disagree or do not understand. A smile may not mean they are happy; rather, that they are embarrassed or concealing anger. Those who arrive in the USA are survivors who have often witnessed extreme violence as they tried to leave their homeland. Often family members have been killed. Adjusting to a completely strange culture after losing so much is extremely difficult.

Southeast Asians have much in common, culturally, with the Chinese. The primary unit in society is the extended family, rather than a nuclear family, or an individual. The most respected member of the household is the oldest male. There is a similar determination to become self-sufficient and to become employed as soon as possible. Like the Chinese, the SEA diet, in its native form, is generally healthful and nutritious. Often their chief dietary problems are those they have adopted from North America!

The Four Food Groups

Dairy. Very few dairy products are used. Most of the calcium in the diet comes from green, leafy vegetables, small fish, fermented fish products, soft shell crabs, bean curd (tofu) with calcium added and, occasionally, fortified soy milk. Children are usually willing to drink milk or eat yogurt. Adults may find the smell of milk nauseating, or may be lactose intolerant. Cheese is completely foreign to the Southeast Asian and is usually unacceptable.

Protein. Fish is eaten more often than meat, with pork the meat of choice. Chicken and eggs were very expensive in Southeast Asia, so they may not be used frequently here. All fish or meat that *is* used is finely chopped and served with rice and sauces.

Fruit/Vegetables. All fruits and vegetables are acceptable. Oranges were a status food in Asia. Many vegetables and fruits common in the USA may look strange to the Asian. He may prefer to buy the more familiar Asian fruits and vegetables, if they are available, even though they are more expensive.

Grains and Cereals. Up to 80% of the energy provided by the Southeast Asian diet comes from rice. Laotian rice is quite sticky, but rice eaten in Vietnam and Cambodia may be more like Western rice; however it often is not enriched. Long grain is preferred to short grain. Bread is usually accepted, but ready-to-eat cereals seem strange.

Seasonings

Many sauces and powders are popular, but most are very high in sodium. The most common sauce is a fermented fish sauce that the Vietnamese call *nuoc nam.* Sauces are served together with rice, meat, and vegetables at each meal.

Beverages

Plain black tea is common, and coffee is served with sugar and cream. Many Asians are easily influenced (at least at first) by Western advertising, and may drink large quantities of soft drinks. Alcoholic beverages are a part of the culture, but not a part of the daily diet. Usually only children drink milk. Many Southeast Asians prefer tea, fruit drinks, soft drinks or juice. Broth made from cooked rice and meat and vegetables is a common drink, believed to be very healthful.

Meal Patterns

Breakfast generally consists of a light soup of greens, perhaps noodles, and broth with rice and egg, meat, or fish. Bread may be included. Lunch and dinner are almost identical. They consist of rice with meat or fish, vegetables, and seasonings. Soup and fruit may be included. Snacks are not part of the typical Southeast Asian diet, although they have become common since the move to the West. Children may learn to snack on typical Western foods such as potato chips, cookies, cereal, and soft drinks.

Infant Feeding Practices

Breast-feeding was common in Asia. However, many women view the bottle as a "superior" status symbol. Those who do bottle-feed may be unsure of how to prepare formula. Consequently, infants may be fed sweetened condensed milk or rice gruel instead of formula.

As with the Chinese, infants may not start solids until 18 months to 24 months. When they do, they may begin with "status" sweets, rather than fruits, vegetables, cereals, and meat.

Practices will differ, and so it is important to talk with individuals.

Common Nutrition Problems

Most nutrition problems relate to the move to the West. Limited language ability and cultural understanding make shopping difficult and Western advertising very convincing. Asians have trouble finding foods familiar to them, either because they are unavailable, or because the foods are packaged in a different way. During their first months in the West, Southeast Asians usually are on welfare and food stamps, while they learn English and search for jobs. So their finances are limited. They may want to try an inexpensive American food, but do not know how to prepare it. They may be unsure of how to use an oven or a toaster. Pictures, home visits, consistent and regular friendly support can help to overcome some of these problems.

Many Southeast Asians follow the Hot – Cold theory in treating disease, and during pregnancy and the postpartum period.

SOUTHERN (USA)

Highlights

Food is an important part of social life everywhere, but this is especially true in the southeastern United States. Many cultures live in this section of the country: Cajun French, black Americans, Spanish, Cuban, and others. Within these cultures, the "soul food" cooking of most black Americans (and some white) is the most prevalent and most commonly called "Southern" by outsiders. The extended family is a close unit, and lots of food is essential at family gatherings.

The Four Food Groups

Dairy. Evaporated milk is most common among adults, and is especially used in coffee. Buttermilk ("clabbermilk"), cheese, and ice cream are also popular. Other calcium sources include small whole fish, greens, and broccoli.

Protein. Pork is the most popular meat, and pork parts rarely served anywhere else in the USA are eaten in the South. These include the pig's intestines (*chitterlings*), its stomach, feet, ears, jowls, hocks, heart, and, of course, its ham. The meat may be boiled, rolled in flour or cornmeal and fried, or baked. Also used regularly are fresh water fish, chicken, eggs, sausage, and lunchmeats. Black-eyed peas are served as a vegetable. Nuts grow well in the South and are used frequently.

Fruit/Vegetables. Greens of the mustard, turnip, spinach, swiss chard, beet, or collard plant are boiled with bacon fat and are the most popular vegetables. Sweet potatoes are cooked with sugar, boiled, or baked. Okra, lima beans, corn, tomatoes, white potatoes, and yams are all accepted and most available fruits are used freely.

Grains and Cereals. Rice, cornmeal, cornbread, hominy grits (also made of corn), biscuits, and white bread are the most common grain products found in the diet.

Seasonings

Bacon and salt pork (called fat back by some) are generously used for flavoring. Most meats, and often potatoes, are served with gravies.

Beverages

Coffee with evaporated milk and sugar is popular, as is iced tea, buttermilk, lemonade, sugared fruit drinks, and soft drinks, but few drink milk. (Many black Americans have a mild lactose intolerance.) Alcoholic beverages are not usually served with meals. How much they are consumed at other times depends on the individual.

Meal Patterns

These vary with the individual. Usually at least one large meal is served each day. Portions are usually large, and desserts are common, and high in sugar and fat.

Infant Feeding Practices

Many persons who have used canned milk in the past want to use it to feed infants, rather than to use formula. Canned milk is cheap, and many feel that children grow best on it. If finances are a problem, the family should be referred to the local Women, Infants and Children's (WIC) program, where iron-fortified infant formula is free to all eligible infants.

Solids are often introduced earlier than necessary. Baby cereal, in varying amounts, may be commonly added to the bottle. Sugar drinks may also be given in the bottle, instead of juice or plain water. Few women actually breast-feed, although many may be interested in doing so.

Common Nutrition Problems

Overweight is the predictable result of regular large portions of food. Also, the diet in the South is high in saturated fat, cholesterol, sodium, and sugar, while it is low in fiber. Diabetes, hypertension and/or heart disease may develop after years of body stress caused by the diet and by excess weight. Iron-deficiency anemia is also common.

VEGETARIANS

Highlights

A *vegetarian* is "one who eats no meat."[4] Vegetarians can be divided into two general categories, the *lacto-ovo* who includes dairy products and eggs in the diet, and the *vegan* who does not do so. A true vegetarian will not eat the flesh of any land or sea animal.

People may choose vegetarianism because of health concerns and/or environmental concerns, or because of religious beliefs. For example, Seventh Day Adventists are lacto-ovos; some members of Far Eastern religious sects are strict vegans. Other individuals may avoid meat because it takes more of the world's available ecologic energy to produce than do the plant sources of protein (see Chapter 3).

The Four Food Groups

Dairy. Lacto-ovo vegetarians use all dairy products, although some may avoid hard cheeses that have been made with rennet (which comes from the cow's stomach). Vegans may drink "soy milk" to obtain their calcium, since it contains no dairy product, and is made from soybeans. If they are not allowed to drink cow's milk, children of vegan parents should be given soy milk fortified with calcium. Regular, unfortified soy milk contains almost no calcium.

Protein. Lacto-ovo vegetarians will eat eggs. The other protein foods that are used include legumes, nuts, and seeds, each combined with grains, dairy products, or with each other to make a "complementary protein."

Fruit/Vegetables. All fruits and vegetables are readily accepted.

Grains and Cereals. For the most part, all grains and cereals are accepted, although many vegetarians abstain from foods made with white flour and sugar.

Vegetarian beliefs and meal patterns vary widely. Some beliefs will be discussed in the chapter on "Food Fads and the Health Food Store."

Seasonings and Beverages

These categories also vary widely, depending on the individual, his habits, and his reasons for the vegetarian diet. Many vegetarians drink herb teas, grain beverages, and fruit or vegetable drinks, as well as water. Stimulants such as coffee, tea, and sometimes alcohol are often used very little if at all.

Infant Feeding Practices

Frequently, vegetarian mothers breast-feed for 6 months to 12 months or more, because of a strong belief in doing what is "natural." Solids introduced at 4 months to 6 months may include cereals, juices, mashed beans, fruit, or rice. These are all appropriate "baby" foods for this age. However, if a parent is relying on adult, hot cereals, the infant may not be acquiring enough iron, which would be provided by infant cereals.

If vegan infants are not breast-fed (and they usually are), a commercial soy formula is the second best choice. Plain (or calcium-fortified) soy milk is not acceptable for an infant. It will not contain the nutrients the infant needs to grow well.

Common Nutrition Problems

Most of the problems of the vegetarian diet stem from a lack of knowledge or because of poor menu planning. Many vegetarians are in excellent health. A lacto-ovo diet can be quite adequate, nutritionally, and the vegetarian diet in general has the additional benefits of being low in cholesterol and saturated fats, and high in fiber.

Vegans and their children are the vegetarian group at highest nutrition risk. The vegan diet is low in its content of kilocalories (or energy). This means a child has to eat great quantities of food in order to get the energy needed for normal growth. Rickets and other bone problems may develop without sufficient calcium or vitamin D. The vegan diet provides little or no vitamin B_{12}. The body may take 2 or 3 years to "run out" of its stores of this vitamin, but the vitamin is essential and must be replaced. Some fermented products and yeast products may contain vitamin B_{12}, but this depends on the individual food. One other way to get B_{12} is through supplementation, which the vegan may or may not feel is "natural."

Protein may also be a problem with young vegan children, although it need not be so if the existing protein sources are combined effectively. (See Chapter 23 for a further discussion of protein complementation.)

STUDY QUESTIONS

1. What are four essential qualities for counseling an individual who comes from another culture?

2. A 74-year-old woman is assigned a visiting nurse who comes to her each week. The woman speaks no English. The nurse does not speak the woman's language. What are some ways the nurse could try to change the woman's eating habits?

3. Which of the four food groups is often lacking in a Southeast Asian or a Chinese diet? What foods would persons from this culture accept as a substitute to provide the necessary nutrients?

4. A postpartum Asian woman has refused most of her first meal in the hospital after delivery. Her husband requests hot broth for her, and nothing else. When this occurs at the next two or three meals, the medical staff becomes alarmed. What may be the problem? Explain your answer.

5. What is kosher meat?

6. What does "pareve" mean?

7. What are some common problems for immigrants as they make food choices in an American grocery store immediately after their arrival in this country?

8. Choose three cultures and describe their infant feeding practices. What practices are recommended? Which are not? Why?

9. For each item or items below, identify the cultural food pattern:
   - The sign "U" or word "pareve" on commercial foods
   - Milk and eggs as the only animal products this group will use
   - Tortillas and rice
   - Soy milk used instead of cow's milk
   - Rice, beans, and sofrito
   - Chitterlings, fat back, and bacon
   - An acceptance of obesity since food is considered a vital expression of love
   - Milk and meat never served at the same meal
   - Fish sauce
   - Coffee is half milk
   - Health is a balance between universal, opposing forces present in the body

10. What is one culture that has influenced your food preference? What part(s) of your diet reflects this influence?

11. Choose a cultural food pattern. Compare it with each of the "Dietary Guidelines for Americans" described in Chapter 12.

REFERENCES

1. Manderson L, Matthews M: Vietnamese attitudes toward maternal and infant health. Med J Aust 1:70, January 24, 1981
2. Go K, Moore I: The food habits and practices of Southeast Asians (primarily Cambodians and Laotians). Public Health Service, Alameda County (CA) Health Care Service Agency. August 1979. Unpublished paper
3. Exodus 23:19
4. By permission. From Webster's New World Dictionary 1973 by G. and C. Merriam Company, publishers of the Merriam Dictionaries

BIBLIOGRAPHY

Other sources used for material in this chapter:

American Dietetic Association: Cultural Food Patterns in the USA. Chicago, American Dietetic Association, 1969, 1976

Barer-Stein T: You Eat What You Are: A Study of Ethnic Food Traditions. Toronto, McClelland And Steward, 1979

Erhard D: The new vegetarians. Nutrition Today, pp 4–12, November–December 1973

Food and Nutrition Service: Southeast Asian American Nutrition Education Materials. Washington, US Department of Agriculture, 1981

Massachusetts WIC Program: Ethnic Food Patterns. Unpublished

Moore-Lappé F: Diet for a Small Planet. New York, Ballantine Books, 1975

Understanding the Puerto Rican Food Habits. Storrs, Conn., University of Connecticut. Unpublished paper

Worthington B et al: Nutrition in Pregnancy and Lactation, pp 80–85. St. Louis, CV Mosby, 1977

Yogai F: Dietary patterns of Spanish speaking people living in the Boston area. J Am Diet Assoc 71:273–275. September 1977

CHAPTER 19

Food Economy

OBJECTIVES

1. To discuss the application of nutrition principles to the purchase of food
2. To provide guidelines that will enable the reader
   a. To set goals before shopping
   b. To choose economically those foods high in essential nutrients
   c. To interpret labels
   d. To choose fresh, safe products
   e. To help prevent food spoilage after purchase
3. To discuss the rationale for these guidelines

Often, a health care provider is a resource for topics as basic as buying food. Since food and health do go together, nutrition principles must be translated into edible food to have any effect. No one really benefits from *knowing* what foods can supply needed nutrients unless he actually *buys* and *eats* those foods. This chapter and the next will help the reader apply the preceding chapters to regular food shopping. It will discuss some practical guidelines for buying—and storing—the most nutritious foods for the lowest prices. These are guidelines that shoppers can use in supermarkets, food cooperatives, farmer's markets, and even health food stores.

Buying from a health food store, will be covered in greater detail in the next chapter.

Economical food shopping involves five basic skills. The shopper must be able to

1. Prepare to shop
2. Choose the best nutrition values at the store
3. Interpret labels
4. Choose safe foods
5. Keep them safe at home

These are skills that can help anyone get the most for her money.

PREPARE TO SHOP

"Impulse buying" is what happens when shoppers do not plan ahead. Food bought on impulse is usually expensive, unnecessary, and may only have many "empty" calories and taste good. Many impulse foods are not particularly healthful and may leave less money for foods that are actually necessary.

Advance planning is the best way to prevent impulse buying. Some people plan menus for an entire week, then buy according to their menu. Others simply make lists of the foods they want and plan the menu later. The person who does not make a list before going to the store usually spends more money on food than necessary, and may even forget important items. When that person returns to the store to buy the foods he forgot, he may buy a few more unplanned items, once again, on impulse.

So economy shopping starts at home. It starts

with planning. A good shopping plan should consider

a. Who will eat the food, and their preferences

b. Available food coupons from newspapers or magazines, for foods the family actually uses. To save money, these should be the foods that the shopper would buy even if a coupon were not available

c. What leftovers are on hand

d. How much storage space is available

e. What foods are in season or on sale

f. What stores have the best selection and prices

g. How much preparation time will be available; convenience foods usually cost more, but may be worth the amount of time they save

h. Are there special events on the calendar that will need certain foods or ingredients

i. What recipe ingredients are needed

j. How much money is available for food

To best avoid impulse buying, NEVER shop on an empty stomach!

GETTING THE MOST FOR THE LEAST

How does the shopper make the best choices at the store? This may not be easy. There are different forms of foods and different brands within each form. There are different sizes, prices, and claims. Some foods are at eye level and easy to reach. Other foods that are just as nutritious (or more so) are displayed on higher or lower shelves.

Here are some general principles for the wise selection of food in the store.

a. Check and compare the prices of different brands and sizes. Unless one brand has been fortified with some nutrient, it will be nutritionally equal to another brand of the same form of the food, no matter what the label looks like. Generic or store brands may be just as nutritious as national brands. They are almost always cheaper.

b. Food that is highly processed and prepared (for example, bakery goods, deli goods, and frozen convenience foods) will be highly priced. In general, the simpler forms of a food are cheaper.

c. Fresh foods that are in season or grown locally are cheaper than foods imported or available off-season. In-season foods may also be more attractive and taste better.

d. Buy the largest size that can be stored and consumed easily. A 10-pound bag of potatoes is usually cheaper (per pound) than smaller amounts or potatoes bought separately. But a person buying for one may not be able to use all ten pounds quickly enough and may find buying a small amount more practical.

e. Read *unit pricing* labels wherever they are available. These are labels posted on the shelves that tell the price per pound of each item on the shelf. Unit pricing can be very helpful when packages have different weights and the comparative price is hard to determine.

f. Shop with a calculator. It can help the shopper keep track of accumulating costs. Calculators can also help determine what the relative costs are when unit pricing is not available.

g. Buy on sale, whenever possible. The shopper should be ready to substitute foods similar to those on her list that are on sale and cheaper.

Listed on pages 156 and 157 are some very specific tips to help the shopper choose from different food groups. On page 158 is an example of how to calculate the unit price by weight of eggs. More in-depth resources are listed at the end of this chapter.

READ LABELS

Food containers are required by law to provide consumers with essential information. The specific information depends on the food and the laws protecting that food. The label identifies the food, its brand name, and the name and address of the producer. It may also provide

Net weight. This is the weight of the food itself. Net weight of a food packed in liquid means the weight without the liquid.

Dates. This may be *open dating* (that is, easy to read and interpret), such as dates on bread or dairy products that specify the end date by which the food must be sold or used, or *coded dating.* Coded dates are stamped on the bottom or top of the container, and they may be a series of letters and numbers that the shopper cannot easily interpret. A coded date tells where, when, and in what batch a food was made. Sometimes manufacturers will send consumers information to help them interpret the codes of a particular product, if a consumer requests this information.

Grades or quality statements. These may be letters or numbered grades (A, AA, U.S. No.1) or descriptive words such as "choice," "fancy," "93 score" or "utility." These grades have nothing to do with the actual nutrients in the food. They simply describe its appearance. A lower "grade" food is just as nutritious as a higher "grade" food. In fact, low grade meats tend to have a lower fat content than top grade meats. The shopper must decide how much he is willing to pay for appearance. Grade differences are often hard to determine from a sight-check.

Nutrition information per serving. Illustrated on page 158 is a typical cereal label. It lists calories, protein, carbohydrate, fat, and sodium found in each serving. The label defines serving size in terms of both weight and volume. It also informs the shopper of the nutrients in a serving of the food to which milk has been added.

Percentage of the US Recommended Daily Allowances. (See Chapter 12 for a description of the US RDA.) The US RDA are usually higher than a person's needs, and can best be used to compare similar foods. The nutrients circled are those for which the government requires information or specifics. The others are optional. Choose the foods with the highest percentage of the US RDA at the best price.

Ingredients. These must be listed in descending order by weight. For the sample label, wheat bran is the ingredient used in the greatest (weight) amount. Sugar is second, and barley flour, third. The ingredients with the least weight in this cereal were the vitamins used to fortify it.

Carbohydrate information. This is usually listed on cereals. It helps the shopper learn how much and what kind of carbohydrates are in the cereal, and the information can also be used to calculate the percentage of sucrose or table sugar in a cereal.

Special nutrition claims. Law requires that all foods making special claims on the label list the nutrient content of the food. This informs the shopper who may need to choose certain foods or to avoid certain ingredients. It protects against fraud. The sample cereal makes a claim about fiber, so, therefore, must list its fiber sources and the amount of fiber contained in each serving.

CHOOSE SAFE FOODS

Federal laws were developed in the first few decades of the 20th century to protect the safety of almost all foods. The *Food and Drug Administration (FDA)* regularly inspects foods and manufacturing plants to make certain that specific standards are being met. This does not guarantee a 100% safe food supply, but it prevents most contamination, fraud, and adulteration.

Food can become unsafe in many ways. The three major culprits that make food unfit are "natural" ones: bacteria, yeasts, and molds. Insects and rodents carry bacteria. Yeasts and molds grow wherever moisture is present. Preservatives help prevent food from spoiling in these natural ways. Insecticides and sprays help inhibit insects. While most preservatives are considered safe, insecticides and sprays are not. Yet without the insecticides, the food may be totally destroyed, that is, eaten by animals and insects, with the remains unsafe for humans. Fruits and vegetables that have been sprayed should be peeled and scrubbed in the home before they are eaten.

SHOPPING TIPS

Dairy Products

Whole, low fat, skim milk, buttermilk and yogurt all have the same amounts of the same vitamins and minerals (although buttermilk and some low fat milks may have more sodium than whole milks and yogurts). The major difference is their calorie content.

Powdered nonfat dry milk is cheaper in bulk than fresh milk.

Yogurt made at home from milk is cheaper than prepared yogurt.

Sharp and aged natural cheeses are more expensive than milder cheeses or processed cheeses.

Protein/Meat Products

Meat

Compare "price per pound" on packaged labels of meat.

"Cheap" meats with a lot of bone may not be a good buy. Most of the cost may be for the bone.

Low grade meats may need more cooking, but often are cheaper and have the same quality of protein as higher grade meats.

Eggs

Eggs are graded AA, A and B. Grades A and B are cheaper and have the same nutrient content as grade AA.

There is no nutritional difference between brown and white eggs.

Eggs come in different sizes. It is possible to save money by buying eggs by size. Price per dozen divided by ounces per dozen (see the example on page 158) equals price per ounce. Compare before shopping or shop with a calculator.

Fish

Fish with a strong smell is too old.

Less popular fish (such as pilchards, which are often used instead of tuna) are often cheaper than more well-known fish.

Poultry

Whole birds are cheaper per pound than packaged, cut-up pieces.

Larger birds have more meat per pound than smaller birds. Birds with very small bones have a high percentage of bone to meat.

Save leftover scraps and odd parts for soups.

Dry Peas and Beans

These are nutritious, cheap protein sources high in fiber and other vitamins and minerals. They should be served with grains, dairy products, or meat in order to permit the body to make the best use of their protein.

Cold Cuts

Such products are expensive and usually are high in fat and sodium.

Nuts and Seeds

Also expensive, they are a protein source similar to dry peas and beans and should be combined with other, complementary protein sources. While dry peas and beans contain very little fat, nuts and seeds are high in fat, and therefore high in calories.

In General

Frozen dinners that list an ingredient other than pure meat as the first ingredient on the label are poor sources of protein.

Never refreeze a protein food that was once previously frozen.

Fruits and Vegetables

Fresh

Bruised or very soft fruit will spoil quickly. It may only be a good buy if it will be cut up and used immediately.

Discoloring (such as yellow spots on broccoli) or thin, wilted leaves may be signs that a vegetable is too old.

Buy what is in season and what is grown locally. It is usually cheaper than out-of-season food that has been shipped a great distance.

Canned

Heavy syrup may be more expensive than light syrup. The cost difference pays for extra sugar.

Store and generic brands are cheaper than national brands and the nutritional quality is usually the same. Check to see if store or national brands have been fortified with any particular nutrient that might give them a slight nutritional advantage. The extra price may not be worthwhile if the diet is already adequate in that nutrient.

Fruits and vegetables sold as irregular or cut up pieces (such as mushroom stems and pieces, chopped broccoli) are usually cheaper than the whole or intact forms of the same food.

Most canned goods will keep, unopened, for one year.

Fruit juices containing 100% juice are a better buy, nutritionally, than mixes, punches, or fruit "drinks" that boast "10% fruit juices."

Frozen

Frozen goods can be stored in a deep freeze for up to eight months without affecting nutrient quality.

Cut or chopped vegetables are cheaper than whole and leaf forms.

Plain vegetables are cheaper than those in a butter or a cheese sauce. Save money by adding butter or cheese at home.

Frozen vegetables are exposed to less heat than canned vegetables. This means they may have a slightly higher content of certain vitamins that may be destroyed by heat processing.

Grain Products

Buy "enriched" rice, bread, and cereals. The nutrients that "enrich" them are essential and the enrichment process is not expensive.

Whole grain products may naturally contain the nutrients that must be added (as "enrichment") to refined grain products. This means whole grain bread and brown rice contain (naturally) slightly more essential vitamins and minerals than white bread and white rice contain. Whole grain products are also much higher in fiber. After enrichment, the difference in vitamins and minerals may be minimal, although the fiber has been removed. If the whole grain product is much more expensive than the refined enriched product, the latter may be the best source of the nutrients for the price.

Dark breads are not always more nutritious than white or light breads. For example, caramel coloring is sometimes the only ingredient that makes one rye bread darker than another.

Day-old bread and bakery products are often cheaper than fresh ones. They may be just as acceptable after heating as their fresh counterparts.

Fat, Sugar, and Alcohol

These contain calories but few other nutrients. They add taste but little else.

Butter and margarines all have the same amounts of fat and calories. The *source* of fat is all that differs.

Baked goods and candies are usually cheaper if they are homemade or bought in bulk.

Bacteria in food is often destroyed by heat. *Pasteurized milk* is an example of this safe process. Heat can also inactivate the natural enzymes contained in fruits and vegetables. If they are not inactivated, these enzymes will continue to ripen the food until it spoils. (The natural enzymes in fresh fruits and vegetables are also destroyed by the acidity of the stomach.) Many other preservation processes are also used to help prevent foods from turning brown or going rancid before being consumed.

Here are some hints to help a shopper choose safe foods:

1. Check the dates on containers. Never buy food that is outdated.
2. Check cans for bulging ends, leaks, visible rust, or severe dents. These may be signs that the seal has been broken and the food may not be safe.
3. Avoid buying seeds, nuts, and grains from open bins. Open bins provide more opportu-

EXAMPLE OF UNIT PRICING: EGGS

Federal regulations establish that one dozen eggs must weigh:

Type	Weight
Jumbo	30 oz
Extra large	27 oz
Large	24 oz
Medium	21 oz
Small	18 oz

If XYZ Supermarket has eggs on sale, with 1 dozen jumbo at $1.32 and 1 dozen extra large at $1.23, how do you get the most for your money?

Use a calculator:

$1.32 ÷ 30 oz/doz equals 4.4¢ per ounce
$1.23 ÷ 27 oz/doz equals 4.55¢ per ounce

So the jumbo eggs are slightly cheaper by weight.

(From: American Home Economics Association Handbook of Food Preparation, p 33)

nity for exposure to insects and rodents than the same products when packaged.

4. Check dates on fresh meat and fish packages. Do not buy them if they have a strong odor or look old.
5. Avoid deli or buffet foods made with cream sauces or mayonnaise, espcially if they are high protein foods. These foods may be high in bacteria if they are not prepared and stored very carefully, at a low temperature. It is safer to make them at home.
6. If a purchased food smells or looks strange when it is opened at home, return it. NEVER taste it. Canned food that "squirts out" when it is first opened is not safe. The "squirt" is a sign that bacteria in it have been busy producing by-product gases.

KEEP SAFE FOODS SAFE

There are high government standards for institutions that store and serve food. However, the FDA cannot regulate the safety of foods at

SAMPLE FOOD LABEL (HIGH FIBER CEREAL)

The nutrients circled are those that must be listed when a food makes any special health-related claim.

Brand Cereal Name

(Special claim: high fiber; no artificial colors, flavors, or preservatives)

NUTRITION INFORMATION PER SERVING

Serving Size:	½ cup (1 oz.)
Servings per Container:	16

	1 oz.	With ½ Cup Whole Milk
Calories	70	150
Protein	3 g	7 g
Carbohydrate	21 g	27 g
Fat	2 g	6 g
Sodium	190 mg	250 mg

PERCENTAGE OF U.S. RECOMMENDED DAILY ALLOWANCES (U.S. RDA)

Protein	4	10
Vitamin A	*	2
Vitamin C	45	45
Thiamine	45	45
Riboflavin	45	60
Niacin	45	45
Calcium	2	15
Iron	15	15
Vitamin B_6	45	45
Vitamin B_{12}	45	50
Phosphorus	30	45
Magnesium	30	35
Zinc	10	15
Copper	15	15

*Contains less than 2% of the U.S. RDA of these nutrients.

INGREDIENTS: 100% Wheat Bran, Sugar, Malted Barley Flour, Salt, Fig Juice, Prune Juice, Ascorbic Acid (Vitamin C), Niacinamide, Pyridoxine Hydrochloride (Vitamin B_6), Thiamine Mononitrate (Vitamin B_1), Riboflavin (Vitamin B_2), Vitamin B_{12}

CARBOHYDRATE INFORMATION

	1 oz	With ½ Cup Whole Milk
Starch and Related Carbohydrates	6 g	6 g
Sucrose and other Sugars	6 g	12 g
Dietary Fiber	9 g	9 g
TOTAL CARBOHYDRATES	21 g	27 g

Values by formulation and analysis

BRAND
City, State, Zip
Made in USA /year

home. The way to keep foods safe at home or in an institution is by proper storage. Foods must be stored at the right temperatures and handled in the safest ways possible to prevent spoilage.

Safe Temperatures

Figure 19-1 illustrates safe temperatures for the storing of fresh foods. Standard refrigerators store food at 45°F or lower. The coldest part of the refrigerator is at the back (usually beneath the light), since the light is off when the door is shut. Perishable foods that do not need freezing (such as milk, eggs, and meat) should be stored there.

Bacteria can grow at almost any temperature. But the colder the environment, the slower they grow. When food is warmed several times, bacteria multiply quickly. This is why leftovers should be warmed up only once (twice at most), and meats that have been frozen and thawed should never be refrozen. The bacteria are not dead; they are waiting for another chance to warm up and grow!

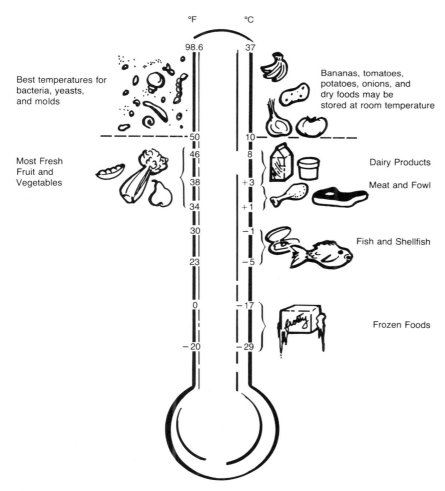

Figure 19-1
Recommended temperatures for safe storage of fresh food. (Adapted from West, Wood, Harger, Shugart: Food Service in Institutions, 5th ed, p 194. New York John Wiley & Sons, 1977)

Foods that spoil very easily (such as fish) should be used within one or two days.

Canned goods, once opened, should be refrigerated.

Safe Handling

The hand and the tongue are two parts of the human body that always carry many bacteria. When they come in contact with food, the food may become contaminated easily. That is why food must always be prepared with hands as clean as possible, in clean containers, with clean utensils. Here are other guidelines for handling foods safely:

- Never "taste test" with a utensil that will go back into the food after the tasting. Taste food with a clean utensil. Use it once, then wash it.
- Never let pets or children sniff, handle, or taste food that will be served to someone else.
- Jewelry and fingernails may also carry bacteria.
- Store foods in containers that will keep out any insects or rodents that may be present.
- Keep dry food dry. Once dry food is exposed to steam or other moisture, it spoils more easily.

Nutritious food that is bought, prepared, and handled appropriately will remain nutritious. Mishandling food can contaminate it and make it a carrier of disease. It is up to those who buy and handle food to make the choices that will keep food safe, attractive, and nutritious.

STUDY QUESTIONS

1. Why should a health care provider know how to buy food and keep it safe?

2. How does prudent shopping begin? List at least four things to consider at this stage.

3. What is "impulse buying?" How can it be prevented?

4. True or false. Explain your answer:
   - Generic brands have better nutritional qualities than national brands.
   - Buying loose onions usually costs more per pound than buying a 5-pound, prepackaged bag of onions.

- Low grade indicates a poorer appearance in a food but not a poorer nutrient content.
- Foods can be refrozen as many times as necessary, as long as the freezer is kept at a very low temperature.
- Some convenience foods may be cheaper than raw ingredients, if labor cost is considered.
- Dark breads are more nutritious than light breads.
- Ingredients are listed on food labels in order of descending volume.
- Open dating means a food is good indefinitely.
- A person must get 100% of the US RDA each day to be adequately nourished.
- Freezing does not kill bacteria.

5. What is unit pricing? Why is it helpful?

6. List and describe at least four items of information that may be found on a food label.

7. What is the purpose of pasteurization?

8. What is the highest safe temperature at which to store perishable food? What happens above this temperature?

9. Where in the refrigerator should milk, eggs, and meats be stored?

10. List at least three principles for choosing safe food and for handling food safely.

SUGGESTED READING

American Home Economics Association: Handbook of Food Preparation. Washington, 2010 Massachusetts Ave NW, Washington DC, 20036

Cooperative Extension Services (available locally throughout each USA county) usually provide valuable consumer information on foods and nutrition

Goldbeck N D: The Supermarket Handbook: Access to Whole Foods. New York, Signet Books/New American Library, 1976

Meal Planning Guide, available from the Office of Consumer Affairs, Grocery Products Division, PET Inc., 400 S. Fourth St., St. Louis, MO 63166

Your Money's Worth in Food, USDA Home and Garden Bulletin No. 183, Feb. 1982 revision. US Government Printing Office, Washington, DC 20402

CHAPTER 20

Food Fads and the Health Food Store

A food fad is a practiced belief that a particular dietary pattern, or the use of a certain nutrient-based substance, will serve as a short cut to certain health or diet goals. Food fads are fads because they are scientifically unfounded. When tested in a tightly controlled setting, the belief does not prove to be true. It may be found false or dangerous, or both.

Two examples of popular food fads include

1. The belief that calcium pangamate ("vitamin B_{15}") prevents heart attacks. In fact, calcium pangamate is not a vitamin. It is a type of drug that cannot be sold legally in the USA. Pills labeled B_{15} may contain almost anything.[1] There has not been the opportunity to prove scientifically and carefully that this substance alone prevents anything.
2. The belief that grapefruit cuts body fat. In fact, grapefruit (and any other food about which the same claim is made) is subject to the same natural laws of digestion as other foods. No food, even in capsule form, can cut or reduce body fat.

It is totally impossible to identify all the food fads. They often make their teachers rich, but rarely make anyone thinner or healthier. Some work, usually because they result in a lower calorie intake, and not for the reasons they claim. Some, however, lead to illness and a few have resulted in death from their toxic action and/or prolonged use. This chapter will outline some principles for identifying food fads and responding to the persons who believe in them. The health food store, which often is a key market for these fads, will also be discussed.

FADS AND CRASH DIETS

Crash diets are fads. The quickest crash diet is the *fast*. To fast is to abstain from all foods and beverages that contain calories, and to drink water only. A "modified fast" is one that includes a small amount of food, and should be closely monitored by a physician. For centuries, Christians, mystics, and other religious groups have practiced fasting for spiritual reasons. Since a true fast includes water only, fasting, especially when it is prolonged or used as a weight loss technique, requires close medical supervision. A prolonged fast can be dangerous. Children, pregnant women, and lactating women, as well as any person on medication, should never fast. Others should check with their physician before beginning any fast.

Other crash diets may not be much safer than fasting, since they are usually some type of prolonged, modified fast. Often a crash diet involves eating only one or two foods or food groups for days or weeks. Crash diets do not solve the real problem. The dieter loses water (which comes back quickly) and a little muscle as well as fat. But long-term eating habits usually do not change.

Overweight is usually a result of long-term excessive eating and inadequate exercise. As a crash diet becomes more and more boring or socially inconvenient, the only alternatives the dieter knows are his old eating habits. They are still a familiar part of the lifestyle, and most crash diets end with a return to these poor eating habits. So when the diet ends, the weight problem goes on. This is rather like a small child who learns to use a life preserver and then believes he does not need to learn to swim. Why put all the effort into swimming lessons when he can depend on the life preserver? Eventually he deceives himself into thinking he really can swim. The crash diet can be the same kind of crutch. A dieter may never learn good eating habits, never learn the value of a balanced diet, because of his dependence on crash diets. And, unlike life preservers, crash diets may not always support life well.

So how can a consumer identify a crash diet and avoid food fads? How can he easily judge the weight loss programs on the market and choose the well-founded ones? Listed on page 163 are some guidelines to help evaluate the programs available and to help clients find a nutritionally balanced program that will fit their lifestyles.

HEALTH FADS

What about the claims that certain nutrients will heal or prevent diseases? What about the self-proclaimed "nutritionists" (who often have no formal education in nutrition or nutritional biochemistry from an accredited institution)? What about salespersons who criticize doctors for dispensing medicine, then claim the same health benefits from their own (vitamin or mineral) pills? These persons often believe what they say and practice what they preach. How is the consumer to know what to believe? The critical aspects involved in understanding and responding to these ads are discussed below.

Sales Techniques

The people who push these substances have certain characteristics in common in the way they propagate them. They usually

1. Appeal to a person's fears about health and the food supply
2. Appeal to a person's hopes for health and a long life
3. Sell pills, liquids, or powders, not food
4. Claim that "natural" is better than man-made. They may hint that man-made substances are harmful
5. Believe that diet alone causes and/or cures disease
6. Quote many personal testimonies. Usually the scientific studies they mention have never been published in standard medical journals, or are serious misinterpretations of articles that have been published
7. Criticize conventional nutrition and medicine
8. Have little or no formal education in nutrition from a reputable institution

Health Fad Dangers

There are many dangers inherent in health fads. The dangers of a vitamin or mineral overdose have been discussed in Chapters 6–8. Given the way the body functions (outlined in Chapters 1 through 10), it is often physically impossible for

FINDING THE RIGHT WEIGHT LOSS PROGRAM: QUESTIONS TO ASK

- How SAFE is the program?
Is an M.D.'s approval required? Long-term weight loss can lead to many body changes, and a physician will best know what this means for the individual. Safe programs will require a physician's approval.
- How much EXERCISE is involved?
Again, the physician should be consulted to see if the exercise program is right for the individual.
- How FAST should I lose weight?
No more than 1 or 2 pounds a week. The first large weight loss is water. These pounds usually come off in the first week or two. After that, more than 2 pounds per week means needed water and muscle are also being lost. Regular, strenuous exercise may help the person lose more quickly. Slow, steady weight loss helps the person learn new eating habits.
- Is the diet WELL BALANCED or too strict?
A diet which omits one (or more) of the four food groups is too strict, and may be harmful. Diets below 1200 calories per day for women and 1800 calories per day for men need close medical supervision. A well-balanced diet includes foods from all four groups in a pattern that can be lived with for a lifetime.
- Does the diet use LIQUID FORMULAS?
Diets made up primarily of certain liquid formulas have led to serious health problems for many and even death for some. Their safety depends on how they are used. If the person's doctor approves, these substances should be used only in combination with the usual, daily food intake (unless the person is hospitalized for weight loss).
- Are DRUGS used?
Drugs that suppress the appetite do not help long-term weight control. They also may have many undesirable side-effects.
- Does the diet make SENSATIONAL CLAIMS?
There is no magic cure or short cut for overweight which allows a person to forget will power and "eat all he wants." Statements that claim this are misleading.
- What does the program COST?
Is it worth it? Can the person afford it? Are there hidden costs (such as books, supplements, drugs, etc.)?
- Is it a plan the individual CAN LIVE WITH for six months (or more)?
It should fit into his lifestyle as well as his feelings and beliefs about weight control. For example, if a person feels strongly about private, individual counseling, he may not want to join a weight control group, and vice versa. The actual weight control plan should fit his personality, his schedule and his budget.

(Adapted from Questions for Judging Weight Loss Programs © 1981 by Massachusetts Nutrition Resource Center, Boston, MA)

these health fad products to do what is claimed for them. However, they often act in other ways that may result in unpleasant or harmful side-effects.

Diet plays a very small role in the cause and cure of most diseases. Persons who believe food or a vitamin will cure them may stop seeing their doctor and stop taking necessary medicine. This deliberate neglect (which has happened, for example, among cancer patients taking laetrile) often makes the illness much worse, or fatal.[2] A person may die from something that could have been prevented if early medical care had been sought and provided.

Many products "naturally" contain trace minerals that can be dangerous. Lead has been found in bone meal tablets and arsenic has been found in kelp.[3] Peach and apricot kernels naturally contain the deadly poison, cyanide.[3] "Natural" substances are not always safe. It is ironic that many persons who are afraid of chemicals they believe have been added to their foods will freely accept chemically formulated and laboratory produced tablets, liquids, and powders simply because it is claimed they are made with *natural* ingredients. The human body cannot distinguish between chemicals naturally present in food and identical chemicals produced in a laboratory.

Another problem with these products is their cost. They are expensive. The people who are most likely to buy them may be elderly or ill, and have only a small income. The same nutrients can be found in fresh food from the grocery store. Moreover, they will be cheaper, and taste better!

Responding to Claims

Health fads may always be with us. But while they are and while persons are being deceived and sometimes harmed, there are ways to respond. The first step is to become informed.

It is perfectly legal for a proponent to claim anything about his product — as long as he does not print this claim on the product itself. It is perfectly legal to write an article for publication that praises a product as a cancer cure. It is legal to take three pages of advertising for that product in the same journal in which the article appears. It is *not* legal to make the cancer claim in the ad.

So question the proponents about these claims. What kind of *formal* nutrition education do they have? What degrees do they hold, and from where? Reputable nutrition degrees include Registered Dietitian (R.D.), Bachelor of Science (B.S.), Master of Science (M.S.), or Doctor of Philosophy (Ph.D.) *in nutrition* from an accredited university. Some doctors of medicine (M.D.) have specialized in nutrition. Persons with these degrees will be the most reliable resources for reputable, well-founded nutrition information. Find out what organizations the proponents of health fads have joined. Ask what they think of conventional medicine and dietetics. Scorn may indicate a lack of knowledge.

Find out what the critics say about these health fad claims. Check with persons who *do* have the qualifying degrees (listed above).

Health fad beliefs are often emotional issues. It is sometimes hard to persuade someone that what he has been led to believe is not true. The beliefs may be harmless, but if they are not, and if someone is spending money on a product that has no proved benefit, or that may be dangerous, he has the right to know. He has the right to obtain correct information. It is the health care provider's responsibility to have this information readily available, or to make appropriate referrals.

The Health Food Store

A "health food store" is a broad term describing any store that claims to sell nutritionally "superior" products or products that are more "healthful" for various reasons. Salespersons in these stores and product advertising make similar claims: The products have no artificial additives. They were not treated with chemical pesticides. They may come in brown bottles to keep out the light, and often have not been heat-treated. They are promoted as products containing nutrients that can change a person's quality of life. They are supposed to cure diseases and, supposedly, they have amazed many doctors with their effects.

A health food store does not necessarily sell *health food.* Sometimes there is little *food* actually sold. Many of these stores specialize in pills, powders, capsules, and liquids. Salespersons may say that most persons do not eat properly, so their products, when taken in addition to meals, help "balance out" the body and make up for poor eating habits. They may rarely talk about foods without including a reference to pills or nonfood products. It seems ironic that many health food stores do not seem interested, above all else, in teaching people to eat nutritionally adequate foods.

These stores usually have a section in which books and magazines are sold that teach and promote current health fads. Authors often have degrees and training that sound credible, but that may not stand up under careful inspection. Many authors are "directors" or "doctors" of their own "nutrition institutes." Store shelves may also be filled with beauty aids made from "natural" products.

The claims promoted in these stores often deceive concerned consumers. Many persons try to learn about good nutrition through these stores. These are the clients who may later ask the conventional health care provider what he thinks about certain beliefs or practices.

But the health food store should not simply be dismissed as useless, and then avoided. To the thoughtful critic, these stores can become good resources. The health care professionals can use these stores to prepare for clients and their questions. Here is where the fads are taught openly. The health food store is *not* a place to learn about good nutrition. It is the place to critically evaluate health claims in the light of what is known to be good nutrition. It is a place to meet faddists on their own ground and evaluate critically the current health fad literature.

Compare the contents of vitamins being sold with the Recommended Dietary Allowances. Ask questions. Review the chapters on vitamins and minerals, and compare this information with what is available at the health food store. Many stores *do* sell foods, and make special claims about them. Learn to respond to these claims. Some such claims, and suggested responses, are discussed on pages 166–167.

Nor are all health food stores useful only as enemy territory for nutrition "spies." Many sell large quantities of food and a few sell more food

than pills and powders. Used selectively, these stores may be helpful supplements to supermarket shopping. For example, odd and foreign foods may only be available in the "natural foods" store. Some stores have regular sales of their food products to attract new customers. Vegetarian staples such as honey, nuts, seeds, rice cakes, and whole grains may be cheaper because they are available in bulk (although prices may be even lower through a food coop). Sometimes spices are cheaper. Persons who want to avoid government-approved additives can usually find foods they want.

But there are drawbacks to using these stores. Foods here are NOT more nutritious than foods found in the supermarket, and identical foods are usually more expensive. Fresh produce may be quite ripe and spoil quickly, or the item may be small, uneven, or not as colorful or attractive as in a grocery store. Usually the foods will be described as "chemical free," but this is not always true. Even when a farmer has not added chemicals, residues in soil or wind may result in the same levels of a chemical in the food.[4]

One problem in using a health food store is knowing what to believe. Fad proponents — and misinformed people — claim many things about foods that simply are not true. Popular advertising hints that certain products will make us more attractive, outstanding, or beautiful. Usually we realize these brand-specific claims are not true. But health food advertising is harder to disbelieve. Such advertising frequently implies that the most "natural" form of a food is the most healthful. Processing and additives are not "natural," therefore, they are "bad." Because we have heard so much in the media about potentially harmful additives, it is easy to believe what the health food stores want us to believe.

However, persons who make these claims often have little or no objective, scientifically tested evidence to support the claims, although they are often adamant about their "truth." Each claim, however, can be countered with known facts.

While incorrect, many of these beliefs are harmless. The major problem with food practices as taught in the health food store (if they are relatively harmless) may be the price. Foods

SAMPLE HEALTH FOOD BELIEFS, WITH RESPONSES

Belief	Facts
Honey is more nutritious than white sugar.	• Honey has more energy (64 calories per tablespoon) than white sugar (46 calories per tablespoon). • Like white sugar, honey is a combination of fructose and glucose. • Honey may be more cariogenic than sugar because it can cling to the teeth longer. • The minerals in honey are present in such small amounts that they are not nutritionally significant.
Brown rice is better than white rice.	• Brown rice has more fiber and minerals than white rice. • Enriched white rice has more iron and fewer calories than the same amount of brown rice. • Brown rice contains more trace minerals than white rice.
White flour is harmful to the health.	• White flour has less fiber and trace minerals than whole grain flours, but it is usually "enriched" with certain key nutrients. • There is nothing intrinsic in white flour that makes it dangerous for the average North American to consume.
Raw milk is better than pasteurized milk.	• "Raw" milk is milk that has not been heat treated (pasteurized) to kill bacteria. Even if it comes from cows that are regularly examined by the State Board of Health, the possibility of disease-carrying bacteria is higher than in pasteurized milk. • It is possible that the proteins in raw milk are slightly more digestible than those in heat-treated milk, but this has never been proved.
Canned vegetables are not nutritious.	• These vegetables were exposed to high temperatures during the canning process. The vitamins in them sensitive to heat may have been destroyed. But not all vitamins are heat-sensitive (see Chapters 6 and 7). • Canned vegetables usually contain less fiber than fresh vegetables.
"Natural" vitamins are better than chemically synthesized vitamins.	• The body cannot tell the difference. The vitamins in both have identical structures when seen under a microscope. This structure determines how the body uses the vitamin. Tests have shown no difference. • "Natural" vitamins are often much larger than commercial brands, harder to swallow, and more expensive.
Preservatives are harmful and unnatural.	• Preservatives make it possible to have fresh foods out of season. This prevents the deficiency diseases discussed in Chapters 6–8. • Preservatives are often substances that occur naturally, such as citric or acetic acid, salt, sugar, and antioxidants.

Additives like nitrites, BHA, BHT (used to preserve food) cause cancer.	• Preserved foods travel without spoiling, so a balanced diet is possible in all climates of the country, year 'round.
	• Preservatives in use have been tested by the government and declared safe.
	• Certain pesticides have been found to cause cancer. They are usually tightly controlled and not meant to be consumed.
	• Nitrites, which prevent botulism (a fatal food poisoning) in cured meats, can cause cancer in laboratory animals.
	• There is no indication that BHA causes cancer.
	• BHT is still controversial. The Food and Drug Administration says it may cause liver cancer in rats, but the National Cancer Institute says no.[5]
	• Many naturally occurring substances are more potent carcinogens than these additives.
"Organic" food is better than food not grown organically.	• *"Organic" foods* are those grown in soil which has had only "natural" fertilizers added. There is no nutritional advantage to them. They may have just as much pesticide residue on them as foods grown with chemical fertilizers and pesticides.[4] This is because pesticides and chemicals stay in the soil for decades. They also travel in the wind and may settle on these fields.
Poor ("depleted") soil produces foods lower in nutrients than well-fertilized soil.	• This is not true. The major nutrients in foods come from the seeds and sun, not the soil.
	• Soil may produce a smaller harvest (quantity) if it is depleted (just as a poorly nourished woman may produce a smaller infant). Major nutrients (quality) are not affected by the condition of the soil.
	• Trace mineral content may be affected by the soil, however. Soils rich in iodine or selenium will produce vegetables that contain these nutrients.
	• The mineral content usually depends on geography, not on fertilizers. Long-term studies have not been able to prove that "organic" foods are more nutritious (or safer) than foods grown in soil using chemical fertilizers.

grown in small gardens are more expensive, since these farmers need a higher profit to make ends meet. These foods have the same nutritional benefits as their supermarket counterparts. Persons who buy from the health food store more frequently than from the supermarket are spending more money than necessary for good nutrition. They certainly have the right, but they should know that the grocery store provides foods that are equally nutritious, and often equally additive- and chemical-free. When money is tight (as with the elderly, with the poor, and with many students), the health food store may cost more than it is worth.

STUDY QUESTIONS

1. What is a food fad? Give one example.

2. Can you think of a food fad current in your

area that was not discussed in this chapter? How would you respond to a client who held this belief?

3. What is a crash diet? Describe the pros and cons of crash diets.

4. Choose a weight loss program available in your area. Find out about it. Evaluate it according to the criteria listed in this chapter. How nutritionally sound does it seem?

5. List five characteristics of a typical health fad proponent.

6. What is wrong with a health fad?

7. Give one example of a "natural" product that may not be "safe."

8. An ad in a health food magazine claims that vitamin XY can cure leukemia, if it is taken in large enough doses. Two articles in the same magazine tell the stories of people who believe the vitamin cured their leukemia. The daily dosage recommended was 100 times the RDA. Can you trust this claim? Why or why not? Would you tell a leukemic patient about these articles? Why or why not?

9. What does a health food store sell?

10. Where do salespersons in health food stores often receive their nutrition training?

11. How may a health professional best use these health food stores?

12. Are there disadvantages to using these stores? If so, what are they?

13. List five common beliefs "health faddists" may have about food. How could a health professional respond to each belief?

14. Why are foods in a health food store more expensive than foods in a grocery store or food coop? Does this extra expense mean foods are more nutritious? Why or why not?

15. Have you ever been in a health food store? If so
    - What did you buy?
    - Why did you buy it?
    - What special properties or benefits, if any, did you believe this product had that made it better than others from a grocery store?

- Based on what you have learned, was it worth its cost? Why or why not?

REFERENCES

1. Herbert V: Vitamin B$_{15}$: Anatomy of a health fraud. Report from American Council on Science and Health, 1981
2. Young VR, Richardson DP: Nutrients, vitamins and minerals in cancer prevention: Facts and fallacies. Cancer 43:2125–2136, 1979
3. Stephenson M: The confusing world of health foods. FDA Consumer, July–August 1978
4. Gourdine SP, Traiger WW, Cohen DS: Health food stores investigation. J Am Diet Assoc 83(3):285–290, September 1983
5. Lehmann, P: More than you ever thought you would know about food additives, Parts I, II, III. FDA Consumer, No. (FDA) 79–2115, 2118–2119, April–June 1979

SUGGESTED RESOURCES

Books

Brody J: Jane Brody's Good Food Book. New York, WW Norton, 1985

Deutsch R: The New Nuts among the Berries: How Nutrition Nonsense Captured America. Palo Alto, CA, Bull Publishing, 1977

Herbert V: Nutrition Cultism. Philadelphia, George F Stickley, 1981

Whelan EM, Stare FJ: The One Hundred Percent Natural, Purely Organic, Cholesterol-free, Megavitamin, Low Carbohydrate Nutrition Hoax. New York, Atheneum, 1983

Consumer Organizations

(With newsletters responding to food claims and controversies)

American Council on Science and Health (ACSH), 1995 Broadway, New York, NY 10023

Center for Science in the Public Interest (CSPI), 1755 S St., NW, Washington, DC 20009

Environmental Nutrition Newsletter, 52 Riverside Dr., Suite 15A, New York, NY 10024

National Council Against Health Fraud Inc., Box 1276, Loma Linda, CA 92354

SECTION 2

Therapeutic Nutrition

UNIT 3

Nutrient-Controlled Diets

CHAPTER 21

Diet Therapy in a Health Care Facility

OBJECTIVES

1. To introduce therapeutic nutrition

2. To introduce the concept of controlled nutrients in a health care facility

3. To outline sample situations where nutrient control is indicated and to provide a basis for effectively applying therapeutic nutrition

4. To define and describe the staffing and roles of the key members of the health care team

5. To describe the essential interactions among team members in the nutrition support of a hospitalized client

6. To discuss institutional diet therapy in terms of
   a. The diet order
   b. The medical record
   c. Food preparation and delivery
   d. Effective communication among team members

7. To define several common diet orders

8. To enable the reader to locate nutrition resources "on the job"

9. To provide specific guidelines for providing nutrition counseling when a dietitian is not available

The previous chapters have outlined the basic essentials of nutrition. They have discussed why good nutrition is important for health, how the body is designed to use nutrients, and how to apply this information to the life of a healthy consumer or client. Yet this is only half of the science of nutrition. The other half, nutrition in disease (also called *therapeutic nutrition* or *diet therapy*), will be the focus of the remaining chapters.

Therapeutic nutrition or diet therapy involves applying dietary change as a result of illness and/or to encourage independence or improve a handicapped individual's quality of life. Nutrition is rarely the primary treatment. Food is not used as medicine, but is a very important part of medical care. The diet may be changed to help make a certain treatment as effective as possible. Normal nutrition becomes therapeutic nutrition when something goes wrong. The body may become less able to receive, make, use, break down, control, or excrete some nutrient or nutrients. The problem may be caused by disease, allergy, psychosocial questions, a physical handicap, or a combination of factors. It may be caused by a side-effect of necessary medical treatment (for example some cancer therapies cause nausea and vomiting).

A therapeutic diet is one that controls certain nutrients. Some therapies only involve control of one or two nutrients; other therapies require a rearrangement of many factors. Chapters 22 through 28 are organized by nutrients, not diseases, and discuss examples of the first type of therapy. These chapters include examples and guidelines to help a client control a specific nutrient. When a client is placed on a certain diet, it may be of more *immediate* importance to learn exactly what this means, in terms of menu planning, than to fully understand the disease. Once his health stabilizes, then there is time to understand the disease in more detail. Chapters 29 through 41 will discuss examples of the second, more multifactorial type of diet therapy.

APPLYING DIET THERAPY

Therapeutic nutrition usually begins when a client receives some type of medical care. He may not change his normal eating habits (his diet) unless the physician says that change is necessary. Frequently, the first persons to help a client adjust to a new diet are the persons in a health care facility, such as a hospital, health center, residential school for handicapped individuals, or a nursing home. So a consideration of diet therapy must begin with a consideration of the systems for medical and nutrition support. Since the hospital is the most common facility, this chapter will use it as a model. The procedures in other facilities are usually quite similar.

Supportive, optimal nutrition for a hospital client requires good communication between the people responsible for health care. These people make up the *health-care team.* Listed on page 176 are many of the members of a team, their qualifications, and their roles in nutrition support.

The key member of the team is the client or patient himself.*

The physician is the head of the team, the person who diagnoses the client's problem and recommends supportive treatment. The physician orders support care, including the most appropriate diet for the client, often working together with a clinical dietitian to develop the diet. Treatment is adjusted as the client's condition changes.

The clinical dietitian follows the client's progress and works with the rest of the team whenever changes occur. The dietitian is the most important contact person between the client and the kitchen. The dietitian must ap-

prove the client's special requests and make sure they are processed so that the right food arrives in the right room at the right time. Usually a woman, the dietitian works with the client to help him *understand* the diet. She helps the client learn to make changes at home and often works together with the family in the hospital and in community health clinics since a new diet may also affect shopping and meal patterns.

The nurse is another key member of the team. She sees the client more often than either the physician or the dietitian because she is responsible for daily basic care. She may be the first to learn of special problems or concerns the client has about the diet or about medical care. She is responsible for carrying out the doctor's orders for medication, treatments, and feeding. If she communicates well to the other nurses responsible for the client's care and to the rest of the team, the client is most likely to enjoy the best possible care. If she or any other member of the team does not communicate effectively, care may become fragmented and inefficient.

Communication among team members occurs in several ways:

1. Written information in the client's medical record. The latter is a legal document all team members use to help coordinate care by informing each other of their support of the client and of relevant concerns. Good care depends on an up-to-date knowledge of the client and his medical record. The record is also a file of laboratory and test results, surgical procedures, and other essential information. This information is used to plan and evaluate care.

2. Formal meetings of the team

3. Communications, often on tape, used by nursing staff between shifts, where one nurse informs the others of the progress of the clients in her care

4. Informal conversations

All of these communications should include any relevant information about the client's eating habits.

The Diet Order

When the client first arrives, the physician examines him, and a *diet order* is issued. This de-

---

* He should understand his care as much as possible and always have the opportunity to voice opinion, ask questions and request change.

MEMBERS OF THE HEALTH CARE TEAM

Patient or Client — Should be as actively involved in his care and treatment as possible. Not a passive recipient. Should always be informed and feel free to question decisions about his care.

Physician (M.D., with specialty) — Primary responsibility for diagnosis and treatment of medical problem. Orders and oversees all care

Prescribes all medications

Issues order for type of diet therapy required during client's stay in health care facility, often in consultation with clinical dietitian

Orders all laboratory tests

Makes appropriate community referrals for follow-up care

Clinical Dietitian (R.D. = Registered Dietitian)
Has Bachelor's degree in Nutrition, an approved 1–2-year dietetic internship. Has passed registration exam, may have graduate degree — Consults with physician to develop appropriate diet therapy for client

Usually attends patient rounds or meetings with physician to follow medical care and provide input as indicated

Primary responsibility for nutrition education of client

May supervise diet aids and assistants who collect menus and bring food to clients

Makes sure client receives food appropriate to diet order

Registered Nurse (R.N.)
Has completed an approved undergraduate nursing program and passed registration exam. May also have a graduate degree or additional qualifications as a nurse practitioner — Primary responsibility for maintaining appropriate care.

Carries out physician's orders regarding daily care

May keep record of what client will/will not eat or drink

Informs dietitian of problems or concerns with diet or appetite

Licensed Practical Nurse (L.P.N.)
Completed 1–2 year L.P.N. program — Works under supervision of a registered nurse to provide appropriate care

Helps feed client, when necessary, and helps maintain intake/output records

Diet Technician (D.T.) Completed 2-year D.T. program	Works under supervision of a clinical dietitian to provide appropriate nutrition care May teach diet therapy May screen medical records for clients at high nutritional risk
Licensed Social Worker Has Bachelor's Degree and often Master's degree in social work	Works with client to help resolve difficult social, financial, or emotional aspects of disease or problems Makes appropriate referrals to community support agencies before client is discharged; arranges follow-up
Psychiatrist (M.D. specializing in psychiatry) or Psychologist (advanced psychology degree but not an M.D.)	Works with client to help resolve difficult emotional and psychological problems that may or may not relate to disease and/or nutrition
Physical Therapist Has Bachelor's degree in P.T.	Helps client learn to compensate physically for disease or disability. This may include teaching new eating behaviors
Occupational Therapist Has Bachelor's degree in O.T.	Helps client learn specific ways to live with disabilities and remain productive*
Chaplain Has Bachelor's degree plus seminary degree plus chaplaincy training	Provides spiritual support to client as indicated. No direct role in nutrition care

*May teach use of special devices to aid feeding for handicapped, stroke patients and others with permanent or temporary disabilities.

scribes the type of diet the physician feels the client needs. The order is then written on the "Kardexes" (large, flat card files) of the nursing staff and dietary staff. When the diet order changes, the file cards are changed accordingly. The dietitian uses the order to evaluate all the client's menus. She may explain any restrictions or needs to the client and correct choices that are not appropriate for the special diet. The diet order may include

1. An order that certain nutrients be controlled. For example a strict salt restriction may read "1 gram sodium." A mild restriction may say "no added salt." The order lists the nutrient and describes the limit.

2. Method of feeding, especially if a client is unable to eat. This would be necessary if the client were receiving nutrients by a tube into his digestive (alimentary) tract or into a blood vessel.

3. Times and/or frequency of feeding, if the client needs nutrients at specific intervals or not at standard hospital meal times. Tube feedings are often given at specific intervals. A client who can eat may need snacks between meals.

4. Special products to be used, either as supplements or total intake.

A diet order will *not*

1. List all foods the client may or may not eat

2. Describe in detail how to feed the client

3. List hours when the client must eat; it will list frequency, for example "q. 2 hours" ("q" meaning "every").

4. Describe how to prepare special products

The nursing staff and the dietitian must work together to apply the diet order to daily meals and feeding schedules in a practical way. Shown on this page are some common diet orders and what they mean.

After the diet is established, the client receives meals and instructions specific to his order. The menus are given to the client, filled out, corrected, and then sent to the kitchen where the food is prepared. If the diet order changes after the menu goes to the kitchen, the dietitian must be informed immediately so she can contact the kitchen and make the necessary changes for the meal or snack.

Each institution will have slightly different methods for applying diet therapy, but the principles and roles of the members of the medical team remain the same. They should all work together to help the client achieve and keep the best possible level of health. To do this they must communicate well with each other, with the client, with his family, and with any health providers who will care for the client after he leaves the hospital. The best medical and nutrition care may begin in a health care facility, but it should not end at discharge. Therapy will be most effective if the client *understands* why certain changes in his diet are necessary and *knows specifically* how to apply them at home. It is up to the health care team to teach him and his family how to make these changes, and how to make arrangements for follow-up care in the facility or in the community.

COMMON DIET ORDERS

Order	Meaning
NPO	"Nil per os," which means *nothing by mouth.* Client receives no nutrients by mouth; this may or may not include plain water
Clear liquid	All liquids transparent at body temperature are permitted, but no other foods or beverages. Unless a client is receiving hyperalimentation and a special nutrient-rich liquid, this diet may provide sugar as the only source of calories
Full liquid	Only liquids or foods that become liquid at body temperature. Often includes milk products as main source of energy. Clear liquids are also permitted
Soft diet	Foods that require little chewing and are well absorbed in the digestive tract. "Mechanical" soft diet includes all foods the client can chew. This diet may be low in fiber
" (x) "-free diet	Diet which includes no " (x) ". Dietitian applies order and helps nursing staff with list of food to avoid

TEST DIETS

One area in which nutrition may be part of hospitalization is that of the preoperative diet and the test diet.

Preoperative diets may include any sort of diet the physician feels will aid in surgery. Refeeding, discussed in Chapter 39, may be one of these diets. Sometimes overweight persons are told to lose weight or are placed on medication and a strict diet to lower blood pressure before surgery in an attempt to minimize risks. The most common presurgery diet prescription, however, is "NPO," also discussed in Chapter 39.

Test diets, however, may not involve surgery or stress. They usually involve controlling or altering some nutrient to test tolerance or to prepare a patient for a medical procedure. There are many different types and reasons for test diets. Whenever a test diet is ordered, the dietitian can help teach the diet to the client and act as a resource to the nursing staff to help translate the diet into practical terms for meals and snacks. Two common test diets are used to test for fat malabsorption and glucose tolerance.

Fat Malabsorption

Fat malabsorption is sometimes tested by a 3-day 100-gram fat diet. The client is given a list of food exchanges, each of which equals 10 grams of fat. He must choose 10 of these each day for three days. The 100 grams of fat can be added to fat-free foods in any desired combination. The stool is collected according to the physician's instructions. The amount of fat found in the stool is then compared to the 100 grams of fat known to be in the diet. If the test proves the client is malabsorbing fat, nutrition and medical care can be altered accordingly. Table 21-1 lists 10-gram fat food portions as well as common fat-free foods.

Glucose Tolerance

Chronic hypo- or hyperglycemia is sometimes tested by a glucose tolerance test, described in Chapter 24. Often a person is instructed to follow a 150-gram carbohydrate diet each day for 3 days before taking this test. This helps to prevent abnormal results, since a very low carbohydrate diet prior to the test can result in an abnormal response curve. The diet may exceed, but it should not be less than, 150 grams of carbohydrate during these three pretest days. Clients may wish to talk with, or be referred to, a dietitian to prepare for this test.

WHEN THERE IS NO DIETITIAN

In many institutions a dietitian is not available full time. She may work as a consultant or, for some other reason, not always be present or available. In some community programs, such as a visiting nurse program or hospice program, federal funds may readily cover nursing care but not allow more than a brief consultation with the dietitian. In many nursing homes, the dietitian is a consultant, available only several days each month. When she is present, she often must spend most of her time planning and adjusting menus and doing the most critical diet teaching.

In some rural or third world health programs, a nurse may be the only trained medical person in 200 miles. This leaves the community worker, nurse, or other members of the staff with the responsibility of

Finding answers to their own and other staff members' nutrition questions, and

Assuming the role of nutrition educator and providing nutrition counseling.

A staff person thrust into these roles—which are not usually a part of her training—must be prepared and know where to go for resources.

Where To Go with Questions?

Every nurse or community worker should have "on-the-job" nutrition resources readily available. Textbooks such as this one—and others that go into much more clinical detail—can help answer quick questions. Many hospitals publish their own "Diet Manual," which has specific instructions concerning how to follow

Table 21-1

10-Gram Fat Exchanges, with Fat-Free Food List

Each of the Portions Below Provides 10 Grams of Fat	*Foods Containing Little or No Fat*
DAIRY:	Coffee
10 oz Whole milk or whole milk yogurt	Tea, regular and herbal
5 oz Evaporated milk (before dilution)	Macaroni, spaghetti
3 oz Sweetened condensed milk	French or Vienna bread
½ cup Ice cream (12% fat)	Rice
1¼ oz American, Swiss, or Cheddar cheese	Fruit juices
1 oz Cream cheese	All fruit except coconut and avocado
MEAT:	All vegetables
2 Medium eggs	Hot cereals
1¼ oz Bologna	Most cold cereals (check label)
3 oz Corned beef hash	All legumes (dry beans and peas)
3 oz Lean ground beef	Air-popped popcorn
4 oz Red salmon	Baked potatoes
3 oz Sardines (in oil, drained)	
OILS:	
2 tsp Vegetable oil or lard	
1 scant tbsp Butter, margarine, mayonnaise	
5 tsp Heavy or whipping cream	
¾ oz Cashews	
2½ strips of Bacon	
2 oz Avocado	
2 tbsp Peanuts	
4 tsp Peanut butter	
BREAD:	
10 Ritz-type crackers	
3½ oz Corn muffin	
MISCELLANEOUS	
1 oz Dry coconut	
1 oz Milk chocolate with almonds	
12 medium Potato chips	

and apply a particular diet order in that institution. Institutions that do not have their own manual may routinely use one published by another institution; these are clear and easy to use. These manuals are usually available from the dietitian and the nursing staff may keep them as well. The Physician's Desk Reference (PDR) is a large manual published yearly with detail on every available drug. It often lists potential drug–food interactions. Nutrition information published by the local heart, diabetes, dietetic, or cancer societies — or the Department of Public Health — may help answer general nutrition questions. Some communities have other reputable nutrition resources available by telephone.

The best source of all, however, is the dietitian. She is trained to be an educator, clinician, and administrator and she should be the key nutrition resource for staff as well as patients (see Figure 21-1). She alone can tailor nutrition information to the individual or the institution.

Other nutrition personnel who may also be available include diet technicians and sometimes dietetic interns, both also educated in nu-

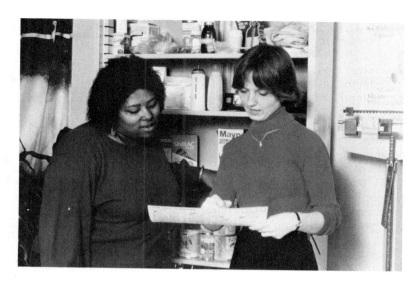

Figure 21-1
Nutrition counseling is a sensitive combination of listening, assessing, and teaching. As part of the health care team in most institutions as well as in the community, the dietitian is primarily responsible for nutrition counseling in both normal and therapeutic nutrition. (Photo courtesy Massachusetts Department of Public Health. Used with permission)

trition who work under the dietitian's direct supervision.

NUTRITION COUNSELING

Counseling is a fine art. It is not just teaching and it is not simply listening, but rather is a sensitive combination of both. Effective counseling takes months and even years of practice and constant critical improvement.

Nutrition counseling involves three basic skills: assessing, interpreting, and teaching. To be effective and relevant to the client, all three *absolutely* require careful and sensitive listening.

1. *Assessment:* This involves asking unbiased, pointed questions about current nutrition-related practices; generally these should be questions that *cannot* be answered by "yes" or "no." Sample questions that may be part of a nutrition assessment are listed on page 182. These questions might begin with the words, *what, when, where, who,* or *tell me about,* and might involve
   a. Asking the client to explain the recommended diet change. This helps the counselor evaluate the client's understanding or concern, and also helps the counselor

to know where to begin the counseling process.
   b. Asking about specific food preferences and normal eating habits. It is usually helpful to get a "24–hour recall," a detailed history of everything the client ate or drank over the past (or on a typical) 24–hour period. Questions to help with this are on page 183.
   c. Asking about food preparation, the situation at home, and problems relating to the buying of food or that may occur at mealtimes
   d. Talking with family members to obtain a complete understanding of the situation
   e. Learning the client's occupation or general lifestyle and priorities, which usually affect eating habits.

As these questions are answered, the counselor should never say, "good," nor express any kind of disapproval. Value judgments—even when they are very subtle—may cause the client to tell the counselor only what he thinks the counselor will approve.

2. *Diagnosing* (or *Interpreting*): Listen to the client; remember (or jot down) what he says, and especially note potential problem areas in nutrition that will need to be discussed.

NUTRITION ASSESSMENT: SAMPLE QUESTIONS

Why are you here? How can I help you with your diet?

What did the doctor tell you about diet and   (insert nutrition concern or medical problem)   ?

What does your family think about   (diet or nutrition problem)   ?

Are you happy with your weight? Why/Why not? What do you think you should weigh?

How is your appetite?

What medications do you take?

What kind of work do you do? When do you eat?

How many people are in your house? Who does the cooking?

Where do you eat? How is the food prepared? (This is a good point at which to obtain a 24–hour diet recall; see opposite page)

How often do you eat/drink_____? (This is a key question. The counselor may—if there is time—ask this about many different foods, by food group and including "junk" food and beverages. This information helps assess likes and dislikes and can later be used to plan meals)

Do you have a refrigerator? Do you have any problems keeping food in the house?

Do you take any vitamins? What kinds? How much?

Do you smoke cigarettes? How much?

How often do you drink alcohol (including beer or wine)? When? What? How much?

Do you get any exercise? What kind? How often? For how long?

What kind of exercise do you like? How can you do more of it?

Without effective, open listening, it is impossible to interpret the information from the assessment, and counseling and teaching will be irrelevant. Never assume; rather, clarify points by asking more questions. They may be open questions (those described above that can't be answered by *yes* or *no*) or closed, directed questions (which *must* be answered by *yes* or *no*). Assess motivation. Who wants change: the physician, the family, or the client? Why? What are the social barriers and how can they be overcome? What foods will be most acceptable to this individual? Will they be helped most by a general informal discussion with guidelines or do they need very specific instructions? As the counselor listens, she will be able to assess what is best for the client.

3. *Prescribe, Teach and Discuss:* The last and most important part of counseling (since it is the reason for assessment and interpretation) involves teaching, discussing, and reaching an agreement about what the client will do now. In this phase the counselor should

   a. Sum up the most relevant points of the assessment. This is the time to praise any part of the diet that is praiseworthy.

   b. Outline diet recommendations: What needs to be changed?

   c. Explain why these changes are important and why they are recommended for this individual

   d. Discuss the recommendations and translate them into a diet, menu, set of guidelines, or a specific list of foods and behav-

OBTAINING AN ACCURATE 24-HOUR DIET RECALL: SAMPLE QUESTIONS

Introduction: I want to get an idea of what you ate yesterday (or on a typical, average day, if the day before was completely unusual). Start in the morning and go through the day, telling me everything you had to eat and drink.

When did you get up?
What was the first thing you ate or drank? When was that?
How much did you eat? Show me. (Use food models, if possible, or empty bowls, cups, measuring spoons, or plates to assess quantity)
What else did you eat with that?
What was on it?/How was it cooked/prepared?
Did you have anything to drink? What? How much? What brand?
When was the next time you had anything? (NEVER assume someone eats three meals a day, or meals at all, or at regular times.) What did you have? How much?
(Repeat questions from * above for each meal or snack reported. Think of other questions if the information you get is not specific enough to evaluate.)
Did you have anything in between those times?
Do you ever nibble or "pick" at food when you're shopping/cooking/traveling/nervous/angry?
Do you ever get up at night to eat or drink? When? Why? How many times? What do you eat?
Do you eat differently on the weekends? Tell me what is different?

---

iors. Involve the client and/or family or caretaker as much as he is willing to be involved.

e. Place final responsibility on the client and/or primary caretaker. Let them talk. Exactly what will they now do? How often will they do it? What problems do they expect? Why? Will they keep records or measure their progress in some way? Negotiate if necessary. Never judge. A nutrition counselor is an educated advisor; the client has the ultimate right to make or refuse change in his eating behavior. The only changes that will last are the changes in which *he* believes.

The chapters that follow will include guidelines to help a client apply to his lifestyle the nutrition changes and diet necessary for proper medical care.

STUDY QUESTIONS

1. Define diet therapy. In such therapy, what is being controlled?

2. When does diet therapy become necessary? What health professional makes this decision?

3. Who are the members of the health care team? List four (do not include the dietitian) and describe their roles in diet therapy.

4. What is a clinical dietitian? What does she do?

5. Why is effective communication in diet therapy important? How does it occur?

6. What is the diet order? What may it describe? Who prepares this order? Who can change it?

7. What does "NPO" mean?

8. List at least three resources that might be available in a health care institution to help answer nutrition questions?

9. What are the three basic parts of sensitive nutrition counseling? List at least two question you might ask in each phase.

10. A 73-year-old Italian widow comes to the doctor with three of her children. She has diabetes and her children (all adults living on their own) want to know what kind of diet she should follow and how they can help her follow it.

    Your institution has only one dietitian and she called in sick today so the doctor asks you to talk to the family. What might you do?

11. Take an hour with a friend or fellow-student. Allow 30 minutes each; do a nutrition assessment, using the questions on page 182. Afterwards, discuss your experience. What would you do next with the information you now have? What is healthful about the other person's diet? What changes should be discussed? What did you learn about your own eating habits?

CHAPTER 22

Energy-Controlled Diets

OBJECTIVES

1. To review energy and the three energy-containing nutrients
2. To review the role of energy in weight control
3. To provide a prudent framework for energy-controlled diets
4. To define and describe the exchange system as it is used in energy-controlled diets
5. To discuss other methods of controlling energy.
6. Using the exchange system as a guide, to outline diets at energy levels of (a) 1000, (b)1200, (c) 1500, (d) 1800, (e) 2000, (f) 2200 and (g) 2500 calories
7. For each diet, to discuss exchanges, sample meal pattern, and sample menu

Body weight depends, to a great extent, on energy control. A young female athlete who uses large amounts of energy every day must eat foods that provide the same amount of energy she uses or she will lose weight. However if her 50-year-old, nonathletic mother ate the same amount of the same foods, she might gain weight. Her energy *output* is less than her daughter's so she needs an *input* of less kilocalories, or food energy.

Chapter 2 describes the role that food energy plays in maintaining a healthy body. The body needs energy from food to maintain

a. Normal body functions
b. Normal growth and activity
c. Proper use of nutrients
d. Body weight

The body's energy needs vary slightly every day. These needs depend on the many factors listed and discussed in Chapter 2. Energy needs usually fluctuate within a certain range. Most people depend on *appetite* to know when they have eaten enough food to meet energy needs. Extra, unneeded food energy stores itself in the body as fat.

Sometimes it becomes necessary to control energy (or other nutrients) by a defined diet. This might happen in any of the following situations:

1. Months or years of overeating make it necessary to lose weight. Only an altered energy balance (where energy taken in—kilocalories of food—is less than energy used up) will successfully "burn off" the excess fat.

2. Disease changes the body's energy balance so that more energy (and often other nutrients, too) are needed for healing and maintenance.

3. The health and resistance to disease of a severely underweight client is jeopardized by too small a store of body fat and protein.

4. Energy needs suddenly change, as in pregnancy, lactation, a more (or less) physically demanding new job, or sudden immobility.

Food energy is produced in the body by four nutrients: carbohydrates, protein, fat, and alcohol. One gram (there are 28.35 grams in an ounce) of pure protein or of carbohydrate will yield approximately 3 to 4 kilocalories (Kcals). One gram of fat yields 9 Kcals; one gram of alcohol yields 7 Kcals. Of these four nutrients, only alcohol is not needed by the body. Chapters 1 through 5 describe the role of the first three in normal nutrition.

A person who has excess energy stores is overfat. An individual may be overweight (according to the weight charts in Chapter 12) without being overfat. He may have large bones and muscle stores and need more energy than someone of equal weight and greater fat. *Skinfold thickness,* a pinch test measured by calipers, is one technique some researchers use to measure body fat and compare it to standards. Too much body fat can become a health risk at any age. It produces an unnecessary stress on body systems and may lead to the development of heart disease, hypertension, or adult-onset diabetes mellitus.[1]

But severe underweight may also be a health risk. A person whose weight is 10% or more *below* the established standards is considered *underweight.* This person has too few fat stores. Low stores of fat may indicate long-term undernutrition. The person may have a low resistance (immunity) to diseases because of poor protein intake. A severely underweight woman may not have enough body fat to allow normal ovulation and menstruation. And if an underweight person becomes ill, the body will quickly use up its meager stores of nutrients in an effort to fight the disease. This may mean trouble, nutritionally. Recovery may take longer. These are some of the reasons energy and weight balance are important.

ENERGY-CONTROLLED DIETS

A diet that controls energy must also be balanced in all the other essential nutrients. This is most easily done in two steps:

1. Allotted Kcals are divided (or budgeted) into each of the three energy-producing nutrients: protein, fat, and carbohydrates, in the proportions advised by the physician *or* those recommended by the Recommended Dietary Allowances (RDA—see Chapter 12). Since physicians' diet orders rarely include a specific ratio of these three substances, this chapter will use the RDA as the standard.

Figure 22-1 illustrates the recommended balance of Kcals from the energy-producing nutrients in an adequate diet. This balance may be changed in certain diseases. Those given are the *general* recommendations, not the *averages.* Many North American diets are much higher in fat and lower in carbohydrate (especially fiber) than the RDA recommends. Other cultures throughout the world may have other variations, but these are recommendations that could be used in diet therapy and normal nutrition in any nation, using indigenous (native) foods.

2. The other step in designing a controlled but adequate diet is to provide enough variety

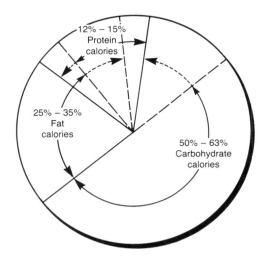

Figure 22-1
Recommended dietary allowances–proportions of energy-producing nutrients. (From information from Food and Nutrition Board, National Academy of Sciences, National Research Council: Recommended Dietary Allowances, 1980)

within the structure of the diet to meet all other essential nutrient needs. This may be done, for example, by encouraging a variety of vegetables, grains, fruit, or various types of protein in the diet.

THE EXCHANGE SYSTEM

The most common method employed to illustrate or teach energy-controlled diets used in health care is the *exchange* system. In diets that use *exchanges,* foods are grouped in categories, for example: Milk, Meat, Fruit, Vegetables, Starchy Vegetables, Breads and Cereals, Fats, Free Foods (permitted in unlimited amounts), and Forbidden Foods. All the foods within each group are listed by specific portions. Illustrated on page 188 is a sample of the bread group in one such diet. One portion of one food within a group is an "exchange." Each of the exchanges in the group (in the portion sizes listed) has roughly equal energy values. They can all be substituted for each other.

The diet is controlled by budgeting the client a certain number of exchanges every day from each of the groups (except those Free or Forbidden). The client has freedom to choose from whatever foods in each group he likes best. For example, he may dislike bread and always "use up" his bread exchanges by choosing to eat crackers or enriched rice or pasta.

Exchange diets have benefits *and* problems. They may confuse a person who is not used to categorizing foods. They require measuring, weighing, and recordkeeping. Planning menus and keeping track of allowed and used exchanges is important, since a diet will only work if it is followed. But the biggest advantage of an exchange diet is that it allows for personal, individual preferences. Choices can be adapted to fit different cultures. An individual who does not want to learn the entire system may do well using several sample menus, based on their present eating habits. Sample menus are often most practical for the older person with consistent, predictable meals. With exchange planning, meals can also be designed to fit the irregular lifestyle. Eating at parties or special events—even eating out—can be easy when it is food groups that are controlled and not individual foods.

SEVEN SAMPLE ENERGY-CONTROLLED DIETS

Pages 189–193 show seven sample diets that control energy through an exchange diet, based on the RDA for protein, fat, and carbohydrate. They range from 1000 Kcals to 2500 Kcals per day. No one should follow the 1000 Kcal diet for more than a few days without the approval of a physician because it does not meet all the essential nutrient needs. The outlines are just that: *outlines, guidelines, aids* to help work with the physician and dietitian in developing energy-controlled diets. The sample meal divisions and menus shown are provided to illustrate the variety possible on an exchange diet. Low fat milk is recommended in most of the diets in order to keep them within the RDA recommendation of 25%–35% Kcals from fat; some individuals may want to give up margarine and choose whole milk. A client who wants more fat in the diet should work with a local dietitian after checking with his physician. Whole grains are recommended as carbohydrate sources because they provide necessary fiber. The three highest calorie diets are probably not appropriate for an ill or undernourished client because these diets may provide more bulk than is realistic for such a client. But they may be suitable for some large men who are in otherwise good health and who do not need to lose weight.

The exchange quantities are taken from the booklet, "Exchange Lists for Meal Planning," published by both the American Diabetes Association and the American Dietetic Association.[2] Sample copies of this booklet may be available from a local dietitian or can be ordered from either of these organizations.

OTHER ENERGY-ALTERED DIETS

Exchange diets may not be appropriate for everyone who needs more or less calories than usual. Some clients prefer tight, regimental diets. Others may be able to alter their diet by using simple guidelines. And some may prefer fad diets, which are *never* recommended.

SAMPLE OF BREAD EXCHANGES

You are allowed _____ each day. One exchange of bread contains 15 grams of carbohydrate, 2 grams of protein, and 70 calories. Starchy vegetables are included because they contain the same amount of carbohydrate and protein as one slice of bread.

Bread

White (including French, Italian)	1 slice
Whole wheat	1 slice
Rye or pumpernickle	1 slice
Raisin	1 slice
Bagel	½ small
Muffin, English	½ small
Roll, plain, bread	1
Roll, frankfurter	1
Bun, hamburger	½
Bread crumbs, dried	3 tbsp
Tortilla (6″)	1

Cereal

Bran flakes	½ cup
Cereal, ready-to-eat (unsweetened)	¾ cup
Cereal, puffed (unsweetened)	1 cup
Cereal, cooked	½ cup
Cornmeal, dry	2 tbsp
Flour	2½ tbsp
Grits, cooked	½ cup
Pasta, cooked	½ cup
Popcorn, popped (no fat added)	3 cups
Rice or barley, cooked	½ cup
Wheat germ	¼ cup

Crackers

Arrowroot	3
Graham (2½″ sq)	2
Matzoh (4″x6″)	½
Oyster	20
Pretzel sticks (3⅛″x⅛″)	25
Saltines	6
Soda (2½ sq)	4
Wafers, rye (2″x3½″)	3

Dried Beans, Peas, Lentils

Beans, peas, lentils (dried, then cooked)	½ cup
Beans, baked (canned, no pork)	¼ cup

Starchy Vegetables

Beans, lima	½ cup
Corn	⅓ cup
Corn, on the cob	1 small
Parsnips	⅔ cup
Peas, green (canned, frozen)	½ cup
Potato, white	1 small
Potato, mashed	½ cup
Pumpkin	¾ cup
Squash, winter, acorn, butternut	½ cup
Yam or sweet potato	¼ cup

(From American Diabetes Association/Amerian Dietetic Association: Exchange Lists for Meal Planning. New York, American Diabetes Association, 1976. Chicago, American Dietetic Association, 1976)

1. A regimented diet spells out exactly what and how much food should be consumed at every meal. This is the kind of diet often published in women's magazines or available from certain drug companies. These diets allow for little freedom in food choices or in meal times. They may be used for the client who does not want to plan or is unable to do so. When these diets are used at home, it is assumed the client can afford all the

KCAL EXCHANGE DIETS

1000 Kcals

Composition:
54% Carbohydrate (129 g)
23% Protein (54 g)
23% Fat (22 g)

Sample Division:

Breakfast
1 Milk
1 Protein
1 Fruit
1 Starch

Exchanges:

Skim milk	2
Fruit	3
Starch	5
Protein	4
Fat	2
Vegetable	2

Lunch
1 Protein
1 Fruit
2 Starch
1 Vegetable
1 Fat

Snack
1 Fruit

Dinner
1 Milk
2 Protein
2 Starch
1 Fat
1 Vegetable

Sample Menu:

Breakfast
1 Egg, soft boiled
1 slice Toast
½ cup Unsweetened
  applesauce
8 oz Skim milk

Lunch
Sandwich of:
2 slices Bread
1 oz Chicken
1 tsp Mayonnaise
1 Nectarine, small

Snack
Small orange

Dinner
Chili of:
½ cup Cooked beans
2 oz Diced lean beef
  on ½ cup Rice
½ cup Broccoli
1 tsp Margarine
Salad with lemon and vinegar
1 cup Skim milk

1200 Kcals

Composition:
54% Carbohydrate (159 g)
24% Protein (72 g)
22% Fat (28 g)

Sample Division:

Breakfast
1Protein
1 Fruit
1 Starch

Exchanges:

Low fat Milk	2
Fruit	4
Starch	5
Protein	6
Vegetable	4
Fat	2

Lunch
2 Protein
2 Starch
2 Vegetables
1 Fat
1 Fruit

Snack
1 Milk

Dinner
3 Protein
1 Starch
2 Vegetables
1 Fat
1 Fruit

Snack
1 Starch

Sample Menu:

Breakfast
- ¼ cup Cottage cheese
- 1 slice Toast
- ½ cup Orange juice

Snack
- 3 Rye Krisp crackers

Lunch
- 2 slices Wheat bread
- 2 oz Turkey
- 1 tsp Mayonnaise
- 1 Orange
- 1 cup Carrot sticks

Snack
- 1 cup Plain, low fat yogurt

Dinner
- 3 oz Broiled fish w/lemon
- 1 Baked potato, small
- 1 tsp Margarine
- 1 cup Steamed summer squash
- ½ cup Pineapple slices (fresh, water, or juice pack)

1500 Kcals
Composition:
52% Carbohydrate (198 g)
24% Protein (92 g)
24% Fat (40 g)

Exchanges:

Low fat Milk	2
Fruit	4
Starch	8
Protein	8
Vegetable	2
Fat	2

Sample Division:

Breakfast
2 Starch
1 Fruit
1 Milk
1 Vegetable

Snack
2 Protein
1 Starch

Lunch
1 Protein
2 Starch
2 Fruit
2 Fat
1 Milk

Snack
1 Starch

Dinner
5 Protein
2 Starch
1 Fruit
1 Vegetable

Sample Menu:

Breakfast
- 1 cup Cooked cereal
- 1 cup Low fat milk
- ½ cup Vegetable juice cocktail
- ½ Banana in cereal

Snack
- 2 oz Low fat cheese
- 6 Saltines

Lunch
- 2 slices Wheat bread
- 2 tbsp. Peanut butter*
- 1 Banana
- 1 cup Plain, low fat yogurt

Snack
- 3 cups Dry popcorn

Dinner
- 5 oz Lean pork
- ⅔ cup Corn
- ½ cup Steamed cabbage
- ¾ cup Fresh strawberries

1800 Kcals
Composition:
49% Carbohydrate (221 g)
21% Protein (95 g)
30% Fat (60 g)

Exchanges:

Low fat Milk	3
Fruit	6
Starch	7
Protein	7
Vegetable	4
Fat	3

---

* Peanut butter is high in fat; 2 tbsp count as 1 protein and 2 fats.

Sample Division:

Breakfast
1 Milk
1 Fruit
2 Starch
1 Fat

Snack
1 Fruit
1 Starch

Lunch
2 Protein
2 Fruit
2 Starch
2 Vegetables
1 Fat

Snack
1 Milk
1 Fruit

Dinner
4 Protein
2 Starch
1 Milk
1 Fruit
1 Fat
2 Vegetables

Sample Menu

Breakfast
1 Bagel
1 tbsp Cream cheese
1 cup Low fat milk
1 Tangerine, medium

Snack
2 Graham crackers
⅓ cup Apple juice

Lunch
1 Hamburger bun
2 oz lean ground beef
½ cup Sliced tomatoes, onions, mushrooms in salad
½ Cantaloupe, small
½ cup Vegetable juice
1 tbsp Italian salad dressing

Snack
1 cup Low fat yogurt
10 Fresh cherries

Dinner
3 oz Fish
1 oz Cheese
½ cup Steamed sweet potato
1 cup Spinach in salad with 1 tsp oil and 2 tbsp raisins vinegar (free)
1 cup Low fat milk

2000 Kcals

Composition:
55% Carbohydrate (273 g)
21% Protein (107 g)
24% Fat (53 g)

Exchanges:

Low fat Milk	4
Fruit	7
Starch	9
Protein	7
Vegetable	4
Fat	4

Sample Division:

Breakfast
1 Milk
1 Fruit
2 Starch
1 Vegetable

Snack
1 Fruit
2 Starch
1 Fat

Lunch
2 Protein
1 Milk
2 Fruit
2 Starch
1 Fat

Snack
1 Milk
1 Fruit
1 Starch

Dinner
5 Protein
2 Fruit
2 Starch
2 Vegetable
2 Fat

plus 1 Milk throughout day in hot beverages

Sample Menu
½ cup Bran flakes
½ Banana
¼ cup Wheat germ
1 cup Low fat milk
4 oz Tomato juice

1 English muffin
1 tsp Margarine
¼ cup Grape juice

1 small Frankfurter
1 Hot dog roll
1 oz Low fat cheese
1 cup Plain yogurt
  with 12 Chopped
  grapes
½ cup Orange juice

1 cup Low fat milk
  blended with
¾ cup Frozen
  thawed
  strawberries
2 Graham crackers

4 oz Shrimp, steamed with
1 oz Cheese, grated
1 cup Noodles
½ Steamed broccoli
½ Sliced tomato
1 cup Fresh, cut fruit
2 tsp Margarine

2200 Kcals
Composition:
50% Carbohydrate (273 g)
20% Protein (114 g)
30% Fat (74 g)

Exchanges:

Whole milk	4
Fruit	7
Starch	9
Protein	8
Vegetable	4
Fat	4

Sample Division:

Breakfast
1 Milk
2 Fruit
2 Starch
1 Vegetable
1 Protein

Snack
2 Starch
1 Fat

Lunch
2 Protein
1 Milk
2 Fruit
2 Starch
1 Fat

Snack
1 Milk
1 Fruit
1 Starch

Dinner
5 Protein
2 Fruit
2 Starch
2 Vegetable
2 Fat

plus: 1 Milk throughout the day or as an evening snack

Sample Menu
1 Egg, scrambled
  with ½ cup
  Chopped green
  pepper
  inside an English
  muffin
½ cantaloupe, small
1 cup Whole milk

1 Bagel, small
1 tbsp Cream cheese

2 oz Roast beef
  on Bulky roll
1 tsp Mayonnaise
8 oz Milk
1 Banana

1 cup Plain yogurt
½ cup Blueberries
3 Rye wafers

5 oz Broiled lamb chops
1 cup Noodles
1 tsp Margarine
½ cup Chopped cucumbers,
  mushrooms, tomatoes
½ cup Steamed spinach
1 tbsp Italian dressing
4 Apricots, canned in water
  or juice

2500 K cals

Composition:
49% Carbohydrate (303 g)
19% Protein (118 g)
32% Fat (89 g)

Exchanges:

Whole milk	4
Fruit	8
Starch	10
Protein	8
Vegetable	5
Fat	7

Sample Division:

Breakfast
1 Fat
1 Milk
2 Fruit
2 Starch
1 Vegetable
1 Protein

Snack
2 Starch
1 Fruit
1 Fat

Lunch
3 Starch
2 Protein
3 Vegetable
2 Fruit
2 Fat

Snack
1 Milk
1 Fruit
1 Starch
1 Fat

Dinner
5 Protein
2 Fruit
1 Vegetable
2 Starch
2 Fat

Plus 1 Milk throughout the day in hot beverages or as an evening snack (buttermilk or sugar-free hot chocolate*)

Sample Menu

Mini-pizzas of:
1 English muffin, toasted
1 tsp Margarine
1/4 cup Plain spaghetti sauce
1 oz Mozzarella cheese
8 oz Grapefruit juice
8 oz Whole milk

1/3 cup Apple juice
1 Corn muffin (high in fat)

Chowder of:
1 cup Milk
2 oz Clams
1 Potato
2 tsp Butter
8 Soda crackers
12 oz Vegetable juice
1 whole Grapefruit

1 cup Plain yogurt
10 Cut-up cherries
5 Round, butter-type crackers
1 tsp Margarine

5 oz Lean, broiled beef
1/2 cup Mashed potato
1/2 cup Steamed broccoli
1 Corn on cob, small
2 tsp Margarine
Fruit mixture of:
3/4 cup Strawberries
1/2 medium Banana

*Regular hot chocolate adds calories and carbohydrate but may be preferred and acceptable if the goal is to gain weight.

IDEAS TO HELP WEIGHT GAIN

1. Snack regularly on high-calorie, vitamin-supplemented formula beverages, such as
   (a) Commercial canned beverages
   (b) Milk blended with Instant Breakfast powders

2. Add fats such as cream cheese, butter, margarine, sour cream, oil, and peanut butter to vegetables, breads, and any other foods desired. Never eat these foods without adding some type of fat.

3. Add sweeteners such as jam, jelly, honey, and sugar and syrups whenever possible.

4. Mix whole milk (1 quart) with nonfat dry milk powder (1 cup). This is called "double strength milk" and provides twice the protein and 1½ times the calories of regular milk.

5. Blend double strength milk with
   (a) Eggs, vanilla, sugar
   (b) Fruit juices or jams
   (c) Peanut butter melted in sweetened condensed milk

6. Make sure all foods and beverages contain as many calories as possible. For example, instead of water, drink milk or juices; instead of plain celery add peanut butter or cream cheese.

7. Eat four to six small meals (that is, every 3 or 4 hours) instead of a few large meals. Try to eat something often.

---

foods listed, and the diets may not include suggestions to help use up leftovers. To be most useful, a regimented diet should be "custom-designed" for each person and include several options for sample menus.

2. General guidelines list only the foods to avoid and those allowed in unlimited amounts. They may include tips, recipes, methods, or suggestions for "behavior modification" to help the client change eating habits, but they may not provide a specific level of energy or balance of nutrients. They may be helpful for individuals who have little control over their meals, and for persons who are highly motivated to make changes on their own initiative. Guidelines are helpful when energy intake is not extremely important; they may be used simply to help a client identify and limit (or avoid) foods high in some nutrient or substance (such as sodium or saturated fats). They may be helpful when a client does not need (or refuses) to follow a controlled plan. A sample of some ideas for weight *gain* is shown above.

3. Fad diets limit energy by severely limiting (or entirely omitting) certain food groups (often carbohydrate or fats), and recommending others in unlimited amounts. These diets are not nutritionally sound, are often deficient in major nutrients, and may lead to rapid but temporary and unhealthy weight changes. A commercial product sometimes takes the place of some meals or foods. A physician and dietitian should be consulted if a client is thinking about this type of diet.

STUDY QUESTIONS

1. Why is energy an important nutrient?

2. In what situations might an energy-controlled diet be necessary?

3. From what four food categories does energy come? Of these four, which are necessary for health?

4. A person overweight because of excess fat has a higher-than-normal risk of developing what diseases?

5. Is underweight a health risk? Why or why not?

6. In any nutritionally adequate diet, including a weight loss diet, what percentage of energy should come from protein? From carbohydrate? From fat?

7. What is an exchange diet?

8. What other types of diets may control energy? How do they differ from an exchange diet?

9. Choose one of the sample exchange diets shown on pages 189–193. Match each allotted exchange with the corresponding foods listed in the sample menu.

10. List all the foods you ate yesterday. Using the chart on page 188 as a guide, how many bread exchanges did you have?

11. Benjamin is a 19-year-old college student, whose height is 6 feet, 2 inches. He is in good health, but weighs only 155 pounds. What are at least two ways he might increase the concentration of calories in his diet to try and gain weight?

REFERENCES

1. CME Communications: Clinical Implications of Overweight: Positive Management Techniques, New York, CME Communications, 1980. (Available from Merrell-National Laboratories, Cincinnati, Ohio 45215)

2. American Diabetes Association/American Dietetic Association: Exchange Lists for Meal Planning, New York, American Diabetes Association, 1976. Chicago, American Dietetic Association, 1976.

CHAPTER 23

Protein-Controlled Diets

OBJECTIVES

1. To review briefly the role of protein in normal nutrition
2. To discuss general indications for a protein-controlled diet in terms of physiological problems
3. To discuss briefly the interrelationship between protein and other nutrients in normal and clinical nutrition
4. To discuss the basis for strict protein control in treatment of
   a. Liver disease
   b. Kidney disease
   c. Phenylketonuria (PKU)
   d. Protein-sparing modified fasts
5. To discuss the basis for increasing protein in the treatment of
   a. Protein-calorie malnutrition
   b. Gastrointestinal diseases and malabsorption syndromes
   c. Cancer
   d. Burn or trauma
   e. Kidney disease
6. To outline current beliefs about diet therapy for gout

As explained in Chapter 3, protein is the most essential—and the most costly—energy-containing nutrient for growth and development. Man can live on a low fat diet. He can even live for months, as in the Arctic, on a diet low in carbohydrates. But if he begins to live for an extended period of time without enough protein, he suffers. This is best seen in the disease of kwashiorkor. In kwashiorkor, infants and children acquire sufficient energy from their diets but not enough protein. They become malnourished and listless. The lack of protein leads to many other imbalances in their bodies and untreated, they die.

Protein is the nutrient that is essential in the manufacture of muscles, hormones, antibodies, enzymes, and to carry many other essential nutrients. Protein in the diet breaks down in the body to amino acids. These are further broken down in the liver, kidneys, muscle, and brain. Ammonia and urea, toxic substances in large quantities, are two of the major by-products of protein breakdown. The extra nitrogen molecules not used in the normal metabolism of the day (that is, the leftover nitrogen) is formed into ammonia and urea. Ammonia is broken down into urea in the liver, and from that point, blood carries it to the kidneys. The healthy kidneys filter out the unnecessary urea. This process helps maintain nitrogen balance in the body. Enzymes and molecular reactions—usually in the liver—convert the remaining proteins into the various forms needed. In order to have sufficient protein to meet all of these requirements, the average adult needs about 0.8 grams of protein (in food) for every kilogram of body weight.

If any of these systems malfunctions, protein metabolism is upset. Malfunction may occur because of

a. Genetic defects

b. Disease, and/or

c. Sudden acute trauma

When protein balance is upset, a physician may order a protein-controlled diet as part of medical treatment.

A diet controlling protein can fit into one of two categories:

1. It may *restrict* protein severely, at or below the Recommended Dietary Allowances (RDA), or more moderately in a tight range slightly *above* the RDA. Protein restrictions are used to keep a particular balance and/or to prevent the harmful, excessive buildup of ammonia, urea and/or other by-products.

2. Or it may be a *high-protein* diet, designed to help replace the protein lost in

   a. Acute stress and *hypermetabolism* (for example, from burns, cancer, or kidneys damaged so that they are losing too much protein)

   b. Disease (for example, anemia or malnutrition)

   c. Abnormal digestion or absorption that causes protein loss

The same disease may require a different level of protein control at different stages. For example, an alcoholic with *hepatic encephalopathy* (delirium resulting from liver damage) is usually put on a protein restricted diet. But a malnourished alcoholic who shows no sign of encephalopathy may be allowed more protein to help correct the malnutrition. The diet order depends on the state of the disease.

Whenever protein is controlled because of disease, trauma, or genetic defect, the degree of diet control is usually prescribed by the physician and worked out, practically, with the dietitian. No one should ever arbitrarily put himself on a strict protein-controlled diet, whether it is a diet far above or below the RDA. The body is a fine-tuned organism. If it receives too much or too little of a nutrient, the balance of the other

nutrients may be affected. This is especially true with protein in disease. Protein imbalance in disease may also affect the balance and need for other nutrients such as sodium, fluid, phosphate, potassium, and energy. Because of the relationship between these nutrients, a client may need more time to learn a protein-controlled diet than one that alters another nutrient.

The following is a more detailed description of some of the diseases for which physicians often order a diet controlling protein.

WHEN PROTEIN IS RESTRICTED

Liver Disease

Protein metabolism leads to the production of ammonia. The liver converts ammonia to urea. When the liver malfunctions, ammonia may build up in the blood. This can be toxic. An alcoholic who is severely disoriented (as in hepatic encephalopathy, described above) because of high ammonia levels is often put on a severely low-protein diet until the symptoms improve. Clients who have liver disease resulting from acute viral hepatitis may also be protein-restricted during the most severe phase of the disease. More protein is usually added to the diet after this phase is controlled.

Kidney Disease

Kidney disease may be the most common cause for a long-term protein-controlled diet. Because of the many functions of the kidney diet therapy in kidney disease is very complex. Diet therapy can help a client to live as well as possible with the disease, but it cannot cure it.

The nephrons (tubules) in the kidney's elaborate network help to filter out wastes from the body and convert them into urine. The major ingredient in urine is urea. Kidney disease may affect the filtering and excretion of urea in two ways:

1. The nephrons may become indiscriminate that is, unable properly to *prevent* nutrients from being filtered out. When this happens, nutrients and electrolytes that would normally be conserved, returned to the blood, and used again, are lost.

2. Or the filtering system begins to shut down. Waste products are not efficiently filtered out and they build up in the body.

Renal (kidney) disease may begin with the first filtering problem but lead quickly to the second. When urea begins to build up in the blood (measured as BUN or blood urea nitrogen), protein—and other nutrients—are commonly restricted. If there is no restriction, toxic build-up may poison the body. Diet is one of the most important treatment controls. Some physicians recommend that a mild protein restriction begin in the very early stages of renal disease.[1] They believe this helps to "spare" the kidneys and postpone the need for dialysis. Dialysis is the artificial filtering of the blood by a machine (hemodialysis) or a hyperosmolar solution (peritoneal dialysis). Dialysis treatments in kidney failure usually begin when the kidneys can no longer function well enough on their own to maintain body balances. If dialysis of some kind does not take over when the kidneys fail, the client will die. Dialysis in kidney disease will be discussed in more detail in Chapter 28.

Phenylketonuria (PKU)

PKU is a genetic defect that can be detected 3 days after birth. It develops as the genetic result of an enzyme (phenylalanine hydroxylase) that is either missing or inadequate. Because of this genetic deficiency, the body cannot convert *phenylalanine,* an amino acid, to tyrosine. Consequently, phenylalanine builds up to high levels in the blood. Unless this condition is controlled, PKU children become permanently mentally retarded. Fortunately, though PKU is not curable, the potential retardation can be prevented by diet. A diet that tightly controls the amount of phenylalanine the child receives will help that child grow up normally, with average or above average intelligence.

In the diet that controls PKU, the necessary protein is supplied by special products that are low in phenylalanine. Some phenylalanine is necessary for normal functioning. (See Chapter 3; phenylalanine is one of the essential amino acids.) All foods that provide any protein contain phenylalanine. This makes diet control more complicated.

Because of the success of careful medical and diet therapy in PKU, many normal women with the defect are now old enough to have children. When a woman with PKU becomes pregnant, her phenylalanine levels must be very tightly controlled; high blood levels may damage her unborn child.

A low phenylalanine diet is a difficult one for a child to accept because it differs so widely from the average diet. Shown on page 199 is a sample of a PKU diet for an 8-year-old-boy. In this diet, Phenyl-free formula is the only significant source of protein. This formula contains all the essential amino acids except phenylalanine. The phenylalanine that the child needs to meet the RDA and to use protein properly comes from "exchanges" of other "normal" foods. The diet is especially hard to learn and follow because almost all foods (including fruits and vegetables) include some of the amino acid. Only jams, jellies, oil, syrups, cornstarch, tapioca, molasses, and sugar are completely free of phenylalanine.

There are still many questions concerning the length of time a child must stay on the tightly restricted diet. Frequent blood tests and counseling with physician and dietitian are an essential part of maintaining health care for the PKU child (and support for his parents) as he grows and his needs change. Some resources are listed at the end of this chapter.[2,3]

Protein-Sparing Modified Fast (PSMF)

The *protein-sparing modified fast* is a diet used with close medical supervision for morbidly obese individuals. On this diet calories are severely restricted to a small quantity of high quality protein each day. This diet is a modified fast that includes some protein to "spare" the body's protein stores. It must only be used in a careful, clinical environment under the care of a trained medical team. Popular diets that use the PSMF principles over a long period but without careful

SAMPLE DAILY DIET OF AN 8-YEAR-OLD CHILD WITH PKU

Breakfast:
1 Slice Toast
1 tbsp Grape jelly
Phenyl-free Formula* with 1 tbsp coffee syrup for flavoring
Lunch:
1 Raw green pepper, large
1 Raw carrot, large
9 Potato chips
6 oz Hi-C
Afternoon Snack:
Phenyl-free Formula with 1 tbsp coffee syrup
½ cup Popcorn with salt
4 oz Hi-C
Supper:
Phenyl-free Formula with 1 tbsp coffee syrup
Salad of:
    1 oz Lettuce
    ½ Raw pepper
    5 Olives, medium
    ⅓ Raw carrot
    2½ tbsp Raw onion
    4 tbsp Cabbage
    4 tbsp Wax beans
    2 tbsp Italian dressing
⅔ cup Applesauce

---

*Total of 20 scoops per day, mixed with water to desired thickness.

---

medical supervision may cause needless death as a result of sudden imbalances in the body.

Even when a diet is low in protein, some protein is necessary. If a diet is too low in protein, the body will break down muscle and other protein stores. Some body muscles (such as the heart) must work well for survival. When protein stores are broken down, nitrogen is freed, ammonia is then produced, and urea must be excreted. So in some diseases protein must be very carefully balanced, since both too much and too little will cause excess waste production.

WHEN PROTEIN NEEDS INCREASE

Protein-Calorie Malnutrition *(PCM)*

PCM is most common in children living in chronically deprived conditions. This malnutriton may be either (1) marasmus, characterized by an emaciated appearance and a diet too low in protein and energy, and (2) kwashiorkor, characterized by a puffy or bloated appearance and a diet with enough energy but too little protein. Marasmus develops progressively, as the child starves, but kwashiorkor may develop quickly, sometimes after a stressful condition such as fever or gastroenteritis. The stress drains the body of its last protein stores. Fat is deposited in places it does not belong (such as the liver) and excess fluid (edema) swells the interstitial spaces. Children with kwashiorkor appear listless and have very low measures of blood proteins. Once careful treatment begins, with a diet containing adequate amounts of protein and energy, recovery may be rapid. At first, however, the child may appear to "lose weight," which is only the loss of excess fluid. After the child is no longer edematous (bloated or swollen), underlying malnutrition may be very obvious.

Marasmic children, however, are so severely malnourished that recovery is often much slower than in kwashiorkor. Treatment is adapted to the child's very fragile health, and energy and protein are introduced and increased very gradually.[4]

Gastrointestinal Diseases and Malabsorption Syndromes

In GI diseases, the lining of the intestine may be abnormal. Proteins may be absorbed across the cell wall in an uneven way. Ingested proteins may not be absorbed, and consequently can never reach the blood or the liver. In some GI diseases, intestinal bleeding may occur. When blood is lost, protein is lost. The physician and dietitian can help a client develop a diet that restricts bleeding to the minimum and replaces lost protein. There are many different GI diseases and treatment depends on the particular problem(s).

Malabsorption from GI diseases can affect many nutrients and nutrition is usually a major part of medical treatment. Nutrition in GI disease will be discussed in more detail in Chapter 33.

Cancer

Many persons with cancer lose weight and protein stores. The reasons are still unclear but most authorities agree that protein and energy needs increase in cancer and that nutrition support helps a client come through the disease and its treatments with the best resources possible. The amount of protein a client needs and the way to include it in the diet depends on the type and stage of the cancer. It also depends on individual preferences. Nutrition as it relates to cancer will be discussed in more detail in Chapter 30.

Severe Burns or Injury

Physical stress increases protein needs. Tissue that is directly damaged by burns, accidents, or other injuries needs to be replaced. To replace tissue, the body needs extra protein. Basal metabolism rates also increase. This condition is called hypermetabolism and a client may have very high energy needs for many days or weeks, as the body recovers from trauma. This need for extra nutrition is often complicated by the fact that trauma or burn victims cannot eat normally. Even when they are able to eat, they are usually unable to consume the great amount of food needed to meet their high needs. For this reason, they are often fed by a *nasogastric tube* (a thin, spaghettilike tubing that goes through the nose and down the esophagus into the stomach). Or they may be fed intravenously with solutions that enter their blood directly. These methods of feeding are called *hyperalimentation,* and are discussed further in Chapter 38. Whatever feeding methods are used, protein must be a key nutrient in the diet. It works both to heal and restore tissues damaged or lost in trauma and to help maintain resistance to

infection—a very high risk for the client with burns or trauma.

Kidney Disease

Many physicians recommend normal or high protein diets for clients with *nephrotic syndrome* or those who are on peritoneal dialysis for kidney failure. In nephrotic syndrome, protein (in the form of albumin) is lost in the urine. The diseased nephrons of the kidney simply permit these molecules to filter out rather than conserve them. Nephrotic syndrome is often an early form of kidney failure, and eventually the nephrons begin to shut down. When this process starts, protein is restricted, and fluid may be restricted as well. (The fluid restriction of kidney disease will be discussed in Chapter 28.)

In *peritoneal dialysis,* a fluid is forced into the peritoneal cavity of the abdomen. There it draws waste products out of the system and into itself. Then it is drained from the body through a surgical opening. Because this is a far cruder method than the kidneys' natural dialysis, substances that would otherwise be conserved are often lost. For instance, large amounts of protein are lost in the drained peritoneal fluid. This protein must be replaced by diet or the client will become undernourished and less able to resist infection and disease. The types of peritoneal dialysis will also be outlined in Chapter 28.

Gout

Gout is a disease that results in high levels of uric acid. Persons with gout often develop painful deposits of sodium urate in their joints, as well as uric acid kidney stones. Because uric acid is produced from substances called purines, treatment used to include a low-purine diet. Physicians now realize that diet does not play a very important role in the disease. Purines are made naturally in the body and dietary sources contribute a minimal amount. Drug therapy, not diet is most important in the control of gout today.

However, some physicians do recommend that a client with gout avoid foods that are very high in purines. This mild diet control, coupled with good drug control, can help keep the symptoms of gout to a minimum. Foods very high in purines include liver, kidneys, sweetbreads, brains, hearts, anchovies, sardines in oil, meat extracts, consommé, gravies, caviar, and herring.[5] Alcohol and fatty foods may also be restricted. Clients with gout may be overweight, so gradual weight loss is often part of treatment. Rapid loss would cause a high release of purines into the blood and may aggravate the symptoms.

STUDY QUESTIONS

1. What body organs help break down proteins?

2. List two by-products of protein breakdown that can build up to toxic levels in some diseases.

3. Why might protein metabolism be upset? Give at least two possible reasons.

4. What is the main purpose of restricting proteins in some diseases?

5. What is PKU?

6. Diseases that affect protein metabolism may also affect what five other nutrients?

7. What might happen to protein balance in a client with renal disease?

8. What is a protein-sparing modified fast?

9. What disease and conditions often are treated with a high protein diet? List at least three and explain why extra protein is needed.

10. What substances build up in gout? What is the role of *medicine* in its treatment? Of *diet*?

REFERENCES

1. Brenner BM, Meyer TW, Hostetter TH: "Dietary protein intake and the progressive nature of kidney disease: The role of hemodynamically mediated glomerular injury in the pathogenesis of glomerular sclerosis in aging, renal ablation, and intrinsic renal disease. N Engl Med 307(11):652–659, September 9, 1982

2. Acosta, PB et al: Parents' Guide to the Child with PKU. Atlanta, Emory University, 1980. (Available from the Programs in Dietetics, Division of Allied Health Professions, 2040 Ridgewood Drive NE, Emory University, Atlanta, GA 30322)

3. Flavin E, Ampola M, Doyle M: Low Protein and Low Phenylalanine Food List. 1979. (Available for $5 per copy from Dr. Mary Ampola, Pediatric Amino Acid Laboratory, New England Medical Center Hospital, 171 Harrison Ave., Boston, MA 02111)

4. Solomons, NW: Rehabilitating the severely malnourished infant and child. J Am Diet Assoc 85(1):28–39, January 1985

5. Thomas CL (ed): Taber's Cyclopedic Medical Dictionary, 13th ed, p 172. Philadelphia, FA Davis, 1977

CHAPTER 24

Carbohydrate-Controlled Diets

OBJECTIVES

1. To review briefly the role of carbohydrate in normal nutrition
2. To discuss situations where carbohydrate-controlled diets may be necessary:
   a. To control blood sugar
      (1) In diabetes
      (2) In hyperinsulinism/hypoglycemia
   b. In carbohydrate malabsorption or enzyme deficiency syndromes, such as
      (1) Disaccharidase deficiencies
      (2) Celiac sprue
      (3) Galactosemia
   c. To control dietary fiber in
      (1) Gastrointestinal disorders
      (2) Diabetes
      (3) Coronary artery disease
      (4) Constipation
3. For each of the above to explain
   a. The rationale for control
   b. Problems associated with control.
      and to provide sample menus or a list of foods containing the carbohydrate involved
4. To define and describe the "glycemic index" of carbohydrate foods
5. To define and discuss the disadvantages of popular low-carbohydrate reducing diets

Carbohydrates are a major source of dietary energy. As discussed in Chapter 4, they are read-

ily broken down in the digestive tract, readily absorbed (except for fiber), and well metabolized. Their presence stimulates the pancreas to release *insulin* into the blood. Insulin then helps carry the carbohydrate (in the form of glucose) into the cells, controlling the level of glucose in the blood. Excess glucose (the result of the breakdown of excess carbohydrate, protein, or fat) is stored in the cells as fat; it is not excreted in the urine, like nitrogen. "Sugar in the urine" is a sign of disease.

Carbohydrate intake is controlled by a special diet when the body, for some reason is unable to

1. Properly control blood sugar and insulin secretion (as in diabetes and/or *hyperinsulinism*)
2. Adequately or properly digest particular carbohydrate(s), for example in malabsorption syndromes, carbohydrate intolerances, or hypersensitivities; or when
3. Carbohydrate control is believed helpful in the treatment of a disease (for example, high fiber diets used for *diverticulosis*)

Carbohydrate may also be controlled in weight loss diets, along with protein and fat control. This was discussed in Chapter 22.

DIABETES MELLITUS

Diabetes Mellitus is a disease for which "treatment" is a lifelong diet controlling total carbohydrate, protein, fat, and energy intake, and monitoring insulin needs. It is a complex disease involving many factors and, for this reason, it will not be discussed in this chapter. (See Chapter 31.)

Some of the other common situations in which carbohydrate is often controlled are listed below.

HYPERINSULINISM

As its name implies, hyperinsulinism means that, in response to carbohydrate, the pancreas releases too much insulin into the blood. This overreaction causes glucose to be carried into the cells too quickly. The result is a temporary low blood sugar, or hypoglycemia.

Simple hyperinsulinism without any underlying cause is rare. The symptom may appear as

DISEASES THAT MAY INCLUDE CARBOHYDRATE CONTROL AS PART OF MEDICAL TREATMENT

A. To Control Blood Sugar
- Diabetes: Type I (insulin-dependent)
- Diabetes: Type II (noninsulin dependent)
- Hyperinsulinism/Hypoglycemia

B. To Normalize Digestion and Absorption
- Disaccharidase deficiency
  -lactose intolerance
  -sucrase deficiency
  -maltase deficiency
- Celiac sprue (gluten enteropathy)

C. To Control Fiber
- Low fiber: Diverticulitis
  Crohn's Ileitis
- High fiber: Diabetes
  Diverticulosis
  Coronary Artery Disease
  Constipation

an early sign of diabetes and is also called *reactive hypoglycemia.*[1] Persons with reactive hypoglycemia may complain of weakness, perspiration, anxiety, nervousness, and mental confusion several hours after eating a high carbohydrate food or meal.[1] These individuals may fit into one of two groups:

- Older people with mild diabetes. Their hypoglycemia is called *reactive hypoglycemia secondary to (2°) mild diabetes*
- Young people (often thin young women) with a high sensitivity to insulin and thus an "alimentary" or "functional" hypoglycemia

True hypoglycemia is diagnosed by a 5 or 6 hour *glucose tolerance test* that measures blood sugar after drinking a concentrated glucose beverage. Figure 24-1 illustrates these blood sugar levels for a normal person and for one who is hypoglycemic.

Diet treatment usually includes small, frequent high-protein meals and snacks, and a reduction and change in the type of carbohydrate. Illustrated on page 204 is a sample diet for an individual with functional hypoglycemia.

Hypoglycemia is a popular term and too often persons may attempt to diagnose the condition themselves without consulting a physician. If they put themselves on too restricted a diet, it is possible that they will not obtain certain nutrients. Some persons may comment

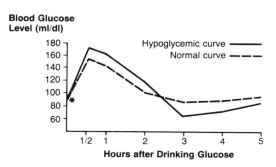

*Normal fasting blood sugar is between 80 mg/dl and 120 mg/dl (mg.%).

Figure 24-1
Blood sugar curves after glucose tolerance test (GTT).

SAMPLE MENU FOR INDIVIDUAL WITH FUNCTIONAL HYPOGLYCEMIA

Meals

Breakfast
½ cup Orange juice
2 Soft-boiled eggs
½ slice Toast
1 tsp Margarine
1 cup Decaffeinated coffee
(artificial sweetener)

Lunch
3 oz Chicken
¼ cup Rice
½ cup Tomato juice
½ slice Bread
2 tsp Margarine
½ cup Fresh cut fruit
Unsweetened decaffeinated coffee

Dinner
3 oz Sirloin steak
½ cup Cooked carrots
¾ cup Tossed lettuce salad
1 tbsp Mayonnaise
2 halves Unsweetened pears
½ cup Milk
Decaffeinated coffee

Snacks

Mid-morning
3 oz Sliced cheese
3 Saltines
½ cup Milk

Mid-afternoon
2 oz Cold sliced beef
½ slice Bread
1 tsp Margarine
½ cup Milk

Evening
2 oz Chicken
½ slice Bread
1 tsp Margarine
½ cup Milk

(Adapted from University of Iowa Hospitals and Clinics, Nutrition Department: Recent Advances in Therapeutic Diets, 2nd ed, p 113. Ames, Iowa State University Press, 1973

that "junk foods" (candy bars, cake, soda) seem to relieve the symptoms of hypoglycemia. They should be advised to avoid these foods; if true hypoglycemia exists these very foods may set them up for another reaction and become part of a vicious cycle. But any *strict* diet should begin only after a medical checkup, a positive glucose tolerance test, and the recommendation of a physician.

The Glycemic Index

Carbohydrate foods do not all cause identical blood sugar and insulin responses. Different types of carbohydrates have different weights, molecular forms, and thus are absorbed in different ways in the body. Carbohydrates that can enter the blood quickly (for example, fluids that contain glucose) give the blood a (temporarily) higher concentration of blood sugar (glucose) than those carbohydrates that are digested and absorbed more slowly (such as lentils, or dry, cooked beans that are high in fiber). Many factors affect the rate of digestion and absorption: fiber, protein, fat, disease, metabolism, and the form of carbohydrate. Some persons who have trouble controlling blood sugar may want to increase the proportion of carbohydrate foods that may help them minimize daily changes in blood sugar. The presence of other types of nutrients may change the rate of absorption in other ways. This relative measure of how quickly a carbohydrate food causes increased blood sugar is called the *glycemic index*. It compares foods to some established standard, usually glucose or white bread. Table 24-1 lists the foods that have been tested and compared with the glycemic index of white bread. The carbohydrate foods *least* likely to cause a fast, high blood sugar are the legumes.

The specific usefulness of the glycemic index is still a subject of controversy. In general, foods with the lowest glycemic indices are not com-

Table 24-1

*Glycemic Indices of Some Common Foods
(compared with white bread)*

Food Group	Food*	Average Glycemic Index (G.I.)†
Bread	White	100
	Whole wheat	99
	Wholegrain rye	58
Cereal products	Millet	103
	Brown rice	96
	Sweet corn	87
	White rice	83
	Wholewheat spaghetti	61
Breakfast cereals	Cornflakes	119
	"Weetabix"	109
	Porridge Oats	85
	All Bran	73
Starchy vegetables	Instant potato	116
	New, boiled potato	81
	Frozen peas	74
	Sweet potato	70
Legumes	Dried, green peas	56
	Kidney beans	54
	Chickpeas	49
	Red lentils	43
	Dried soybeans	22
Fruit	Raisins	93
	Banana	79
	Orange juice	67
	Orange	66
	Apple	53
	Pear	47
	Grapefruit	36
	Plum	34
	Cherries	32
Sugars	Maltose	152
	Glucose	138
	Honey	126
	Sucrose	86
	Fructose	30
Dairy products	Yogurt	52
	Ice cream	52
	Whole milk	49

* All foods were tested in 50 g carbohydrate portions
† Glycemic Index (G.I.) = (blood glucose area of test food/b.g.a. of reference food) × 100.
(From: Jenkins. DJA et al: The glycemic response to carbohydrate foods. *Lancet:*August 18:388–391,1984)

mon daily staples in the average American diet. Perhaps they should be. The American Diabetes Association's policy statement on the glycemic index recommends that diabetics choose the carbohydrate containing foods that are *least* likely to raise blood sugar levels.[2]

DISACCHARIDASE DEFICIENCIES

Lactose Intolerance

One of the most common food tolerance problems is an inablility to digest milk readily. It is usually lactose, the sugar in milk, that causes the problem. Persons who do not manufacture high levels of *lactase* (the enzyme that breaks down milk sugar into glucose and galactose) cannot tolerate large quantities of *lactose*. When there is not enough lactase, the undigested lactose continues on through the intestines and causes gas, cramps, and diarrhea. The condition is called *lactose intolerance*.

Lactase deficiency is more common among people of African or Asian descent (70%–95%) than Caucasians (6%–10%), occurs in all parts of the world, and is more common in adults than in infants.[3a]

Some persons can produce small amounts of lactase and so can digest some lactose-containing foods. They may be able to drink a half cup of milk with no complaints, but develop severe gas pains after drinking a larger amount. Sometimes a lactose intolerance develops after an intestinal illness, or while someone is on a medication that causes intestinal changes. Antibiotics may destroy natural bacteria and other substances in the small intestine that help break down nutrients, including lactose. Usually this type of intolerance is only temporary. After the intestine returns to normal, so does the activity of the lactase enzyme.

Lactose intolerance is not the same as milk allergy. Persons with a lactose intolerance can eat foods that contain milk products only if there is little *lactose* in the product or if the product has been treated to break down the sugar. Milk is composed of casein ("curds") and whey; the whey contains most of the lactose. Cheese is made by coagulating the casein and draining off the whey. Thus natural cheeses are very low in lactose. Processed and soft cheeses, on the other hand usually have milk solids (with lactose) *added* so are not recommended for individuals with lactose intolerance.

Milk can also be *treated* with lactose, the enzyme that is commercially available in drugstores as "Lact-Aid." Several drops are added to each quart of milk and it is then allowed to sit, refrigerated, for 24 hours while the enzyme breaks down the lactose. Lact-Aid-treated milk can usually be used without causing gastrointestinal upset. This type of milk is also available commercially with 70% of lactose treated and can be used immediately. Because of the sugar breakdown, it tastes a bit sweeter than regular milk but contains exactly the same amount of carbohydrate, now chiefly glucose and galactose.

How much lactose is allowed in a diet depends on how much a person can tolerate. Milk, buttermilk, yogurt, kefir (a bacteria-cultured milk similar to yogurt), unripened cheeses (such as ricotta, and cottage cheese), sour cream, ice cream, and cream cheese all contain lactose, but in varying amounts. Hard cheeses do not contain lactose. Many persons can tolerate cheeses and fermented dairy products even though they contain some lactose. Yogurt contains as much lactose as milk, yet it is often well accepted. This may be a result of lactase-production by the yogurt culture (bacteria) itself.[4]

Heating milk does not change the amount of lactose in the milk, or the form of the lactose.

Persons with lactose intolerance still need calcium. They may need to acquire calcium from sources other than milk and may need to work more consciously to acquire a sufficient quantity.

Sucrose and Maltose Intolerance

Sucrase is the the enzyme that breaks sucrose down into glucose and fructose. Sucrase deficiency is a rare genetic defect that may be combined with a deficiency in dextrinase or maltase (the enzyme that breaks down maltose).[3b] Diet treatment may require only the simple elimination of table sugar and other products that contain these sugars. These enzymes are not commercially available.

Sometimes these enzymes are deficient because of an acute disease that has temporarily destroyed the enzyme's activity. Cholera, gastrointestinal flu, or a chronic problem such as an irritable bowel syndrome, or a shortened intestinal tract (the result of surgery) may lead to a sucrase or maltase deficiency. Because the disaccharidases are active in the jejunum (see Figure 1-2), any damage to this part of the intestinal tract will affect sucrose, maltose and lactose absorption. When healing occurs (as a result of medication, diet, and/or other treatments), the enzyme activity may return in whole or in part.

Diet treatment depends on the disease or condition involved and may require nutrients other than these specific carbohydrates. Sucrose and maltose are added to many foods, and are contained naturally in many others.

Celiac Sprue

Celiac sprue is also called gluten-sensitive enteropathy or nontropical sprue. It is a lifelong hypersensitivity to the substance called gliadin, which is a part of the composition of *gluten*.

Gluten in the diet—even in a very small amount—causes a good deal of damage to the absorptive surface of the small intestine. The villi or or hairlike surface where nutrients are absorbed (see Figure 1-3) are destroyed. The results are malabsorption, enzyme deficiencies, diarrhea, and steatorrhea (diarrhea caused by fat malabsorption). The most effective treatment is a lifelong diet absolutely free of gluten.

Gluten is found in wheat, rye, oats, and barley. Many gluten-containing substances (listed below) are added to processed foods. Therefore, it is difficult to maintain a gluten-free diet. Since processed cereal and convenience foods usually contain some form of gluten, the client with

FOODS THAT CONTAIN GLUTEN

All purpose flour
Apple-flavored vinegar
Barley
Beverages made with grain alcohol (includes most alcoholic beverages)
Breaded foods
Brewer's yeast (some)
Buckwheat groats
Bulgar wheat
Caramel coloring
Cereal (except 100% corn or rice or special prepared gluten-free cereal)
Cereal beverages (including Postum, Ovaltine, cocoa mixes)
Cream sauces
Emulsifiers
Flour
Gluten
Gluten stabilizers
Graham flour
Hot dogs and other processed meats (many)
Hydrolyzed vegetable protein
Kasha

Luncheon meats
Malt and malt drinks (*e.g.*, beer, malted milk)
Malt flavoring
Malt syrup
Malt vinegar
Millet
Modified starch
Oat bran
Pasta
Processed cheese and cheese food products
Rye
Rye flour
Semolina (couscous, a form of wheat)
Soy sauce (some)
Stabilizers
Triticale (mix of wheat and rye flour)
Vegetable gum
Wheat
Wheat bran, germ, gluten, and starch

Some medications may also contain wheat or other gluten-containing substances

(From Midwestern Celiac Sprue Association: Gluten-Free Diet. Des Moines, Midwestern Celiac Sprue Association)

celiac sprue must strictly control the consumption of all grain products and carefully check labels for foods that might contain even a trace of gluten. The person just beginning a gluten-free diet may still have damaged intestines unable to tolerate lactose and often other gluten-free substances. Often, however, after a week on the diet, the villi return and the surface may be healed sufficiently to introduce these particular foods once again.

Medical care and diet counseling are critical in celiac sprue. It is most important for the client with recurrent symptoms, anyone having trouble planning an adequate diet, or the newly diagnosed individual. A national celiac sprue organization exists for support and education. The address of the national organization is listed under "Resources" at the end of this chapter. Local branches are listed in most telephone directories. Special gluten-free products are available in some pharmacies. Specific information about these or other local resources is available from these organizations or from a local dietitian. A sample menu for a client with celiac sprue is shown below.

Galactosemia

Galactosemia is an inborn error of metabolism that will be discussed in Chapter 34.

FIBER-CONTROLLED DIETS

The types of carbohydrates that make up dietary fiber are often increased or decreased in the treatment of certain complaints and diseases.

When the intestines are sensitive, inflamed or diseased, low-fiber diets may be necessary to help avoid further irritation of the area. This occurs in Crohn's disease or Crohn's ileitis (see Chapter 33). In Crohn's disease, the entire gastrointestinal tract is very easily damaged. A low-fiber diet may help minimize this damage. Fiber may also be restricted in *diverticulitis.* Diverticuli are forced pouches created in the intestinal wall. A person who develops these pouches is said to have *diverticulosis.* When the pouches become inflamed and very painful (sometimes because food particles become trapped in them), the condition is called *diverticulitis* or inflammation of the diverticuli. Low-fiber diets help reduce the irritation to a minimum.

Low-fiber diets may also be called low *residue* diets. *Mechanical soft diets* or "liquid" diets may also be low in fiber and be designed for the client who has trouble chewing or swallowing. (Chapter 35 discusses diet control by texture.)

Fiber has many benefits in most diets, however, as was discussed in Chapter 10. This is why high-fiber diets may be part of current medical treatment for diabetes mellitus, coronary artery

---

SAMPLE MENU FOR GLUTEN-FREE DIET

Breakfast	*Lunch*	*Dinner*
Apple juice	Chicken	Broiled fish
100% Cream of rice cereal	Rice	Butter
	Broccoli	Lemon juice
Milk	Butter	Baked potato
Soft-boiled egg	Lettuce–tomato salad	Carrots
Special gluten-free bread	Mayonnaise	Salad with permitted dressing
Grape jelly	Canned peaches	Jello with cream
Coffee with milk/ sugar		Coffee with milk/ sugar
	Snack	*Snack*
	Flavored yogurt	Puffed rice bar
		Milk

disease and some gastrointestinal diseases such as diverticulosis, as well as constipation and hemorrhoids.[3c,5,6]

Fiber is recommended in diabetes because fibrous foods are digested more slowly than lower-fiber carbohydrates. In the gut, fiber seems to prevent rapid absorption of other foods as well. This slowed release of glucose from the diet into the blood may help control blood sugar levels.

Some medical authorities believe fiber may help lower blood lipids (cholesterol, lipoproteins) by binding with them in the digestive tract and preventing complete absorption. This may help slow or prevent coronary artery disease. The evidence is not yet conclusive. However, high-fiber foods are very low in fat and cholesterol. They could certainly be added to the diet if a person with coronary artery disease wanted more fiber, and they may be good substitutes for high-fat, high-cholesterol foods.

Fiber is most clearly beneficial in certain gastrointestinal problems. A high fiber diet in diverticulosis helps to keep the diverticuli clear of food particles and perhaps helps minimize the risk for further infection. The pouches them-

Table 24-2

Guide for a Fiber-Controlled Diet

Food Group	Lower Fiber Foods	Higher Fiber Foods
Dairy products	All	None
Protein	Meat,* Fish, Poultry, Eggs*	Dry beans and peas Seeds, Nuts* Peanut butter*
Fruit	Canned, cooked fruits except prunes and figs Avocado* Apple juice†	Dry fruits Raw fruits Prune juice
Vegetables	Peeled, cooked or canned vegetables, seeds removed Vegetable juices†	All raw, steamed or stir-fried vegetables Vegetable peels, seeds
Grains and cereals	White (bleached or unbleached) flour Breads and cereals made from white flour and free of "high-fiber" ingredients (seeds, dry fruits, whole grains)	Whole grains (wheat, oats, rye, barley, corn, *etc.*) Flour, Cereals, Breads and Crackers made from whole grains Bran products Wheat germ Cracked wheat Kasha (buckwheat groats)
Condiments/Beverages	Oils,* Catsup, Mustard, Horseradish, Seasoning mixes, Vinegar, All herbs and spices except seeds All alcoholic beverages	Pickles, Relish, Hot peppers, seeds Persons on a high-fiber diet should get enough fluid to help elimination of the increased bulk

*May be high in fat

†These foods contain dietary fiber but are sometimes permitted on low-fiber diets because they do not irritate the digestive tract

(Note: This list is only a general guideline. Any client on a specific, fiber-controlled diet should receive individual diet counseling)

selves may be created by the pressure of a low-fiber diet, in which residue forces itself slowly through the intestines. A high-fiber diet must also include plenty of fluid. Since fiber absorbs water, stools will be softer, will move more quickly, and will create less pressure on the intestinal walls.

Constipation is also usually treated with fiber, either from medication, diet, or both.

Table 24-2 provides a guideline for a fiber-controlled diet.

LOW-CARBOHYDRATE DIETS FOR WEIGHT LOSS

Chapter 4 briefly discussed the effects of a low-carbohydrate diet. These diets are common. They usually restrict all grains, cereals, fruits, and milk and may allow unlimited quantities of meat, fish, poultry, and often hard cheeses, some vegetables, and most fats and oils. These diets promise fast weight loss and appetite control. However, they are not nutritionally sound for several reasons:

Water Loss. Initial weight loss is a result of water loss, not fat loss. Fat is lost only when the energy output exceeds the energy input. When the diet returns to normal, much of the water lost is often gained again.

High Fat. These diets are often extremely high in fat content. Depending on the type of fat, blood cholesterol levels may increase. Large amounts of fat are not recommended (see Chapter 5). Blood lipids may increase on such diets.

Ketones. When dietary carbohydrate drops below a certain level, the body starts to burn fat for energy. This fat comes from the diet or the stores of fat in the cells. By-products of this fat breakdown, *ketones,* are then produced and excreted in the urine. Ketones compete with uric acid (a by-product of protein breakdown; see Chapter 23); the kidneys will excrete ketones first. Thus, the uric acid level of the blood may rise,[7] and individuals susceptible to gout may suffer.

The presence of ketones does not necessarily mean the body is breaking down its fat stores. If the diet is high enough in energy to maintain weight, the ketones in the urine may be from the fat in the food consumed.

Any person who is not on a low carbohydrate diet but detects ketones in the urine should consult a physician immediately, since this is a sign of disease.

Nutritionally Inadequate. The low-carbohydrate diet omits entire food groups and, therefore, many essential vitamins and minerals. It is also low in fiber, so may lead to constipation.

Poor Endurance. Muscle is burned, as well as fat. The result is less body muscle and a decrease in physical endurance.

STUDY QUESTIONS

1. What is the relationship between insulin and blood sugar?

2. When might a physician want to place a person on a carbohydrate-controlled diet?

3. A woman says she is *hypoglycemic.*
   - What does she mean?
   - What test will determine if she is truly hypoglycemic?
   - Does this mean she has diabetes?

4. What is the "glycemic index" of foods?

5. Rate the following foods 1 – 7, with 1 being the food which causes the most rapid rise in blood glucose:

_____ Soy beans	_____ Orange juice
_____ Honey	_____ Brown rice
_____ Whole wheat bread	_____ Fructose
	_____ Sweet potato

6. What causes lactose intolerance?

7. What foods contain lactose?

8. In what conditions might sucrose and/or maltose intolerance occur?

9. What is the most important diet restriction in celiac sprue? List at least five foods which must be eliminated from the diet.

10. Why is dietary fiber sometimes restricted in a diet?

11. What foods are high in fiber among the
    - Protein foods
    - Grains and cereals?

12. Tina is on a low carbohydrate diet, trying to

lose weight. Each day for the past week she has eaten only broiled fish, broiled chicken, hard cheese, salad with sour cream dressing, and coffee. She says she has lost 5 pounds but always feels nauseous and has little energy.

- What are some of the problems of her diet?
- What would you tell Tina?

REFERENCES

1. Joslin Diabetes Foundation: Reactive Hypoglycemia. Boston, Joslin Diabetes Foundation Inc., 1972.
2. Council on Nutrition of the American Diabetes Association: ADA issues policy statement: Glycemic effects of carbohydrate, Diabetes Forecast. 37 (3): 20–21, May–June 1985
3. Goodhart RE, Shils ME: Modern Nutrition in Health and Disease, 6th ed, pp a, 492; b, 105; c 1048. Philadelphia, Lea & Febiger, 1980
4. Olson, RE (ed): *In vivo* digestion of yogurt by lactase. Nutr Rev 42:216–218, 1984
5. Fiber and the Patient with Diabetes Mellitus: An Annotated Bibliography. Chicago, American Dietetic Association Council on Practice, 1980
6. Burkitt D: Fiber as protective against gastrointestinal diseases. Am. J. Gastroenterol 79(4): 249–252, 1984
7. Worthington BS, Taylor LE: Balanced low calorie vs. low-protein low-carbohydrate reducing diets. J Am Diet Assoc. 64:52–55, January 1974

RESOURCES

Celiac Sprue Association—USA, 2313 Rocklyn Drive, Des Moines, IA 50322
Lact-Aid Inc., P.O. Box 111, Pleasantville, NJ 08232

CHAPTER 25

Fat-Controlled Diets

OBJECTIVES

1. To review briefly the role of fat in normal nutrition
2. To discuss national recommendations for dietary fat and cholesterol reduction
3. To discuss situations in which a lipid-controlled diet is sometimes indicated:
   a. The high fat diet
   b. Coronary artery and peripheral vascular disease
   c. Hyperlipidemias
   d. Gallbladder dysfunction
   e. Pancreatic insufficiency
4. For each of the above, to explain the rationale and provide practical guidelines to help clients follow a diet

Chapter 5 described the many types of fats or lipids found in foods and in the body. It identified the major dietary sources of fat and discussed their importance. It outlined the different types of lipids in the blood and their role in energy production and storage. A good understanding of the role of fat in normal nutrition is necessary to understand the major circumstances that require fat or lipid control.

Fats are an easy, concentrated energy source because they provide twice as many calories (9 per gram) as the same amount of carbohydrate or protein (4 per gram). High-fat diets are rarely recommended by physicians except to increase the concentration of calories when a client is severely underweight. A high (100 gram) fat diet is sometimes used as a test diet when a physician feels a person may not be absorbing fat sufficiently. The diet is followed for several days, with the client including 100 grams of fat in the diet each day. Fat absorption is tested by measuring how much fat is lost in the stool. The details of this diet may vary from one health care facility to another.

Most fat-controlled diets limit or lower dietary lipids. The Dietary Guidelines (see Chapter 12) recommend a diet providing 30% of total daily calories from fat, including 10% from saturated fats and daily cholesterol intake of less than 300 milligrams. The American Heart Association's recommendation for blood lipid control also suggests limiting fat to 30% of calories with 10% each from polyunsaturates and monounsaturates and 8% from saturated fat. They recommend limiting cholesterol to 250 milligrams per day; salt, to 4 grams per day, and advise that individuals eat more unrefined carbohydrate (whole grains, legumes, fruits and vegetables).[1] Much research has been conducted and controversy has developed over a possible link between a high-fat diet and certain types of cancer, resulting in recommendations for a diet lower in fat.[2,3] Fats, like protein and carbohydrate, are controlled in the treatment of some diseases. These diseases will be the focus of this chapter.

Diets may be fat-controlled for several reasons:

Lipids in the blood can build up, creating "plaque" or thick deposits on the walls of the blood vessels and eventually blocking the passage. This is called *coronary artery disease* when it occurs in the blood vessels of the heart. When it occurs in blood vessels in other, more distant parts of the body, it is called peripheral vascular disease. Coronary artery disease *(CAD)* may lead to heart attacks or stroke. When the flow of blood is restricted, even for a limited amount of time, the cells, which cannot get food and oxygen from the blood, will die. A fat-controlled diet is sometimes used to help prevent or slow the accumulation of plaque deposits.

Lipids, together with medication, are sometimes controlled to help limit or lower blood cholesterol or triglyceride levels.

Because lipids are concentrated sources of energy, a low-fat diet is often part of a weight-loss program.

Fat-controlled diets are also used to test, prevent, or treat a problem with fat digestion or absorption.

CORONARY ARTERY DISEASE

As mentioned above, CAD is a general term for the thickening of the blood vessels by deposits of fat, primarily cholesterol. The deposits, called *plaque,* build up inside the vessel walls. The channel for blood flow becomes narrower and narrower. The lipids that build these thick deposits come from the very blood flowing through the channels. Medications, along with a fat- and cholesterol-restricted diet are often used to try to minimize the risk of further disease and to prevent the vessels from closing entirely by stopping or reversing the buildup.

Fat is not the only substance that must be controlled in CAD. Energy may be controlled to help the client lose weight. Sodium or other electrolytes may be controlled as part of treatment for high blood pressure. The type of carbohydrate and alcohol intake may be controlled to help lower triglycerides and/or to encourage weight loss. A client with CAD who smokes may be told to quit.

Diet control often begins *after* the disease has

already led to a myocardial infarction (MI, heart attack) or a stroke (where a blood vessel in the brain has become blocked, clotted, or erupted). It is frequently accompanied by treatment, including many medications, and often some type of surgery. These treatments may help the client survive, but they do not cure the disease. Diet therapy can help to minimize the risk of further damage. The fewer lipids in the blood, the less likely it is that damage will recur. Diet may have an important role in lowering blood lipids.

In CAD, cholesterol and saturated fats are the lipids that are usually controlled. Total fat may also be limited. Table 5-1 provides a useful list of the cholesterol levels in certain foods.

Cholesterol-free blood is an impossibility. The liver manufacturers cholesterol naturally and this lipid is necessary in normal metabolism. But the liver may produce all the cholesterol needed; "more" is not necessarily better. Diet control may help blood control though some individuals may continue to produce excessive cholesterol. The lower the blood levels of these fats, the less risk of an artery becoming clogged, causing stroke or heart attack.

Saturated fats may also be restricted. As described in Chapter 5, almost all saturated fats are solid at room temperature. Most of them (except coconut oil, palm oil, and hydrogenated vegetable oils) are animal products that may also contain cholesterol. Cholesterol and saturated fats are not the same thing. But a diet high in saturated fats may, for some people, play a role in high cholesterol levels. The U.S. Dietary Goals suggest a national limiting of saturated fats to about 10% of total energy; the American Heart Association suggests 8%[1]. This means that the remaining 20% may come from polyunsaturated and monounsaturated fats — 10% from each. Table 25-1 lists foods high in saturated fats, with acceptable alternatives from poly-or monounsaturated fats.

HYPERLIPIDEMIAS

Hyperlipidemias are, by definition, high blood levels of lipids. A person with hyperlipidemia is at increased risk for heart disease. The type of *hyperlipidemia* (also called *hyperlipoproteine-*

Table 25-1

High-Saturated Fat, High-Cholesterol Foods With Acceptable Alternatives

Food Group	Sources of Saturated Fat	Sources of Cholesterol	↓ Saturated Fat ↓ Cholesterol Alternatives
Protein	Organ meats, Beef, Pork, Lamb, Duck, Goose, Cold cuts, Eggs	Shrimp	Poultry (white meat, skin removed) Fish Shellfish other than shrimp Dry beans, Peas Peanut butter Low cholesterol egg-substitutes
Dairy	Cream, Whole milk and Yogurt Cream cheese Ice cream Hard cheeses Cheeses made with cream, whole milk	Processed baked goods high in butter and eggs	Skim milk, Low fat yogurt Low fat ricotta or farmer's cheese Low fat cottage, mozzarella or other "low fat" cheese product Ice milk Frozen yogurt made with low fat milk
Grain, Cereals	Processed baked goods that include animal or hydrogenated fats		Baked goods made with liquid vegetable oils, Nonfat dry milk solids, which do not contain foods listed at left
Fruits, Vegetables	Coconut	None	All fruits and vegetables served or prepared without extra sources of saturated fats or cholesterol. NOTE: avocados are naturally high in (unsaturated) fat
Fats	Coconut oil Palm oil Hydrogenated oils Lard	Lard Butter Bacon fat All other meat fats	To increase Polyunsatured:Saturated fat ratio, substitute liquid vegetable oils (do not use coconut or palm). Use margarines with labelling information that indicates the P:S ratio is greater than 1:1 To limit total fat, bake, broil, steam or boil foods without adding fat sources; use seasonings low in or free of fat.
Condiments, Desserts, and Snack Foods	Any containing above ingredients Cream-filled cookies, Pastries Ice cream bars Chips, Curls, etc., fried in above fats Chocolate		Gingersnaps, Graham crackers, Fig bars Popsicles Acceptable margarines, Jam, Peanut butter Most condiments, herbs, and spices are low in fat though they may be high in sodium and/or sugar Note: mayonnaise is high in (unsaturated) fat.

mia or HLP) depends on the type and proportion of lipid (carried in the form of lipoprotein molecules) that is elevated. Table 5-2 describes the types of lipoproteins that carry lipids. The lightest carriers are the chylomicrons. The heaviest are the high-density lipoproteins (HDLs). Each lipoprotein carries a particular proportion of cholesterol or triglyceride. When the fat levels in the blood reach too high a level, one or several of the lipoproteins must also increase in number to carry the extra loads of cholesterol or triglyceride. The normal balance and proportion of the four lipoproteins—chylomicrons, very low density (VLDL), low density (LDL), and high density lipoproteins (HDL)—is lost. Further testing (by centrifuging blood to measure the proportions of lipoproteins as they arrange themselves in a test tube from the heaviest to lightest) can help researchers tell which type of HLP is present. Then treatment is planned.

Table 25-2 outlines the major types of HLP. Each type is distinct and involves a different treatment, which may include diet and medication. All types of HLP may develop as a result of genetics, lifestyle (that is, obesity, alcohol, lack of exercise), or disease. Both diet and medications may be the lifelong treatments that help prevent serious complications.

CHOLECYSTITIS

Cholecystitis is the inflammation of the gallbladder. It usually occurs when gallstones have developed in the gallbladder and then have begun to irritate or block the organ's normal bile acid production. This bile production is the main function of the gallbladder. Bile flows from the organ, down the common bile duct (a channel shared by the gallbladder and the pancreas; see Chapter 1), and into the small intestine. Bile production is a normal reflex that is triggered by the entrance of fat into the small intestine. When gallstones block the gallbladder or become lodged in the common bile duct,

1. Bile produced does not reach the small intestine to help break down fat
2. The pressure of bile against the gallstones causes severe pain
3. Fat is not properly digested.

Common treatment for this situation is surgery; the gallbladder is drained and the stones are removed. A low-fat diet is important because very little bile needs to be released if there is little fat in the diet. All types of fats are severely restricted, especially before and sometimes immediately after surgery. Once the client has recovered, most physicians gradually reintroduce fats into the diet.

PANCREATIC INSUFFICIENCY

Pancreatic *lipase* is the key enzyme that breaks down long-chain triglycerides. This enzyme is manufactured in the pancreas and, together with bile, enters the digestive system through the common bile duct. When the pancreas is diseased, blocked, or damaged, there may not be a sufficient quantity of the enzyme to break down the lipids, and malabsorption may occur. This can happen in cystic fibrosis, pancreatic cancer, chronic pancreatitis (an inflamed or infected pancreas), or severe protein energy malnutrition.

When the pancreas cannot produce enough pancreatic lipase, fats are not digested and are lost in the stool. This leads to many problems: diarrhea, weight loss because of the energy lost, and a difficulty absorbing fat-soluble vitamins. The usual diet treatment is to select a source of fat that can be absorbed *without* pancreatic lipase. Medium chain triglycerides (MCTs) are the only fats that do not need this enzyme; MCTs are simply absorbed into the mucosa of the small intestine and carried to the liver through the portal vein. Since they are fats, MCTs contain the same concentration of energy (9 per gram) as long-chain triglycerides, and they can help a client avoid diarrhea and weight loss.

However, there are several problems with MCTs. They are not available in significant quantities in food. Commercial "MCT Oil" is the major source. This oil, which is then used in cooking and food preparation, is expensive. It is available only from a pharmacy and it does not contain the essential fatty acids, which must be provided in some other way. Because it is not metabolized in the same way that long-chain triglycerides are metabolized, it is not a good

Table 25-2

Hyperlipoproteinemias: A Summary

Type	Occurrence	High Lipoprotein	Blood Is ↑ = High ↓ = Low	Complaints, Risks	Role of Diet
I	Very rare; appears in infancy 2° genetics	Chylomicrons	↑↑ TG* maybe ↑ Chol.	Severe abdominal pain, pancreatitis, affects liver, spleen, some need insulin	Low fat diet; maybe MCTs. Alcohol not recommended.
IIa	Common genetic disorder diagnosed in childhood	Low Density Lipoproteins (LDL)	↑ Chol.	CHD may develop early; xanthomas	Fat Cholesterol P:S ratio of 1.0
IIb		LDL and VLDL	↑ Chol. maybe ↑ TG		
III	Uncommon; detected in adulthood	Intermediate Density Lipoproteins (IDLs)	↑ TG ↑ Chol	Early CHD and vascular disease; Obesity, glucose intolerance, ↑ Uric acid in blood; xanthomas	
IV	Common; detected in adulthood May often be related to drugs, disease, obesity, and/or inadequate exercise	Very Low Density Lipoproteins (VLDLs)	↑ TG, maybe ↑ Chol		Achieve normal weight Limit saturated fat, cholesterol P:S ratio of 1.0
V	Uncommon; genetic disorder detected in adulthood Sometimes also related to diabetes, alcoholism, or kidney diseases.	VLDLs and Chylomicrons	↑↑ TG, maybe ↑ Chol.	Obesity; ↑ uric acid in blood, glucose intolerance, xanthomas May have arthritis, dry mucous membranes, fatty, enlarged liver and spleen	Achieve normal weight Limit saturated fats, cholesterol, and simple sugars Alcohol not recommended

* Triglycerides

(From Goodhart RS, Shils ME: Modern Nutrition in Health and Disease, 6th ed, pp 1058–1069. Philadelphia, Lea and Febiger, 1980; Thomas CL (ed): Taber's Cyclopedic Medical Dictionary, 13th ed, p H-74. Philadelphia, FA Davis, 1977; Lipid Disorder. Unpublished notes from Molecular Disease Branch, National Heart, Lung, and Blood Institute, National Institute of Health)

carrier for the fat-soluble vitamins; consequently, physicians often prescribe water-soluble forms of these vitamins.

STUDY QUESTIONS

1. Referring to Chapters 5 and 25, define the following terms:
   - a. Lipid
   - b. Saturated fat
   - c. Polyunsaturated fat
   - d. Triglyceride
   - e. Cholesterol
   - f. P:S ratio

2. 50 grams of fat provide how much food energy?

3. List and explain three reasons dietary lipids might need to be controlled.

4. Plaque, the fatty deposits that build up on the walls of blood vessels, is made up of many substances; what is one?

5. What two types of lipids are often limited in the diet of a client with CAD? List at least three different food sources of each type of lipid.

6. List five foods high in cholesterol or saturated fats. What would be acceptable alternatives (low in cholesterol and saturated fats) for each?

7. What is "hyperlipidemia"?

8. Betty L. has HLP Type IV. She is not overweight but has some signs of CAD and glucose intolerance. Her typical breakfast is: toast with butter and jelly, two scrambled eggs, and coffee with three teaspoons of sugar.
   - a. Why should she change her breakfast and choose different foods?
   - b. What foods would you suggest? Why?

9. Why is a low-fat diet recommended in
   - a. Cholecystitis?
   - b. Pancreatic insufficiency?

10. a. What are MCTs?
    - b. Why are they used in fat malabsorption disorders?
    - c. What are the major sources of MCTs?

REFERENCES

1. Kannel WB et al: Report of inter-society commission for heart disease resources: Optimal resources for primary prevention of atherosclerotic disease. Circulation 70: 191 A, July 1984

2. van Eys J: Nutrition and neoplasia. Nutr Rev 40(12): 353–359, December 1982

3. Gorbach SL, Zimmerman DR, Woods MN: The Doctors' Anti-Breast Cancer Diet. New York City, Simon & Schuster, 1984

CHAPTER 26

Vitamin Therapy in Disease

OBJECTIVES

1. To review the role and identity of vitamins needed in human nutrition
2. To introduce vitamin therapy in disease, with a caution against self-diagnosis and treatment, megadoses, and common beliefs of many "health" proponents
3. To discuss the vitamin deficiency syndromes that may cause disease
4. To discuss briefly some major diseases and social behaviors that may result in vitamin deficiencies
5. To discuss therapeutic treatment

Chapters 6 and 7 defined the two major groups of vitamins (fat- and water-soluble) and explained why vitamins are necessary for health. The 13 vitamins known to be needed in human nutrition are listed at right. Each vitamin has a unique role to play in bodily health and well-being. Each is needed in small quantities at different stages of metabolism. This chapter will discuss what happens when those needs are *not* met or when they change, and why.

Nutrient deficiencies may result when any of the following occurs:

1. Inadequate ingestion
2. Inadequate absorption
3. Inadequate utilization
4. Increased requirement
5. Increased excretion
6. Increased destruction[1a]

Because vitamin balance, like mineral, fluid or electrolyte balance (Chapters 27 and 28), is very fine-tuned and because the Recommended Dietary Allowances (RDA) suggests *more* of each vitamin than many persons truly need, deficiencies are rare if a person is healthy and has some regular source of the vitamin. In fact, in the developed nations today, *overdoses* of vitamins are more likely than *deficiencies*. Health proponents recommending megadoses of vita-

VITAMINS KNOWN TO BE NECESSARY IN HUMAN NUTRITION

Fat-soluble vitamins:
Vitamin A (Retinol)
Vitamin D
Vitamin E (the tocopherols)
Vitamin K
Water-soluble vitamins:
Thiamin (B_1)
Riboflavin (B_2)
Niacin
Pyridoxine (B_6)
Cyanocobalamin (B_{12})
Ascorbic Acid (Vitamin C)
Pantothenic acid (Pantothenate)
Folic acid (Folacin)
Biotin

mins for every potential complaint have influenced many people to take far more of some vitamins than they really need. This is an inappropriate, ineffective use of vitamin therapy and is discussed in more detail in Chapters 6, 7, and 20. Unless they are prescribed by a physician for a specific purpose, megadoses of vitamins have little proven value in medicine and may, at times, be harmful. Until the middle of the twentieth century, however, certain vitamin deficiencies were a common occurrence. They developed because foods high in certain vitamins were not available, long-term, and their importance was not understood. These deficiencies still occur today in similar settings because of limited food supplies, inadequate variety in the diet, problems with storage or transportation, food preparation techniques that destroy the nutrient and/or lack of knowledge. These factors are common in many poor nations and in very poor areas of wealthier nations. But they also occur among the alcoholic, the mentally ill, or among people who have financial resources but who practice imbalanced, unusual food patterns. For these people, deficiency is preventable.

Of the six causes of nutrient deficiencies (listed above), only the first — inadequate ingestion — simply not getting enough of the nutrient in the diet — causes deficiencies in healthy individuals. The other five relate to disease. Disease affects the way in which the body can utilize any nutrient. Certain diseases may act upon a particular nutrient more readily than others. For example, low bile production (from disease or gallstones) leads to fat malabsorption. (This was discussed in the last chapter.) The vitamins carried by fat will be poorly absorbed and deficiency may develop over a period of time, unless some other source of these vitamins is provided.

Nutrient balance can also be upset when an organ or some part of the digestive tract is damaged. Figure 1-2 clearly diagrams the actual area along the digestive tract where the various nutrients are absorbed. If a portion of the intestine is damaged, the vitamin absorbed in that area is affected, even if the rest of the intestine is healthy. The body may not absorb it as well or at all. Deficiency results.

Table 26-1 lists the major vitamins and, when they exist, deficiency syndromes and causes. Each of these will be discussed below.

VITAMIN A

The first sign of vitamin A deficiency is *xerophythalmia* or night blindness. Night blindness occurs when bright, sudden lights in the night cause temporary but severely limiting blindness. The eye's ability to readapt to the darkness again doesn't "bounce back" as quickly as it should. If it continues, especially in children, it can lead to permanent blindness.

This deficiency is most common in underdeveloped nations where the diet has little or no sources of vitamin A, and in young children. Since dark green, leafy vegetables are high in vitamin A, including them on a regular basis in the diet may be one of the most important ways to help prevent this deficiency. When detected at an early stage, it is often treated with cod liver oil or halibut liver oil, which are both very high in vitamin A.

In the more developed nations, vitamin A deficiency is most likely to result from diseases that affect fat malabsorption. This may occur in cystic fibrosis, celiac sprue, jaundice, and hepatitis and is usually treated with medication or special forms of the vitamin, not with foods.

VITAMIN D

In children, vitamin D deficiency leads to rickets; in adults, it leads to osteomalacia. Both are the result of an imbalance in the relationship between vitamin D, calcium, and phosphorus metabolism. Vitamin D helps to mineralize (harden) bone. When the body does not acquire enough vitamin D, bones soften and are easily damaged. Children with rickets are easily recognized by their bowlegs or the prominent bumps on their ribs (referred to as the "rachitic rosary"). Most milk in developed countries today is fortified with vitamin D to help prevent rickets.

Deficiency may also be a side effect of disease. Kidney failure can affect metabolism because vitamin D must be converted to its active

Table 26-1

Vitamin Deficiencies

| | | | | Deficiency May Be Precipitated By: | | |
				Nutritional Problems	*Medical Problems*	*Social Problems*
Vitamin	*Foods Fortified*	*Deficiency Syndrome*				
A	Milk	Xerophthalmia (night blindness)		PCM with low protein intake, long-term Vitamin A deficiency	Fat malabsorption ↓ Bile output	Extreme poverty
D	Milk	Adults: osteomalacia Children: rickets		Lack of Vitamin D from diet and/or sunlight	Genetic defects Kidney disease	Lack of sunlight from urban living Excess clothing No time outdoors.
E	—	Vitamin E deficiency		—	Prematurity, low birth weight Cholestasis Thalassemia	—
K	—	Vitamin K deficiency		Rare; may be 2° gut changes in pellagra	Prematurity Sterile gut Fat malabsorption ↓ Bile production	—
Thiamin	Some grains and cereal products	Beriberi		Subsistent diet of polished rice	Damage to jejunum Chronic vomiting	Alcoholism
Riboflavin	—	Ariboflavinosis		Rare	Needs of growth to repair tissue damage	—

Niacin	—	Pellagra	Diet of primarily maize or sorghum vulgare $\downarrow$ Niacin $\downarrow$ Protein	—	Extreme poverty
Pyridoxine	—	B_6 deficiency	Long-term inadequate diet	Damage/surgery to jejunum	—
Pantothenate	—	Pantothenate deficiency	Rare; usually part of general malnutrition	Genetic abnormalities	Long-term diet of solely processed food with little pantothenate content
Vitamin C	Some fruit juices, fruit drinks	Scurvy	3–5 months without Vitamin C source	Increased needs in trauma; Damage to jejunum	Living in isolated areas during long winter months without fresh produce; Possible in extreme poverty
Folacin	—	Megaloblastic anemias	Months on highly processed foods $\downarrow$ Absorption 2° $\uparrow$ Bean diet	Cancer; Blood loss; Kidney disease; Sprue; Some medications	Lactation; Pregnancy; Alcoholism
Vit. B_{12}	—	Megaloblastic or Pernicious anemia	Chronic vegan diet	Lack of intrinsic factor; Competitive need of parasites and bacterial overgrowth; Damage or surgery to distal ileum; Hyperthyroid; Liver or kidney disease	Pregnancy; Poverty; Food faddism; Alcoholism
Biotin	—	Biotin deficiency	$\uparrow$ Avidin intake from raw egg whites	Inborn errors of metabolism	—

form in the kidneys. Because the balance of vitamin D, calcium, and phosphorus is so precarious, treatment must be carefully supervised.

VITAMIN E

A vitamin E deficiency is extremely rare. Some infants may be treated with parenteral vitamin E to prevent the possible retinal complications that may result from prematurity[2] or as part of treatment for beta-thalassemia, cholestasis, or sickle cell anemia.[3,4] Problems with fat absorption will affect the absorption of this vitamin. Abetalipoproteinemia, the most severe form of vitamin E deficiency, may affect children and young adults.

VITAMIN K

Like E, vitamin K deficiency may occur in premature infants but not in adults except, perhaps, as part of general malnutrition resulting from changes in the intestine. Normally, the bacteria in the intestine manufacture vitamin K, but in an infants's first few days, the gut is sterile (no bacteria). Since the vitamin helps blood to clot, premature infants may be given this vitamin to encourage normal blood clotting until they are developed sufficiently to produce their own vitamin K.

THIAMIN

Thiamin deficiency is common throughout history. Called "beriberi," it was most often seen among Asian people whose diet consisted mostly of polished rice, that is, rice cleaned of its outer (bran) surface. The thiamin in rice is stored in the bran. Because the bran was discarded and used for animal feed, humans became deficient in this vitamin. At the end of the 19th century, it was finally discovered to be a nutrient deficiency, and this discovery made treatment more widely available. Beriberi may still occur however, among infants who may be fed only gruels of white rice (congee) if they have no other food source.

Because the vitamin is absorbed in the jejunum, surgery on that area may increase the risk of deficiency. The poor diet of a chronic alcoholic may also lead to thiamin deficiency.

RIBOFLAVIN

Riboflavin deficiency is rare and occurs only after months with a diet that lacks the vitamin. Deficiency is usually part of general malnutrition and accompanies other nutrient deficiencies.

NIACIN

Called *pellagra,* niacin deficiency was quite common, even epidemic, during the early decades of the twentieth century, especially in the southeastern USA. For centuries it has developed after long-term subsistence on maize or certain types of sorghum.

Pellagra is both a niacin (vitamin) and tryptophan (amino acid) deficiency, because niacin is manufactured in the body by tryptophan. Maize or corn does contain niacin, but it is in a form that is "bound" or not available for absorption. The protein in maize is "limited" or proportionately low in the amino acid tryptophan (see Chapter 3 for a discussion of complementary amino acid balance). So, among the poor in the southeastern USA who ate primarily cornmeal, molasses, and pork fat, the disease, pellagra, afflicted many and led to many deaths. It could have been prevented.

In some nations, maize is treated with alkalies such as lime. Cornmeal treated with lime is called *masa harina* and contains more available niacin, since the treatment "unbinds" some of the vitamin. Ground coffee may also contain niacin and help to prevent pellagra, even though the diet may still be deficient in protein and lead to other deficiency diseases.

Niacin (niacinamide) is one vitamin currently used by many physicians as a pharmacologic agent in the treatment of coronary artery disease and some hyperlipidemias.

B₆

Vitamin B_6 deficiency may result in decreased conversion of tryptophan to niacin. This deficiency is not common but may occur in infancy, in long-term inadequate diets, or after surgery that affects the distal jejunum and proximal ileum where the vitamin is absorbed.

PANTOTHENATE

Deficiency in pantothenate is rare and is usually accompanied by other nutrient deficiencies. Since the vitamin is easily destroyed by processing, it is possible that many months on a highly restricted, highly processed diet may increase the likelihood of a pantothenate deficiency.

VITAMIN C

Scurvy, or vitamin C deficiency, is the best known vitamin deficiency. It takes 4 to 5 months of little to no ascorbic acid in the diet before a deficiency in C will develop but in the eras when fresh fruits and vegetables were available only for certain months of the year, and persons might go for months without them, scurvy was prevalent. It was most apparent in sailors after they had spent months at sea.

The effective treatment was recognized early, although it was not commonly accepted until the eighteenth century. In 1534, Cartier noticed that the diseased improved after eating a concoction of pine needles and bark.[1b] In 1600, lemon juice became one cure for scurvy, and the British navy began to include limes among its ship rations. When artificial infant formulas became more popular in the late nineteenth century, infants on these formulas developed scurvy. This may still occur with infants who are fed only cow's or unfortified soy milk for 4 or 5 months, with no other food or supplement.(Cow's milk is naturally very low in vitamin C; unfortified soy milk is inadequate in many nutrients and is never recommended for infants.)

FOLACIN

Deficiencies of folic acid, (or deficiencies of Vitamin B_{12}, below) lead to the megaloblastic anemias. Anemias caused by B_6 or B_{12} deficiencies are similar in symptoms but respond only to the particular vitamin that is deficient. They may often be mistaken for each other. If one anemia is treated when the problem is actually with the other anemia, temporary improvement may occur, but the real problem will become worse.

B_{12}

Two types of anemia respond to vitamin B_{12}: megaloblastic anemia and pernicious anemia. Megaloblastic anemia results from a long-term dietary deficiency in B_{12}. It may take several years to deplete the body's stores of this vitamin. Since B_{12} is found only in animal and bacterial products, strict vegans may develop B_{12} deficiency. This may be a real risk for the children of strict vegan parents, if the children do not receive vitamin supplements or dairy products. Megaloblastic anemia from B_{12} deficiency may result from surgery or from mucosal damage to the distal (end portion of the) ileum, where B_{12} is absorbed.

Pernicious anemia is caused by deficiency of a carrier protein called *intrinsic factor* (IF). This protein is normally manufactured in the stomach, where it attaches to the B_{12} contained in food. B_{12} is then carried by IF through the small intestine to the distal ileum. There it attaches to the villi on the wall of the intestine, IF breaks off, and B_{12} enters the bloodstream.

When IF is missing, B_{12} can not be absorbed. Diet may be adequate but the vitamin never reaches the blood. Treatment involves lifelong periodic injection of B_{12}.

B_{12} deficiency may also result from certain parasites that enter the small intestines and use the vitamin for their own metabolism or from overgrowth of bacteria in the small intestine. In good health, however, natural bacteria in the intestine usually *produce* B_{12}.

BIOTIN

Biotin deficiency is rare and generally occurs in unusual circumstances. Certain genetic enzyme deficiencies may be responsive to treatment with biotin.[5,6] Avidin, a substance in raw egg white, binds dietary biotin so that the regular use of raw eggs can potentially lead to a deficiency of this vitamin.

MALNUTRITION AND VITAMIN DEFICIENCIES

Treatments for vitamin deficiencies vary, depending on the cause and severity of the deficiency. As discussed, deficiency may be only one part of general malnutrition. Figure 26-1 summarizes the known physical signs of major deficiencies, and lists the causes that sometimes contribute to them.

Symptoms, such as depression, chronic weariness, occasional forgetfulness, anxiety, or appetite changes are *not* included on the list precisely because they are vague and are common complaints. Some individuals may "diagnose" such symptoms as nutrient deficiencies without

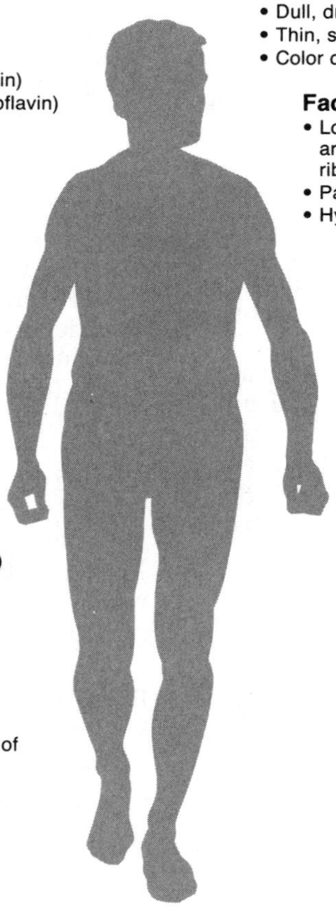

Eyes
- Pale membranes (B_{12}, folacin, iron)
- Night blindness, dull or soft cornea, dry membranes (vitamin A)
- Red and fissures at lid corners (niacin)
- Angular inflammation of eyelids (riboflavin)

Gums
- Spongy, swelling, redness, bleed easily (vitamin C)

Teeth
- Missing or erupting abnormally (general poor nutrition)

Neck
- Thyroid enlargement, symptoms of hypothyroidism (iodine)

Skeletal System
- Demineralized bone (calcium, phosphorus, vitamin D)
- Bowed legs (vitamin D)
- Growth failure in children (vitamin D)

Nervous System
- Listlessness (protein, energy)
- Poor or no ankle/knee reflexes, loss of sense of position and movement (thiamin, B_{12})
- Seizures (magnesium)

Hair
- Dull, dry, lack of natural shine (protein, energy)
- Thin, sparse, loss of curl (zinc)
- Color changes, easily plucked (other)

Face
- Loss of color, dark cheeks, eyes, scaling skin around nostrils (protein, energy, niacin, riboflavin, and/or pyridoxine)
- Pallor (iron, folacin, B_{12}, vitamin C)
- Hyperpigmentation (niacin)

Lips
- Redness, mouth swelling, angular fissures, scars at corners (niacin, riboflavin, iron, B_6)

Tongue
- Purplish color (riboflavin)
- Smooth with small projections (riboflavin, B_{12}, pyridoxine, iron, and/or zinc)
- Sores, swollen, scarlet, raw (folacin, niacin)

Skin
- Slow wound healing (zinc)
- Scaliness (biotin)
- Black and blue marks due to skin bleeding (vitamin C, K)
- Dryness, mosaic, sandpaper feel, flakiness of skin (too much or too little vitamin A)
- Swollen and dark (niacin)
- Edema, lack of fat (protein, energy)
- Yellow color (too much or too little carotene)
- Cutaneous flushing (niacin)

Muscular System
Wasted appearance (protein, energy)
- Calf tenderness, absent knee jerks (thiamin)
- Peripheral neuropathy (folacin, pyridoxine, pantothenic acid)
- Muscle twitching (magnesium)
- Muscle cramps (chloride imbalance)
- Muscle pain (biotin)

Figure 26-1
Signs of nutrient deficiencies. Any of these symptoms may also be a sign of disease other than a deficiency; a physician should be consulted. (Adapted from Powers DE, Moore AO: Food Medication Interactions, 4th ed, pp 165–167. Tempe, AZ, F–MI Publishing, 1983)

a valid, scientific basis. Others may prescribe for themselves high levels of vitamins believing that social factors such as the stress of urban life increase needs. Research that has tested the effect of environmental stress on vitamin deficiencies indicate that it has *no* effect. Vitamin deficiencies developed at the same rate, whether the individual was "under stress" or not. Therefore, vitamins for "stress" have no special benefits.

However, stress caused by *physical* trauma (burns, wounds, or shock) does increase the body's needs for many nutrients, including vitamins. Treatment is usually intense, involving medication, sometimes parenteral nutrition, and close care that is individualized to meet particular needs.

STUDY QUESTIONS

1. Why might nutrient deficiencies develop? (List at least four reasons.)

2. Persons in western developed nations are (more or less?) likely than persons in poorer nations to experience vitamin overdoses. Explain your answer.

3. For what vitamins, if any, have you heard (in the paper, magazines, or from friends) special claims made, *i.e.,* that they prevent or cure certain problems? How would you respond now to these claims?

4. Match the name of the vitamin with its common letter: B_1, B_2, B_6, B_{12}, C, E, or A:
   _____ Cyanocobalamin
   _____ Alpha-tocopherol
   _____ Riboflavin
   _____ Pyridoxine
   _____ Retinol
   _____ Thiamin
   _____ Ascorbic Acid

5. Why might a person have problems following a diet adequate in the essential vitamins?

6. What happens when the walls of the digestive tract are damaged? What might cause damage?

7. Which vitamin deficiency is being described in the following list?
   - British seamen carried limes on ship to prevent it
   - Induced by avidin
   - Induced by a diet high in polished white rice
   - Rare except in premature infants (two vitamins)
   - Epidemic at one time in southeastern USA as a result of an inadequate diet (primarily maize, molasses, and high fat meats).
   - Lack of intrinsic factor
   - Less likely to occur when "masa harina" and coffee are part of the diet
   - Night blindness
   - Ingesting raw egg regularly may lead to this deficiency
   - Bowlegs and soft, easily damaged bones
   - Megaloblastic anemia (2 vitamins)

8. Does stress increase vitamin needs? Explain your answer.

REFERENCES

1. Goodhart RE, Shils ME: Modern Nutrition in Health and Disease, 6th ed pp a, 238; b, 259. Philadelphia; Lea & Febiger, 1980

2. Hittner HM et al: Retrolental fibroplasia: Efficacy of vitamin E in a double blind clinical study of preterm infants. N Engl J Med 305(23):1365–1371, December 3, 1981

3. Giardini O et al: Vitamin E therapy in homozygous β-thalassemia. Letter. N Engl J Med 305 (11):644, September 10,1981

4. Natta CL et al: A decrease in irreversibly sickled erythrocytes in sickle cell anemia patients given Vitamin E. Am J Clin Nutr 33: 968–971, May 1980.

5. Thoene J et al: Biotin responsive carboxylase deficiency associated with subnormal plasma and urinary biotin. N Engl J Med 304 (14):817–824, April 2, 1981

6. Tanaka K: New light on biotin deficiency. N Engl J Med 304(14):839–840 April 2, 1981

CHAPTER 27

Minerals and Trace Elements in Disease Therapy

OBJECTIVES

1. To review and identify the major minerals and trace elements in human nutrition:
   a. Calcium
   b. Phosphorus
   c. Magnesium
   d. Iron
   e. Zinc
   f. Iodine
   g. Copper
2. To outline the major disease and/or deficiency syndromes related to each mineral and to discuss established relationships and the role of diet
3. To describe and discuss in detail the common disorders of osteoporosis and iron deficiency anemia, providing specific guidelines for nutrition support and prevention
4. To list briefly the remaining trace elements for which deficiency in humans is unknown

Chapter 8 described the minerals and trace elements essential in human nutrition and listed some of the major food sources in which they can be found. This chapter will discuss the role certain minerals may play in disease, including the syndromes caused by deficiency. The major minerals and trace elements that may have a role in disease and deficiency syndromes are cal-

cium, phosphorus, magnesium, iron, zinc, iodine, and copper.

CALCIUM

Calcium and phosphorus are the major components of bone. Of the two, calcium balance is most easily upset. Figure 27-1 and Figure 27-2 illustrate the role of the organs and hormones in calcium balance. Many diseases influence calcium balance; the problem that causes the greatest concern to the most people is *osteoporosis*.

Osteoporosis

Osteoporosis, or the progressive loss of bone mass, is a major health problem in the western world today, affecting 15 million to 20 million people in the USA alone. It may cause most of the hip and other bone fractures that occur in the over-45 population.[1]

In healthy bone, the minerals calcium and phosphorus (or phosphate) are constantly being released into the blood and replaced. In osteoporosis, the release of calcium and phosphorus into the blood continues but the reabsorption of calcium *back* into the bone occurs at a slower rate. The result is a net loss of bone mass called *osteopenia* or "too little bone." As bones become thinner, the risk of fracture increases. The quality of the bone does not change; there is simply less bone. This is quite different from osteomalacia (Chapter 26), the disease of "adult rickets" caused by vitamin D deficiency. In osteoporosis the thinned bones break, often causing

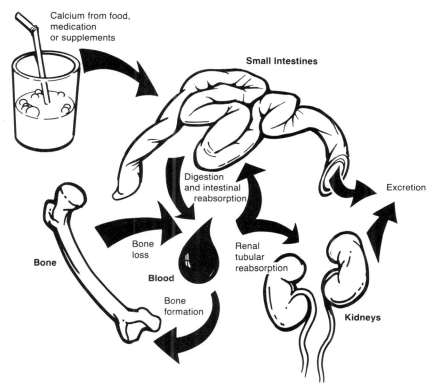

Figure 27-1
Factors in calcium balance.

hospitalization and requiring a long healing period, seriously handicapping an otherwise healthy, mobile, and independent person, usually a woman.

Postmenopausal women are at highest risk. Not only are women's bones thinner than men's bones but the reabsorption of calcium back into the bone seems to decrease automatically after menopause. Thin, small-boned Caucasian women are at higher risk than their overweight, large-boned or Black or Asian counterparts who generally have more bone. It is difficult to diagnose osteoporosis except by special x-ray film, until the bones actually break. In osteoporosis blood and bone tests will all be normal; abnormal results are a sign that something else is wrong. Even the x-ray films are not good detectors of bone loss until 20%–30% of the bone mass is gone.[1] As the disease progresses, vertebrae compress and break, causing back pain, shortening height, stooping posture ("dowager's hump") and sometimes making it difficult to breathe.

Bone loss may begin years, even decades, before menopause. This is why preventive treatment is so important. By age 40 a woman may begin to lose about ½% of her bone each year. After menopause this loss jumps to 1% to 3% each year.[2]

Causes of osteoporosis may include a combination of the following:

1. Normal aging

2. A change in hormone balance, especially estrogens

3. Not enough calcium in the diet

4. Too little exercise

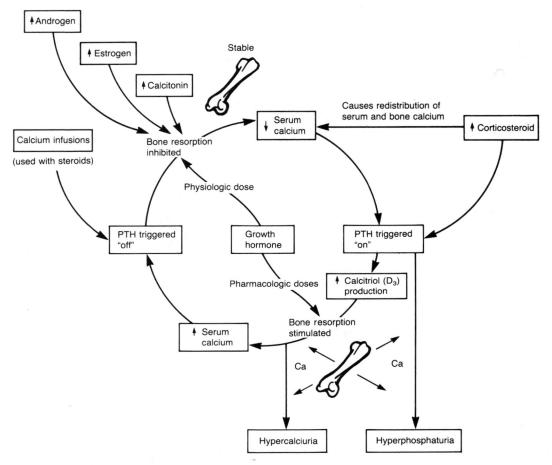

Figure 27-2
Osteoporosis and hormone balance. (Adapted from Gordon GS, Vaughan C: Clinical Management of the Osteoporoses, pp 18–22. Acton, MA Publishing Sciences Group, 1976)

Some researchers have theorized that another cause may be an imbalance between calcium and phosphorus. This has not been clearly proven and evidence is contradictory.[3] Extra vitamin D is not necessary unless there is clear evidence that the person is also deficient in this vitamin.[4]

Treatment and prevention should begin early. This is the recommendation of the 1984 National Institutes of Health Consensus Conferences on Osteoporosis.[1] The report of the conference recommends that high-risk Caucasian women discuss estrogen therapy with their physician (since estrogen therapy may carry a risk of endometrial cancer). It also recommends

1. Daily calcium intake of 1000 milligrams to 1500 milligrams

2. Adequate vitamin D intake (not more than twice the Recommended Dietary Allowances — RDA)

3. Modest weight-bearing exercise, such as walking

Exercise helps prevent bone loss in the bones that bear the weight of the exercise.

Some physicians also recommend sodium fluoride in their treatment of osteoporosis. Fluoride may help in severe cases. It should only be used in such cases and only when a physician has specifically recommended it, since fluoride imbalances can be harmful and the doses usually are much higher than that of fluoridated water and the average diet. In extreme, excess fluoride changes the quality of the bone, creating a coarser structure and perhaps *increasing* the risk of fracture.

Calcium in other Diseases

Calcium may play a role in other diseases as well, as illustrated in Table 27-1. Treatment may include dietary or supplemental calcium, depending on the disease and the physician's recommendations.

Table 27-2 lists the major food sources of calcium. Persons who, for some reason, cannot acquire sufficient calcium from their diet should check with their physician regarding a calcium supplement. These supplements may provide calcium in the form of calcium gluconate, calcium carbonate, or calcium lactate. Any of these can adequately supplement the diet, although each form contains a different concentration of calcium.

Calcium imbalance may also play a part in some hypertension.[5] It is not clear, however, if this is related to a low calcium diet or to a cellular inability to use calcium. A person with high blood pressure should certainly try to meet his RDA for calcium, for the sake of his general health. This may have little effect on hypertension, but research continues in this area.

PHOSPHORUS

Phosphorus has many roles. It is involved in bone formation, carbohydrate, fat, and protein metabolism, electrolyte balance in the body, and the activity of many enzymes.

Its relationship with calcium is complex. Diets too low or too high in phosphates may

Table 27-1

*Diet and Disease Factors in Calcium Absorption**

| | *Effect on Absorption* | |
	Increased Absorption	*Decreased Absorption*
Disease	Idiopathic hypercalciuria Sarcoidosis Hyperparathyroidism	Nontropical sprue Malabsorption syndromes Primary biliary cirrhosis Celiac disease Severe Crohn's disease Chronic renal failure Diabetes Hypoparathyroidism Intestinal surgery
Food Substances	Lactose Medium chain triglycerides (MCT)	Phytate Cellulose Fiber Oxalate Fat (in severe diarrhea) Alcohol Uronic acid Sodium alginate

*Many medications may also affect calcium absorption
(Allen LH: Calcium bioavailability and absorption: A review. Am J Clin Nutr 35:789, 801, April 1982)

Table 27-2

Food Sources of Calcium

Food	Amount	Kcals Energy	Calcium (mg)
Animal Products			
Cheese, American	1 oz	106	174
Cheese, cheddar	1 oz	114	204
Cheese, cottage (creamed)	½ cup	117	68
Kefir,[a] plain	1 cup	160	350
Milk, whole	1 cup	157	288
Milk, 2% fat/milk solids added	1 cup	137	352
Milk, goat's	1 cup	168	326
Sardines, Atlantic in oil, w/liquid, bones	3-½ oz (8 med.)	311	354
Salmon, red canned, w/bones	3-½ oz	170	259
Yogurt, whole milk	1 cup	139	274
Yogurt, low fat, flavored, milk solids added	1 cup	varies	314
Cocoa from mix, water added	1 cup	110	107
Plant Products			
Almonds, shelled, whole[b]	1 oz	176	66
Broccoli, cooked	½ cup	20	68
Chickpeas, cooked[c]	1 cup	290	94
Collard greens, cooked[b]	½ cup	21	130
Kale, cooked	½ cup	22	103
Navy beans, cooked[c]	1 cup	286	138
Pinto beans, cooked[c]	1 cup	262	96
Soy milk, unfortified[c]	1 cup	90	20
Soy flour, whole grain[c]	¼ cup	90	42
Spinach, leaf, cooked[b]	½ cup	24	99
Tahini (sesame butter)	1 tbsp	135	21
Tofu (soybean curd)	4 oz	86	154[d]

[a] Kefir is a cultured milk similar to yogurt
[b] Contains oxalates that may inhibit calcium absorption
[c] Contains phytates that may also inhibit calcium absorption
[d] Calcium in tofu may vary, depending on what is used to coagulate the soybeans
(Truesdale DD et al: Nutrients in Vegetarian Foods. Copyright the American Dietetic Assn. Reprinted by permission from: J Am Diet Assoc 84(1): 28–35, 1985)
(Bowes & Church: Food Values of Portions Commonly Used, 14th ed. Philadelphia, JB Lippincott, 1985)

increase the excretion of calcium. Similarly a very high calcium diet may cause an imbalance in the ratio of calcium to phosphorus and may also lead to bone loss.[6] The RDA suggests a diet containing equal calcium and phosphorus (a 1:1 ratio, 800 mg of calcium to 800 mg of phosphorus for the average adult).

*Hypo*phosphatemia (low serum phosphate levels) is rare because the body tightly conserves phosphate. Only 5%–15% of the phosphate filtered through the kidneys is actually excreted.[6] Renal diseases can cause many imbalances; when kidneys lose their ability to filter nutrients, phosphorus is conserved even more than usual. This altered calcium:phosphorus balance in chronic renal failure can lead to serious bone disorders, so treatment in this disease usually includes a diet low in phosphate and often recommends the use of phosphate-binding antacids.

Kidney diseases that cause the tubules of the kidney to lose excess nutrients (by filtering out too much of them) may cause low phosphate levels. Consistent use of antacids may also lead to low phosphate levels in an otherwise healthy person. Too little phosphate in the system is manifested by weakness, anorexia, aching bones, and general malaise. It may result in problems such as calcium stones in the kidneys (renal calculi), too much calcium lost in the urine (hypercalciuria), and hemolytic anemia.[6]

MAGNESIUM

Like phosphate, magnesium balance is not usually a problem, except in disease. Diseases in which it may be involved include malabsorption syndromes, general malnutrition, malnutrition from alcoholism, tubular dysfunction in renal disease, diabetic acidosis, and trauma-like burns, or severe accidents. Magnesium balance may be upset or body stores exhausted by some diuretics, by a breast-feeding woman whose diet is much too low in the mineral, or by an individual on a parenteral formula that for some reason contains little magnesium.[6] Over one third of all infants born to diabetic mothers show signs of low magnesium levels during their first 3 days of life,[7a] probably a result of poor maternal control of the diabetes during pregnancy.

Magnesium balance affects calcium and potassium metabolism, so deficiency symptoms include hypokalemia (low blood potassium levels), hypocalcemia, and hypocalciuria (low blood and urine calcium levels) as well as anorexia, nausea, apathy, and seizures or other neurologic problems. While a high magnesium diet is important prevention, diet is usually not the first treatment for hypomagnesemia since physicians usually must increase blood and body levels quickly.

IRON

Iron deficiency an*emia* is the most common nutrient deficiency in the world.[7b] To understand why, and how it is treated, it is important first to understand how iron is absorbed, stored, and excreted in the body.

Absorption

Most iron enters the body in the form of food. It may be bound to the protein *heme,* in animal sources, or may be carried in an inorganic (nonheme) form in vegetable and grain sources and in iron-fortified foods. In digestion, iron is changed from its ferric form (Fe^{+3}) to the more absorbable ferrous form (Fe^{+2}). Absorption begins in the upper part of the small intestine.

Iron absorption is highly variable. It depends on the food substances present and on the body's need for "new" iron. Most iron in the body is well conserved, used over and over again. Some estimate that an adult man may acquire 95% of the iron he needs from his body's normal storage pool, since iron is both stored and reused.[8] Only 5%, then, would need to come from the diet. But the effect of conservation on dietary needs depends on growth and storage. A twelve-month-old infant may need 30% of iron from diet. Certain disease states may require a great quantity of iron.

Iron molecules or ions are absorbed into the walls of the small intestine. Absorption depends on need, available iron, and inhibitors or enhancers. Fiber, phytates, oxalates, phosphates, alkali, antacids, rapid transit time (the speed at which food passes through the intestines), or malabsorption can all inhibit iron from being well absorbed.[7c] On the other hand ascorbic acid (vitamin C), amino acids (protein), and sugars help enhance or increase absorption. These are important factors in planning a diet for the iron-deficient client. Since the upper part of the small intestine is where iron is best absorbed, damage to this area may also inhibit iron absorption and place an individual at greater risk of iron deficiency, making the use of enhancers especially important.

Storage

Once absorbed into the mucosal cells that line the small intestine, iron is bound together with various proteins, both in the mucosal cells and in the blood. It then may be used for one of two roles in the body: (1) to help in the transport, storage and use of oxygen, or (2) to become storage iron, maintaining an iron balance in the body. Iron in the forms of *hemoglobin,* myoglobin, cytochromes, and some other proteins form the iron portion of the red blood cells that helps to keep the oxygen : carbon dioxide balance. Ferritin and hemosiderin are the two major forms of storage iron. Listed below are some definitions of the major terms used in iron nu-

VOCABULARY OF IRON METABOLISM AND DEFICIENCY SYNDROMES

Anemia: Low levels of red blood cells or hemoglobin. Anemia may be due to deficiency in iron, certain vitamins, or diseases.

Erythrocyte: Red blood cell.

Erythropoiesis: The formation of red blood cells in the bone marrow.

FEP: Free Erythrocyte Protoporphyrin. Protoporphyrin is a protein carried in red blood cells that combines with iron to make heme..When there is not enough iron to combine with most available protoporphyrin, the result is a higher level of free EP, (a high FEP), indicating possible iron deficiency.

Ferric iron: The Fe^{+3} form of iron, a common form in food.

Ferritin: The nonheme compound in which iron is stored in blood serum, liver, bone marrow, and the spleen.

Ferrous iron: The Fe^{+2} form of iron, produced by digestion.

Hematocrit: Percentage of total blood volume that is made of red blood cells.

Hemoglobin: The iron-containing protein mainly responsible for transporting, storing, and using oxygen throughout the body. Hemoglobin is part of the red blood cell, made with the red blood cell in the bone marrow. It is responsible for carrying oxygen through the blood to the cells and for carrying carbon dioxide from the cells to the lungs. The average lifespan of a red blood cell is 120 days.

Lactoferrin: An iron-binding protein in milk.

MCV: Mean corpuscular volume, or the average volume of red blood cells. When iron is deficient, MCV decreases.

Nonheme iron: Iron that is not in the form of heme; usually refers to iron in foods from plant sources, not carried in the red blood cells of animal products.

Pica: An abnormal craving for nonfood items, which often is part of iron-deficiency anemia. Pica cravings may include clay *(geophagia)*, ice *(pagophagia)* or starch.

TIBC: Total iron binding capacity.

Transferrin: The compound in which almost all serum iron is bound.

Transferrin saturation: A measure of iron stores. Low percentages of saturation of transferrin with iron indicates iron depletion. The degree of saturation is calculated by:

$$\% \text{ Saturation} = \left(\frac{\text{Serum iron concentration}}{\text{TIBC of serum}} \right) \times 100$$

triture and iron-deficiency anemia. Hemoglobin is made in the bone marrow and carried in the blood. Storage iron is found in reticuloendothelial cells (which travel through the body), liver, bone marrow, and spleen. When old cells die and are replaced, the iron portion is usually conserved.

Excretion

As mentioned earlier, very little iron is excreted. Normal iron loss occurs in menstruation, childbearing, minor blood losses in the intestines, and some normal sloughing off (called "desquamation") of the old layers of intestinal mucosal cells.

Iron Deficiency

Iron deficiency is the result of depleted iron stores, depleted transport, and low hemoglobin production. Usually hemoglobin production continues until body stores or reserves become very low. So iron-deficiency anemia in its early stages is hard to measure by hemoglobin. As it progresses, however, several blood tests indicate anemia: low *transferrin* saturation, high *free erythrocyte protoporphyrin (FEP), total iron binding capacity (TIBC),* and low *mean* (average) *corpuscular volume (MCV).* These are defined on the opposite page.

Iron deficiency anemia is usually the result of one of the following:

1. Long-term intake less than total body needs
2. Total body needs more than most diets can meet, such as in pregnancy, in lactation, in women of childbearing age, and possibly during some periods of growth
3. Blood losses from hemorrhage or certain parasites, such as hookworm
4. Insufficient absorption that results from
  a. Pica (defined on page 232)
  b. A diet low in protein (especially animal proteins) and vitamin C
  c. Diet high in iron inhibitors
  d. Surgery affecting the duodenum, where iron is best absorbed

Young children and women of childbearing age are at the highest risk for iron-deficiency anemia. An infant is usually born with a 4-month to 6-month supply of iron (assuming his mother was not anemic during pregnancy). Because they are growing quickly, infants have a high need for iron and usually get it from breast milk, iron-fortified formulas and (later) iron-fortified dry baby cereals. Cow's milk has very little iron and the iron that is present is poorly absorbed. Proteins in cow's milk may also cause minor bleeding in an infant's immature intestines. (See Chapter 15 for a more detailed discussion of infant feeding.) This increases rather than prevents the risk of anemia in the infant and is one of several reasons cow's milk should never be fed to an infant less than 6 months old. While iron-fortified infant formulas contain more iron and and will supply the infant with the RDA for the mineral, breast milk is the most *absorbable* source of iron. The iron content of breast milk is low (0.3 mg per liter; see Fig 27-3) but almost 50% is absorbed.[8] This compares to a 23% absorption of heme iron (the iron in animal products such as meat, poultry, or fish) and the RDA for iron, which assumes that only 10% will be absorbed from foods or supplements. This is why the RDA for a woman of childbearing age is 18 milligrams of iron: Her body needs about 1.8 milligrams but she may be able to absorb only 10% of the iron in her diet.

Treatment of iron deficiency includes supplements recommended by a physician and/or a diet high in absorbable iron.

Figure 27-4 illustrates ways to adapt a diet to absorb nonheme iron more effectively. Nonheme iron is the iron in plant and grain foods such as legumes, enriched cereals, green, leafy vegetables, dried fruit, and molasses. The best absorption is the result of a meal that combines nonheme iron with heme iron *and* some source of vitamin C. Sample meals are described. Because absorption depends so much on the presence of other foods that either enhance or inhibit iron absorption, cultures whose normal diet is high in nonheme iron and in fiber, phytates, or oxalates, including coffee and tea (high in these substances) may be at risk for iron-deficiency anemia even though the diet contains a good deal of iron.[9,10] Adding meat or vitamin

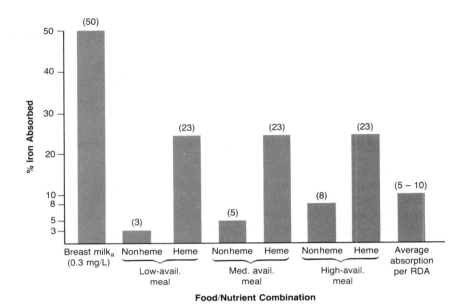

Figure 27-3
Relative absorption of dietary iron. See Fig. 27-4 for explanation. (From Goodhart RE, Shils ME: Modern Nutrition in Health and Disease, 6th ed, p 89. Philadelphia, Lea & Febiger, 1980)

C-containing fruits, vegetables, or juices to these meals would increase absorption and may decrease the risk of anemia.

Individuals with iron-deficiency anemia often complain of chronic fatigue, weakness, shortness of breath, cold or numb hands and feet, pallor, and palpitations. Children with anemia may be slightly less interested in learning than nonanemic counterparts and may have a higher risk of getting infections.[8] Pica seems related to low iron levels, although the relationship is not clear. Pica may interfere with the individual's ability to eat iron-containing foods; he may crave only ice, clay, starch, or some other nonfood substance. A high iron diet is usually not sufficient to improve severe anemia, but an anemic person may be better able to absorb the nonheme iron in the prescribed supplements if the diet is high in iron. So diet is only a part, but it may be a very important part, of treatment for this common problem. Table 27-3 lists the common food sources of iron.

The two most common tests for iron in the blood are the blood tests measuring *hemoglobin* and hematocrit. Authorities may differ about what levels of these two tests indicate iron-deficiency anemia.

Iron Overload

Too much iron in the blood is usually a result of disease. Some diseases, such as liver diseases and perhaps pancreatic insufficiency, cause a high absorption of iron that can lead to stores of iron much higher than necessary. Miners may inhale iron particles from the dust surrounding them. Persons who have a high-iron diet or take iron supplements unnecessarily may develop iron overload. Idiopathic *hemochromatosis* is the hyperabsorption of iron with no known cause. Too much iron in the system is sometimes harmful; it may lead to cirrhosis of the liver, diabetes, hyperpigmentation of the skin and, ultimately in extremely high levels, cardiac failure.[7d] Iron overload can also develop after frequent blood transfusions or after long-term

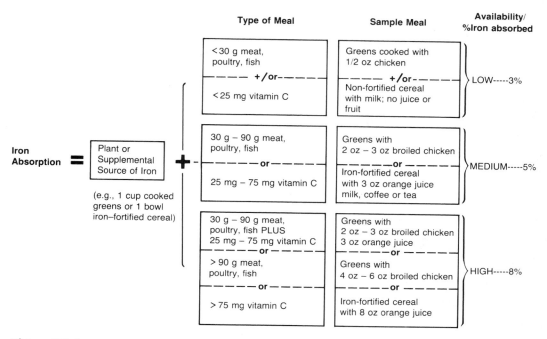

Figure 27-4
The effect on absorption of nonheme iron of protein and ascorbic acid contained
in a meal.

kidney dialysis, and requires close medical attention.

Sickle Cell Anemia

Sickle cell anemia is a genetic anemia that results in defective red blood cells. The hemoglobing in the red blood cells is abnormal and this causes the cell to "sickle," or become sicklelike in shape (like a crescent moon, in contrast to healthy red blood cells that are shaped like disks —thick around the outer edges and thinner in the center, but circular—somewhat like Syrian bread). Because of their long, narrow shape, the sickled cells damage the tissues of the body by blocking the blood channels. When body tissue cannot get blood, it cannot get oxygen the blood is carrying, and it dies. Sometimes these sickle cell blocks cause severe pain and disability; this is called a *sickle cell crisis.*

There is no cure for sickle cell anemia and persons afflicted with it may develop skin ulcers, internal infections, and kidney failure. A nutritionally adequate diet may help the client to resist infection and to recover as quickly as possible from the crises. There are variations of sickle cell anemia that are less severe. The most common, *sickle cell trait,* rarely causes painful crises. Because it is a genetic disorder, some persons simply "carry" the trait. These carriers may pass on to their children the trait or the disease, but they themselves will never suffer from any symptoms of sickling.

Persons with sickle cell anemia are more resistant to malaria. Some scientists believe that this natural "advantage" is part of the reason this debilitating disease is so common among people from parts of the world where malaria is common, especially among Blacks.

Thalassemia

Thalassemia is another genetic defect of the hemoglobin in red blood cells. Severe forms of

Table 27-3

Food Sources of Iron

Food	Amount	Iron (mg)
Heme		
Liver	3 oz	6–18
Lean beef or pork	3 oz	3
Chicken or turkey	3 oz	2
Fish	3 oz	1–2
Frankfurter	1 large	< 1
Cold cuts	2 average slices	< 1
Nonheme		
Iron-fortified cereals (to meet 45% USRDA)	1 cup	8
Beans, dry, cooked	1 cup	4
Blackstrap molasses	1 tbsp	3
Rice, enriched*	1 cup	2
Spinach, cooked	½ cup	2
Prunes	5 large, dry	1
Raisins	½ cup	1.5
Kale, collard or mustard greens, cooked	½ cup	1
Egg	1	1
Whole grain bread	1 slice	1
White bread	1 slice	0.5

* Rice that is not enriched or enriched rice that is washed before cooking will contain very little iron.

(Bowes & Church: Food Values of Portions Commonly Used, 14th ed. Philadelphia, JB Lippincott, 1985)

thalassemia cause death *in utero.* Persons with the most common form, beta-thalassemia minor, may have a normal lifespan. This disease causes anemia and is most common in people of Mediterranean descent (Africa, southern Europe, and the Middle East).[11] Iron treatment has little or no effect.

ZINC

Zinc imbalance is usually a result of disease or malnutrition. Like iron, zinc is better absorbed with protein and less well absorbed with fiber meals.[12] A dietary deficiency in zinc can result from poverty and/or a long-term *marginal* diet.

Genetic zinc deficiency, called "acrodermatitis enteropathica," is one genetic disease that

may be cured by parenteral zinc. Other diseases that may lead to deficiency of the mineral include hemolytic anemias, alcoholic liver diseases, renal failure, and gastrointestinal diseases (including malabsorption syndromes). Intestinal surgery may also affect zinc absorption. Signs and symptoms of zinc deficiency include psoriasis, poor wound healing, anorexia, poor growth in children, less acute sense of taste and smell, and thin, sparse hair. Abnormal zinc levels may affect the immune system, the thyroid and blood lipids.[13–16] A well-planned diet that includes meats, seafood, and whole grains can help prevent marginal deficiencies.

IODINE

Iodine (also called *iodide*) is a trace element used to make the hormones that are essential for the thyroid. Goiter (an enlarged thyroid, see Fig. 27-5) is the classic sign of iodine deficiency.

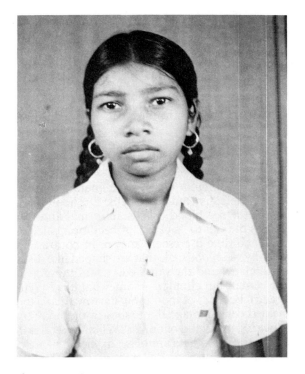

Figure 27-5
Girl with a goiter. (From: Help A Child, Inc. Used with permission.)

Since iodine enters through the soil, goiter occurs where soil contains little iodine, plants in the diet are grown locally (that is, not in iodine-rich soil), and there is no other source of iodine in the diet. Goiter is not as common in the more developed nations as it once was, probably because salt that has iodine added ("iodized salt") is available and can provide the iodine needed in the areas where soil and produce are deficient in iodine, areas once called the "goiter belt."

Goiter and hypothyroidism (underactive thyroid) may also occur when an individual is on thyroid-inhibiting drugs, or has too *much* iodine in the diet. Hypothyroidism (also called *myxedema*) is usually a result of a hormone disorder, not an iodine deficiency. Thus, most physicians treat it with hormones, not iodine. Mistaken laypersons who believe their thyroid is low and self-treat with iodine may cause thyroid imbalance, because the thyroid is a very sensitive organ. Over 200 milligrams daily of iodine may cause this "iodine goiter," a reactive *low* thyroid condition that results in a goiter. This has happened in Japan where seaweed (very high iodine) was a regular part of the diet.[7e]

Other foods that may naturally cause goiters in some sensitive persons include asparagus, broccoli, brussels sprouts, cabbage, kale, and other leafy green vegetables, soy beans, lettuce, peas, spinach, turnip greens, and watercress.[17] These foods are called *goitrogens* and do *not* contain high levels of iodine. Rather they contain some substance ("goitrin") that inhibits thyroid in experimental animals. In humans, they may cause no symptoms of goiter unless they are consumed in very high amounts by persons who live in an iodine-poor area and who have no other dietary source of the mineral.

COPPER

Copper imbalance is very rare. It may occur under the following, special circumstances:

1. In Menke's kinky hair syndrome. This is a genetic defect (kinky hair is one of the side effects) in which the brain and spinal cord degenerate during the first few years of life. Copper in the mother's diet during pregnancy may have some preventive effect.[7f]

2. Wilson's disease, another rare genetic disorder seen in infants. High concentrations of copper are excreted. Certain body organs (the brain, kidneys, cornea of the eye) contain high levels of copper and it causes damage to those organs. Treatment usually includes medication to rid the body of its excess copper.

3. Gastrointestinal malabsorption that results from prematurity, celiac disease, nonceliac sprue, and some rare disorders.

4. Hypochromic anemia, a copper deficiency that develops in malnourished infants given only milk as treatment for kwashiorkor.[7g]

Copper is found in many of the same foods as iron and is stored in the kidneys, heart, hair, and brain. This is why copper deficiency may be seen in diseases of these organs and be manifest in some cases by hair depigmentation. Overdoses of copper (a result of supplements or chronic exposure, as in copper mining) can lead to damage to these same organs.

OTHER TRACE ELEMENTS

Deficiencies of the other trace elements, selenium, molybdenum, manganese, cadmium, and cobalt, are extremely rare if they exist at all. There is no established human need for elements such as tin, nickel, silicon, vanadium, or arsenic. Any supplementaton of these minerals may lead to symptoms of excess and poisoning.

STUDY QUESTIONS

1. The balance of what two minerals is important in healthy bone?

2. Define the following:
   - Osteoporosis
   - Osteopenia
   - Hypophosphatemia
   - Sickle cell anemia
   - Goiter
   - Hypochromic anemia

3. How does osteoporosis differ from osteomalacia?
   - Who is at greatest risk for osteoporosis?
   - How can this group work to prevent or

postpone this disease? Explain and list at least six foods important in prevention.

4. True or False: Explain your answer.
   - Phosphorus is easily lost by the body.
   - Infants of diabetic mothers may be born with low levels of magnesium.
   - Zinc deficiency is the most common nutrient deficiency in the world.
   - Iron is carried by the blood in the nucleus of the red blood cell.
   - Animal sources of iron are more readily absorbed than plant sources.
   - Breast milk has more iron than infant formulas.
   - Underactive thyroid should be treated with iodine.
   - Vanadium, nickel, and tin are not necessary for human nutrition.

5. What influences the absorption of iron?

6. Where is ferritin (a storage form of iron) stored in the body?

7. What causes iron-deficiency anemia? Who is at greatest risk?

8. List eight foods that contain iron.

9. How do abnormal zinc levels affect the body?

10. What nutrient causes goiter?

11. What foods may cause goiter?

12. What are some causes of low serum copper levels?

REFERENCES

1. National Institutes of Health (NIH): Osteoporosis: Consensus conference. JAMA 252(6) 799–802, August 10,1984
2. Whedon GD: Osteoporosis: An editorial. N Engl J Med 305(7):397–398, August 13, 1981
3. Allen LH: Calcium bioavailability and absorption: A review. Am J Clin Nutr 35:783–808, April 1982
4. Slovik DM et al: Deficient production of 1, 25-Dihydroxyvitamin D in elderly osteoporotic patients. N Engl J Med 305(7):372–374, August 13, 1981
5. Henry H et al: Increasing calcium intake lowers blood pressure: The literature reviewed. J Am Diet Assoc 85(2):182–185, 1985
6. Draper HH, Scythes CA: Calcium, phosphorus, and osteoporosis. Fed Proc 40:2436, 1981
7. Goodhart RE, Shils ME: Modern Nutrition in Health and Disease, 6th ed, p a,316; b,327; c,339; d,349; e,401; f,418; g,419. Philadelphia, Lea & Febiger, 1980
8. Dallman PR, Siimes MA, Stekel A: Iron deficiency in infancy and childhood. Am J Clin Nutr 33:86–118, January 1980
9. Morck TA, Lynch SR, Cook JD: Inhibition of food iron absorption by coffee. Am J Clin Nutr 37:416–420, March 1983
10. Acosta A et al: Iron absorption from typical Latin American diets. Am J Clin Nutr 39:953–962, June 1984
11. Fishman MC et al: Medicine, p 348. Philadelphia, JB Lippincott, 1981
12. Sandstrom B et al: Zinc absorption from composite meals: 1. The significance of wheat extraction rate, zinc, calcium, and protein content in meals based on bread. Am J Clin Nutr 33:739–745, April 1980
13. Sullivan et al: Enhanced lipid peroxidation in liver microsomes of zinc-deficient rats. Am J Clin Nutr 33:51–56, January 1980
14. Chandra RK, Au B: Single nutrient deficiency and cell-mediated immune responses: 1. Zinc. Am J Clin Nutr 33:736–738, April 1980
15. Morley JE, Gordon J, Hershman JM: Zinc deficiency, chronic starvation and hypothalamic-pituitary thyroid function. Am J Clin Nutr 33:1767–1770, August 1984
16. Crouse SF et al: Zinc and lipoprotein levels. JAMA 252(6): 784–787, August 10, 1984
17. Powers DE, Moore AO: Food Medication Interactions, 14th ed, p 160. Tempe, AZ, F-MI Publishing, 1983

CHAPTER 28

Fluid- and Electrolyte-Controlled Diets

OBJECTIVES

1. To review the relationship between normal fluid and electrolyte balance
2. To define and describe acid-base balance
3. To discuss causes and general treatment for
   a. Dehydration
   b. Edema
   c. Acid-base imbalances
4. To list and explain several common examples of fluid- and/or electrolyte-controlled diets, as in
   a. Diarrhea of malnutrition
   b. Congestive heart failure
   c. Ascites due to liver diseases
   d. Renal disease
   e. Hypertension
5. To define and discuss briefly the now-outdated acid/ash diet
6. To provide specific guidelines and resources to help a person live with a fluid, sodium, and/or potassium-restricted diet

The body's normal balance of water and the electrolytes was discussed in Chapter 9, as was the role of the essential electrolytes and their balance in the different fluid compartments of the body. Listed here, as a review, are the sub-stances in the blood that most depend on a stable balance of fluids and electrolytes.

Water balance is carefully controlled by thirst, by the adrenal gland, the hypothalamus and the kidneys. This balance of mechanisms, hormones, and renal blood pressure as illustrated in Table 28-1. Water balance and sodium balance are closely related, because body water must always contain a certain concentration of sodium. The more sodium the body holds, the more water it must also hold. This is part of normal balance.

When sodium, the other electrolytes, acids, or bases lose their proper balance in the body fluids, a life-threatening emergency can quickly develop. These imbalances usually occur in diseases and treatment depends on the disease. Fluid and electrolyte imbalances can result in or be caused by dehydration (too little water) or edema (extra water held in parts of the body where it does not belong). They can also lead to an imbalance in acids and bases in the body.

SUBSTANCES AFFECTED BY FLUID AND ELECTROLYTE BALANCE

Bicarbonate	Organic Acids
Calcium	pH
Chloride	Potassium
Glucose	Proteins
Lipids	Sodium
Magnesium	Sulfate

There is some evidence that an electrolyte/fluid imbalance may play a role in the development of cataracts.[1]

ACID-BASE BALANCE

Substances are acidic or basic, depending upon how they affect body fluids electrically. Electrolytes, acids, and bases all have a charge; it may be positive (+) or negative (−) (see Fig. 28-1). When (+) substances combine with (−) substances, the result is *neutral*. In acid-base balance, the acids are the positive (+) substances because they contain hydrogen ions (H^+). Bases are the substances that receive the hydrogen ions. The balance between acids and bases is called the *p*H balance. Figure 28-2 illustrates the possible *p*H ranges within the body.

A *p*H ranging from 0 to 6.9 indicates that the substance is acidic. Foods such as lemon juice, vinegar, and citrus fruits are acidic. The acid in the stomach is even more acidic. Between 7.1 and 14, the *p*H range is basic or alkaline. Substances such as baking soda (sodium bicarbonate), lye, and most tap waters are basic. A *p*H of 7.0 is neutral.

Acids and-bases must be kept in balance in the body. Within that balance there is room for many variations. But if the balance swings too far in one direction or the other, stability is lost and danger signals appear. Balance may be restored naturally, or with much outside help. If

Table 28-1

What Happens when Water/Sodium Levels Drop*

Stimulus	*Mechanism*	*Response*	*Comments*
Total body water content drops 1%–2%	Thirst	Water is consumed	
Extracellular fluid volume drops	Sensed by cells in hypothalamus	Release of antidiuretic hormone (ADH)	ADH causes the kidneys to conserve sodium and water. These substances are then reabsorbed back into the body.
Blood pressure in the kidneys drops	Sensed by cells in the kidney	a. Enzyme *renin* is released	
		b. Renin makes *angiotensin*	Angiotensin causes the tubules in the kidney to narrow. This increases renal blood pressure.
		c. Angiotensin triggers the adrenal glands to release the hormone *aldosterone*	Aldosterone causes the kidney to save sodium. The increased osmotic pressure† causes water also to be conserved.

* These are mechanisms that turn "on" when water and sodium levels are low. They turn "off" automatically (except in disease) once balance is restored to a certain point.
† See Chapter 9 for explanation.

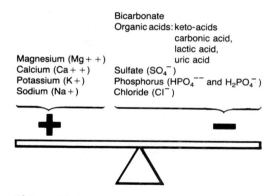

Figure 28-1
Blood serum balance.

have a pH between 7.3 and 7.4.* If the body becomes too acidic, the condition is called *acidosis*. If it becomes too basic, it is called *alkalosis*. Systems and substances that make it hard for the pH to change and thus help maintain the balance are called *buffers*. When acidosis causes the body pH to drop below 6.8, or when alkalosis causes it to rise above 7.8, death results. This is why buffers are so important in acid-base balance. Figure 28-2 lists the major causes of acidosis or alkalosis and ways in which the body tries to compensate, or maintain balance.

Since fluids feed the cells, fluid imbalances can cause great damage to cells. This is why the

the imbalance continues the extreme may eventually cause great damage and even death.

Most body fluids outside the digestive tract

---

* A narrow range when compared to the pH of digestive fluids: saliva (6.0–7.0); stomach acid (1.0–3.5); bile (7.8), and pancreatic juices (8.0–8.3). (Guyton AC: Textbook of Medical Physiology, 6th ed, p 803. Philadelphia, WB Saunders, 1981)

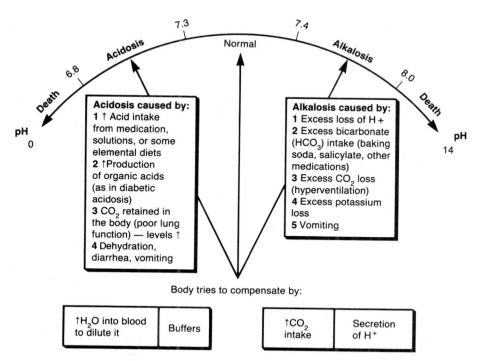

Figure 28-2
pH and acid-base balance. (From Taber's Cyclopedic Medical Dictionary, pp A–25, A–55; wheel adapted from McClintic, JR: Basic Anatomy and Physiology of the Human Body, p 325. New York, John Wiley & Sons, 1975)

balance of a substance in the body is usually more important than its *quantity*. Thus, the body may sometimes excrete water (by urinating or sweating) or carbon dioxide (by rapid breathing) to maintain a balance.

Both acidosis and alkalosis may be either metabolic or respiratory. A metabolic imbalance is the result of something abnormal in the production, ingestion, or excretion of hydrogen (H^+). A respiratory imbalance is caused by an abnormal release of carbonic acid in the form of carbon dioxide from the lungs (hypo- or hyperventilation). Acidosis is most likely to occur in diabetes, renal and liver diseases, and diseases that lower the ability of the lungs to function well. Alkalosis occurs most frequently as the result of hyperventilation or too much base in the system from medication or other substances. Metabolic alkalosis is often common immediately after surgery.[2] Figure 28-2 outlines these causes and ways in which the body tries to compensate for them. Both situations need immediate emergency medical care, since they can worsen very quickly.

Diet may influence acid-base balance in special cases of

1. Renal disease or diabetes mellitus with poor control

2. Chronic vomiting from illness or from eating disorders, such as bulimia

3. Excess intake of acids or bases due to improper administration of a parenteral or elemental diet

4. Starvation

5. Extreme cases of long-term, low-carbohydrate, high-fat diets[2]

DEHYDRATION

Dehydration occurs when the tissues of the body lose needed water. It is one extreme of fluid imbalance; edema (below) is the other.

Water may be lost with or without a loss of the electrolytes. *Hypertonic dehydration* is a condition that occurs when, proportionately, more water is lost than electrolytes. This happens in burn patients, in diabetes, in excessive sweating (as from a fever), or after a long period

without water. The concentration of electrolytes in the blood becomes too high. Muscle weakness, paralysis, and abnormal heart and lung functions are some of the symptoms. Treatment depends on the cause, but will include replacing the lost fluid.

Hypotonic dehydration occurs when, proportionately, more electrolytes are lost than water. This is a result of severe vomiting and diarrhea, some hormone deficiencies, kidney disease, and extreme sodium deprivation. Symptoms depend on the electrolytes most affected but will include muscle changes and sometimes mental disorientation or convulsions.

Finally, *isotonic dehydration* occurs when fluids and electrolytes are lost in the same proportion as they exist in body fluids. This type of dehydration may result from blood loss, or mild diarrhea, or vomiting.

All types of dehydration may quickly lead to serious complications and should receive immediate medical attention.

EDEMA

Edema means *swelling*. In the body, edema means the swelling caused by excess fluid in body tissues. Edema was once called dropsy.[3]

Many conditions may lead to edema. If something goes wrong with the "thermostat" system that regulates fluid and sodium balance (the system described in Table 28-1), the body may conserve more water than it should.

Another cause of edema may be an imbalance in the osmotic pressure. Chapter 9 describes osmolarity in some detail. Briefly, osmotic pressure in the blood, for example, is the pressure needed to retain water *inside* the blood. As the number of particles increases, more water pushes in through the walls of the blood vessels. Water comes from the cells and the interstitial fluid. It helps to keep the concentration of water–to–particles normal throughout the body.

Normal osmotic pressure in the blood is 280 to 290 milliosmoles per kilogram (mOsm/kg) of plasma. Some foods and dietary formulas cause this pressure to rise to over 600 mOsm and this high level can affect fluid balance.

Osmotic pressure is important in every cell of the body. It is dependent on water, but also on the ability of particles to enter or leave the cell. This ability, in turn, depends on the permeability of the cell membrane, that is, the ability of particles to move from one side of the cell membrane to the other. If membrane permeability is damaged, there will be an imbalance in osmolarity. Fluid will accumulate in the wrong areas and edema will result. The damage depends on the cause.

Heart failure can result in edema; *pulmonary* edema (fluid around the lungs) is often part of congestive heart failure and makes it difficult for both heart and lungs to function. Edematous swelling may also occur following infections (fluid surrounds and cushions the affected area), bacterial poisons, venom (from snake bites or bee stings), or electrolyte imbalances that cause the body to hold excess sodium.

Kidney disease causes fluids, which cannot be excreted because the kidneys do not function, to build up in the peritoneal cavity (the between-organ spaces in the abdomen, enclosed by the peritoneal membrane). This type of edema is called *ascites*. Ascites, or excess fluid in the peritoneum, also can result from too little protein in the blood. Osmotic pressure goes down when there is not enough protein, and fluid then seeps from the blood to the interstitial spaces in the peritoneum. This is also common in liver diseases, especially alcoholic cirrhosis.

Treatment for edema varies. Persons with liver damage usually begin a diet that strictly controls electrolytes, fluids, and protein; edema is only one sign of many complex problems. Persons with kidney failure may begin *dialysis* and a diet tightly controlling the same nutrients in slightly different ways. Edema that results from a simple excess sodium content in the body may be treated with a low-sodium diet. Edema resulting from venom or infection usually requires close medical attention, with nutrition playing a lesser role unless malnutrition is also a problem.

Some of the major situations that need a specific fluid- or electrolyte-controlled diet are discussed below.

DIARRHEA OF MALNUTRITION

Malnourished children in poor countries rarely die of their malnutrition. They usually die from diseases or infections that their bodies are simply too weak to fight. In places where water may be contaminated, diarrhea *(gastroenteritis)* is a real risk and can quickly cause death, especially in children, since fluid and electrolyte balance, acid and base balance, are quickly and seriously upset. The World Health Organization (WHO) estimates that at least 5 million children die every year simply from diarrhea. In response, WHO has developed an *oral rehydration therapy* that any trained person can administer to persons with severe diarrhea. It is a mixture of fluid, electrolytes, and sugar that, when mixed and administered to a person, can help restore a normal fluid: electrolyte balance and perhaps save lives. The WHO rehydration solution is a mixture of

3.5 grams (⅔ tsp*) sodium chloride (table salt)

2.5 grams (¾ tsp) sodium biocarbonate (baking soda)

1.5 grams (⅓ tsp) potassium chloride [The primary ingredient in many salt substitutes; also available in pure form from a pharmacist]

20 grams glucose (or 40 grams — 3⅓ tbsp — of sucrose or table sugar)

1 liter of boiled or sterile water [4]

Some professionals recommend that 2 grams of sodium be used in mild diarrhea instead of 3.5 grams.[5] The fluid may help in an emergency, but anyone with severe or chronic diarrhea should receive medical attention as quickly as possible.

CONGESTIVE HEART FAILURE

In congestive heart failure (CHF), the lower two chambers (ventricles) of the heart are unable to

---

* These measures are very close but not totally precise; if it is at all possible the electrolytes and sugar should be weighed rather than measured — or the dry mix obtained in prepackaged form.

work well. They cannot pump blood through the lungs effectively, nor into the aorta (the main blood vessel of the body). Blood flow becomes congested; blood pressure rises, and fluid leaks into the lung cavity. This is called pulmonary (*i.e.*, lung) edema, and it makes breathing difficult.

Treatment includes ridding the body of excess fluids. This is done through medications and, often, by means of a sodium- and fluid-controlled diet. Fluid control will be described below in the discussion of ascites, and sodium control will be discussed in the section labeled "Hypertension."

Since osmolarity also affects water balance, it may play a role in the dietary control of CHF. Treatment depends on the individual and the degree of the disease.

ASCITES

Ascites is a symptom, not a disease. It often occurs, as discussed above, as a result of cirrhosis but also as a result of cancer, the inflammation of some organ in the peritoneal cavity, or kidney failure.

Ascites can cause excess pressure on the vital organs. The heart has to work harder and pumps less, and breathing is also more difficult. Many problems result.

This is why the treatment is often a severe fluid and sodium restriction. Treatment may permit fluid that the client needs in order to take medication, but leaves very little allowance for any liquids in or with meals. This means a person may not be able to have soup, a full cup of coffee or tea, or have a glass of water whenever he is thirsty! The specific restriction is determined by the physician. It is then up to the nursing and dietary staff to work together to help the individual stay within the allowance, yet receive enough fluid for medications and necessary nutrients. Most clients who are on this difficult limitation are in a health care facility, so fluid intake can be monitored carefully. However, clients with kidney failure, may be able to go home as long as they are willing to control their total fluid intake to meet their restrictions. An unlimited fluid intake — without the ability to urinate — may cause great discomfort, and further motivate clients to restrict themselves.

Abstaining from alcohol is an essential, assumed, and sometimes difficult part of treatment of any liver disease. Alcohol is never allowed as fluid for a cirrhotic individual.

RENAL DISEASE AND KIDNEY DIALYSIS

The dietary treatment of renal disease is complex and may involve a tight control of protein and phosphorus as well as control of sodium, potassium, fluid, and calories. The restriction depends on the degree of the disease and on the treatment. Kidney failure may result from complications of heart disease, hypertension, urinary tract infections, and diabetes, as well as kidney disease itself.

Individuals whose kidneys have failed may receive one of three types of *renal dialysis*. Dialysis is the mechanical filtering of waste products from the blood. Usually the kidneys perform this function by producing urine. Without some type of dialysis, a person with renal failure will die from the buildup of these fluids and waste products. Clients who are unable to receive a kidney transplant, or who are waiting for one, must be dialyzed frequently. The major types of dialysis are hemodialysis (direct filtering of the blood), peritoneal dialysis and *continuous ambulatory peritoneal dialysis (CAPD)*.

Hemodialysis is the most common treatment for clients with chronic kidney failure. The client is connected to a hemodialysis machine 2 or 3 times a week for as long as 4 to 6 hours at a time. This treatment is usually done in a hospital or in a special unit, although some persons have the treatments at home. As the person's blood circulates through the hemodialysis machine, the machine filters out the waste products. Costs for the treatment of chronic renal disease are covered by federal funding; however hemodialysis costs the client many hours each week — the time spent attached to the machine.

Hemodialysis clients require a diet that tightly controls their sodium, potassium, protein, phosphorus, and sometimes fluids. The restriction is highly individual and depends on how well the kidneys are able to function, since many clients with kidney failure still can manufacture some urine.

Fluid, protein, and energy control have already been discussed. Phosphorus is usually controlled by medication that binds phosphates.

The potassium restriction is one that often takes a long time to master, and it is hard to follow. If possible, this restriction is not tightly controlled. But when it must be controlled, and is not, hyperkalemia (high blood levels of potassium) can lead to cardiac arrhythmias and complications.

High potassium foods include fruits, vegetables, whole grains, nuts, and seeds. Milk, meat, and beverages (including coffee) also contain potassium, but these substances will be controlled by the protein and fluid restrictions. So it is the fruits and vegetables that the client may not expect to be, but must be, restricted. Many persons with kidney failure already have a poor appetite due to their disease and often experience depression because of it. Fruits and vegetables may appeal to them more than any other foods, making the restriction even more difficult. When it is begun, 1500 milligrams to 2000 milligrams per day is an average allowance. Often this restrictive diet is taught to a client by means of exchanges (see Chapter 22). These are far easier to calculate than the milligrams in each food.

Table 28-2 lists the sodium and potassium content of some high- and low-potassium fruits and vegetables.

Sodium is restricted in kidney disease to help prevent edema. Unlike urination, which rids the body of waste products every few hours, hemodialysis requires a wait of 2 to 3 days. Fluid buildup should therefore be as minimal as possible to prevent discomfort and medical problems. Sodium control is discussed below.

Not all nutrients are tightly restricted in hemodialysis. Many vitamins and often minerals are given as supplements. The diet is so restricted that the client cannot meet the Recommended Dietary Allowances (RDA) for many of these, and many are also lost in the filtering process of the hemodialysis machine.

Peritoneal dialysis is the removal of the excess peritoneal fluid by a dialysate, as in the process of CAPD, discussed below. An opening is made and fluid is released into the peritoneum; after 10 minutes to 60 minutes it is drained by gravity into a bag. However, this type of dialysis is not continuous. It is usually done only in emergencies or at infrequent intervals, and the client cannot be ambulatory. Peritoneal dialysis is done in a hospital.

In *CAPD,* the person is constantly being dialyzed by a hyperosmolar fluid in the peritoneal cavity. The fluid attracts wastes by osmosis. The client has a permanent, surgical opening into the peritoneal cavity where the fluid first enters (from a tube connecting the cavity with a bag of fluid hung above the head), then exits several hours later (by changing the position of the bag and tube, to permit the fluid to flow out of the cavity and back into the bag). Between the time fluid enters and the time it is allowed to flow out, the bag is rolled up, worn around the waist, and the client continues normal life. The fluid is changed every 3 or 4 hours with a new bag of fluid called dialysate. The surgical opening to which the tubes attach must be constantly kept clean or it can become infected. If the peritoneum becomes infected, CAPD must stop and another type of dialysis (hemodialysis) must begin.

Clients on CAPD have few diet restrictions. They are filtering out waste products effectively, so the complication of fluid or electrolyte imbalances are not a problem. The dialysis fluid does contain glucose and there is some evidence that these extra calories may cause a CAPD client to gain weight.[6] Persons who choose a high sodium diet will need more glucose in the dialysate in order to "pull out" the excess fluid they hold. The glucose in the dialysate is absorbed and may lead to elevated levels of triglycerides and not just to extra weight.[7] Persons on CAPD must also be individuals who have a life that is sufficiently ordered and organized to change the dialysis fluid bag regularly, every 3 or 4 hours, and must also be able to keep the area as clean as possible.

Table 28-2

Potassium and Sodium in Fruits and Vegetables

Low Potassium (<100 mg per serving)

Fruit	Amount	Mg Sodium	Mg Potassium
Applesauce, canned	½ cup	2	91
Blueberries, canned	½ cup	4	51
Blueberries, fresh, froz.	½ cup	4	65
Cranberry juice	½ cup	5	30
Grape juice drink	½ cup	tr.	7
Kumquats, raw	1 medium	1	37
Lemon	1	1	80
Lemonade, froz, diluted	½ cup	13	50
Lime-aid	½ cup	tr.	16
Peach nectar	½ cup	9	50
Pear nectar	½ cup	5	16
Persimmons, raw	1	0	78
Raspberries, frozen	½ cup	0	94
Watermelon, fresh	½ cup	1	93

Vegetables	Amount	Mg Sodium	Mg Potassium
Bamboo shoots, canned	½ cup	2	64
Bean sprouts, canned	½ cup	35	98
Beans, green, snap	½ cup	2	95
Beans, yellow wax, canned	⅔ cup	317	100
Cucumber, peeled	½ medium	3	80
Lettuce, raw	1 cup	4	99
Parsley	1 tbsp.	4	73
Peas, canned	½ cup	246	79
Radishes, raw	2 small	3	64
Scallions, raw	2 medium	2	92
Watercress	10 sprigs	5	28

High Potassium (200mg–300mg per serving)

Food	Portion		
Apples, dried	10 rings	56	288
Apricots, fresh	3 medium	1	313
Canteloupe	½ cup	7	247
Elderberries	½ cup	0	203
Guava	1 medium	2	256
Honeydew melon	¼ small	12	251
Kiwi fruit	1 medium	4	252
Nectarines,	1 medium	0	288
Orange, navel	1 medium	1	250
Plums, fresh damson	2	8	226
Prune juice	½ cup	2	235
Strawberries, raw	1 cup	2	247
Asparagus, frozen	3-½ oz	7	271
Broccoli, froz, chopped	½ cup	21	224
Carrots, cooked	⅔ cup	33	222
Collards, cooked	½ cup	25	234
Dill pickle	½	464	290
Eggplant, raw	½ cup	2	214
Spinach, cooked	½ cup	45	291
Sweet potato, canned	½ cup	60	250
Tomato, raw	1 small	3	244
Tomato juice, canned	½ cup	338	299
Vegetable juice cocktail	½ cup	357	264

Very High Potassium (over 300 mg per serving)

Food	Portion		
Apricots, dried	10 halves	3	482
Avocado, fresh	½(150 g)	7	742
Banana, fresh	3-½ oz	1	395
Currants, black dry	½ cup	6	642
Dates, dried	10	2	541
Figs, dried	10	20	1332
Papaya, raw	1 medium	8	780
Peaches, dried	10	9	1295
Pears, dried	10	10	932
Prunes, dried	10	3	626
Raisins	½ cup	9	563
Bamboo shoots, fresh raw	½ cup	0	355
Beet greens, cooked	½ cup	76	332
Lima beans, frozen	½ cup	64	394
Mushrooms, raw	10 small	15	414
Plantain, cooked	1 cup	8	716
Potato, inst., reconst., salt added per directions	½ cup	245	352
Potato, baked w/skin	1 medium	4	503
Spinach, raw	3-½ oz	71	470
Sweet potato, baked	1 small	12	300
Tomato paste, canned	½ cup	50	1120
Tomato sauce, canned	⅖ cup	531	389
Winter squash, baked	½ cup	8	716

(From Bowes & Church: *Food Values of Portions Commonly Used*. 14th ed. Philadelphia, JB Lippincott, 1985)

Table 28-3

Sodium in Sample Condiments

Condiment	Amount	Sodium (mg)
Standard Condiments		
Baking Powder	1 tsp	339
Baking Soda	1 tsp	821
Catsup	1 tbsp	156
Chili powder *	1 tsp	26
Garlic powder	1 tsp	1
Garlic salt	1 tsp	1850
Herbs, spices, no salt	1 tsp	0-25
Horseradish	1 tbsp	198
Lemon juice	1 tbsp	0
Mayonnaise	1 tbsp	140
Monosodium Glutamate (MSG)	1 tsp	492
Mustard	1 tsp	65
Oils	1 tbsp	0
Olives, black	3	96
Olives, green	4	323
Parsley, dried	1 tbsp	6
Pepper, black	1 tsp	1
Pickle relish, sweet	1 tbsp	124
Salad dressing		
French	1 tbsp	214
Italian	1 tbsp	116
Low Calorie	1 tbsp	153
Thousand Island	1 tbsp	109
Salt, Table	1 tsp	1938
Sauce		
Barbecue	1 tbsp	130
Chili	1 tbsp	227
Tabasco	1 tsp	24
Worcestershire	1 tbsp	206
Vinegar	½ cup	1
Wines, cooking	½ cup	657
Yeast, baker's	1 pkg	1
Oriental Condiments		
Miso	1 tsp	112
Sauce		
Brown bean	1 tsp	426
Hot bean	1 tsp	300
Sweet bean	1 tsp	160
Hoison	1 tsp	160
Oyster	1 tsp	260
Satay	1 tsp	65
Shrimp	1 tsp	412
Soy	1 tsp	343
Shrimp, dried, rinsed	1 tsp	22
Shrimp, dried, unrinsed	1 tsp	92

* Check labels. Salt is added to some chili powders

(From Chew T: Sodium values of Chinese condiments and their use in sodium-restricted diets. J Am Diet Assoc 82(4):397–401, April 1983. Greenfield H *et al:* Sodium/potassium content of salt and salt substitutes. Med J Aust 140(8):460–462 April 1984. United States Drug Administration. The Sodium Content of Your Food, Home & Garden Bulletin #233, 1980. United States Drug Administration: Composition of Foods: Spices & Herbs Agriculture Handbook No. 8–2, January 1977)

HYPERTENSION AND SODIUM RESTRICTION

Many physicians recommend a low-sodium diet for clients with hypertension or high blood pressure. A low-sodium diet may help lower the amount of fluids that the body holds. Less fluid in the body could mean less pressure throughout the bloodstream. Other factors (genetics or perhaps a problem with calcium metabolism) may also play a role in hypertension.[8] Research continues. Some authorities believe certain persons are more sensitive to sodium than others. Thus, a sodium-restricted diet may help lower blood pressure for some persons but not others. Still, sodium control does seem to help medication work most powerfully to lower blood pressure.[9] Persons eat far more of this mineral than they need. While sodium may not cause hypertension, it may aggravate it. If uncontrolled, high blood pressure can cause damage to many organs and lead to kidney disease, stroke, and heart attack. Hypertension is often a common and severe problem among the elderly and among the black population who may also have some type of heart or kidney disease, or diabetes.

Many cookbooks and brochures are available to help the public use less sodium, and some of these are listed at the end of this chapter. Some sources of sodium were listed in Chapter 9 (see Table 9-2). The most common source is table salt (made of sodium and chloride) and the condiments added to foods at the table or in processing. Table 28-3 lists many other condiments used in North America, and their sodium content.

Sodium is also "hidden" in many foods. Processing techniques often add substances high in sodium. For example, mono*sodium* glutamate, sodium nitrate, sodium phosphate, "brine," and "soda" are all high in sodium. Food may not taste salty but may be very high in sodium. "Soft" water is high in sodium because sodium is one of the substances used in the "softening" treatment.

Powdered seasonings and herbs or spices that contain salt (celery, garlic, onion salt) are high in sodium. Most natural dried herbs and spices, though, are very low in sodium. Listed on page 250 are three recipes for mixtures that can replace salt (sodium chloride) in the salt shaker.

Some tangy seasonings, such as lemon juice and vinegar, are also good low-sodium alternatives. Alcoholic beverages (except cooking wine or sherries) are usually low, though mixed drinks may contain a lot of sodium, depending on what ingredients are added. Many medications also contain sodium, so a person on a sodium restriction should check with his physician before taking any medication.

Below are some suggestions that may help a client make low sodium choices from each of the four food groups

1. *Meat and other protein foods.* High-sodium meats include those that are cured, smoked, dried, or salted; for example, ham, sausages, corned beef, bacon, frankfurters, chipped beef, and smoked, pickled, canned, or salted fish. Fresh meat, poultry, or fish are naturally low in sodium. Nuts are also low, if they are "unsalted." Eggs are naturally low in sodium, though they contain cholesterol. But egg substitutes, low in cholesterol, are usually very high in sodium! Dry beans are low in sodium. Peanut butters may be high, because of added salt.

2. *Dairy products.* "Milk solids" are concentrated, dry particles of milk. Since milk contains sodium, yogurt and low fat milk products with added "milk solids" will contain more sodium than plain or whole milk and yogurt. Buttermilk may contain added sodium. Cheeses are also naturally high in sodium; processed cheeses are extremely high, since the sodium is added in processing. More and more grocery stores, however, are selling "no added salt" cheeses. Some of these are very low in sodium; others contain the same amount of sodium in an ounce of cheese as is naturally contained in a cup of milk. Nutrient information is available from the companies that manufacture these products.

3. *Fruits and Vegetables.* Fresh fruits and vegetables are naturally low in sodium. Canned vegetables may be high, since sodium is added in processing; choose labels that read "no salt added." Frozen vegetables and al-

"NATURAL" SALT SUBSTITUTES: 3 RECIPES

These recipes can be placed in shakers and used instead of salt:

1. Saltless Surprise*

2 tsp Garlic powder
1 tsp Basil
1 tsp Anise seed
1 tsp Oregano
1 tsp Powdered lemon rind or dry
    lemon juice

Put ingredients into blender and
    mix well. Store in glass con-
    tainer; label. Adding rice will
    help prevent caking.

2. Pungent Salt Substitute*

3 tsp Basil
2 tsp Savory (summer savory is
    best)
2 tsp Celery seed
2 tsp Ground cumin seed
2 tsp Sage
1 tsp Lemon thyme
2 tsp Marjoram

Mix well and then powder with
    mortar and pestle.

3. Spice Mix

½ tsp Tumeric
1 tsp each: Chili powder
            Black pepper
            White pepper
            Ground ginger
            Onion powder
            Celery powder
2 tsp. each:Garlic powder
            Paprika

Mix thoroughly. Use in seasoning
    meats, fish, eggs, soup, vegeta-
    bles.

---

* (From United States Department of Health and Human Services, Public Health Service, Food and Drug Administration: "A Word about Low-Sodium Diets," HHS Publication No. (FDA) 84–2179. Available from Public Health Service, FDA, 5600 Fishers Lane, Rockville, MD, 20857)

---

most all canned or frozen fruits are low in sodium. Any product that is "pickled" contains sodium.

4. *Grains and Cereals.* In general, the less processing done to a grain or cereal, the less sodium it contains. Pancake, muffin and bread mixes, highly processed and almost "instant," are very high in sodium. Sodium in cereals varies widely, but most cereal labels do list sodium content. Crackers are

often high in sodium; choose those with "unsalted tops." (And use butter or margarine that is unsalted on foods from any of the four groups).

As mentioned earlier, the client with cirrhosis or a severe problem with fluid retention may be put on a very strict, low-sodium diet. The severely restricted client may only be able to have 1500 milligrams or less of sodium. Major changes in the diet are needed to bring sodium to this low level. All foods that are naturally high in sodium are omitted or substituted. Low-sodium milk and bread may be necessary. This very low level is a difficult restriction to accept; the physician, dietitian, nursing staff, and family should all work together to help the client adjust to the change required. Most clients on a mild restriction may be allowed 3000 milligrams to 4000 milligrams of sodium per day. Because sodium is contained in so many foods, a person on a "2-gram sodium" diet (commonly recommended for individuals with hypertension) may actually be taking in closer to 3 grams to 4 grams of sodium.

THE ACID/ASH DIET

The acid/ash diet is an outdated therapy based on the theory that certain foods can make urine more acidic than others. Since bacteria cannot survive well in acid, an acidic urine might help treat or prevent urinary tract infections. If diet can help change the *p*H of urine, this might also help in treating certain kidney dysfunctions.

The first list of the theoretical effect of foods on urine *p*H in humans was published by Sherman and Gettler in 1907.[10] The list was developed from mathematical calculations of the net effect of the electrolytes in foods. It was not based on actual testing in humans. In time, other foods were added and the diet was used widely in those years before there were drugs that could specifically make the urine acidic or alkaline.

A recent review of the data has identified many problems and inadequacies of this theory.[11] Diet does seem to influence urine *p*H, but it depends on many known and unknown factors. Three foods: cranberries, prunes, and plums do have a very mildly acidic effect on the urine. The natural benzoic and quinic acid convert in the body to hippuric acid, which is known to acidify urine and may help kill bacteria. This effect may not be relevant, though, unless these foods are taken in large quantities. This could upset other balances in the diet. The mathematical *in vitro* calculations of Sherman and Gettler were not completely accurate and do not necessarily predict what will actually happen *in vivo* in the human kidney; Therefore the acid/ash diet as it currently exists is too imprecise to be used therapeutically. Until research yields more precise data, prescribed drugs are probably the most reliable way to change urine *p*H.

STUDY QUESTIONS

1. What mechanisms control water balance?
2. How quickly must a fluid or electrolyte imbalance be corrected? Why?
3. Are electrically positive substances (+) acids or bases? What makes them positive?
4. What is the average range of *p*H for the healthy body? Is it slightly acidic or basic?
5. Define the following:
   a. Buffer
   b. Acidosis
   c. Alkalosis
   d. Dehydration
   e. Hypertonic dehydration
   f. Edema
   g. Peritoneal dialysis
   h. Pulmonary edema
   i. WHO rehydration therapy
   j. CAPD
6. List at least three disease states which may cause
   • Acid-base imbalances.
   • Fluid imbalances.
   • Electrolyte imbalances.
7. How important is nutrition in treating edema that results from a snake bite?
8. You are in a primitive area in a poor nation with the nearest physician 200 miles away. A local mother brings you her child. The child is obviously malnourished and has severe diarrhea. What would you do?
9. How important is fluid and electrolyte control in congestive heart failure? Explain your answer.
10. How is severe ascites treated?
11. True or false: Explain your answer.

- Alcohol is permitted in the diet of clients with cirrhosis, as long as it is fit into their fluid restriction.
- Hemodialysis patients may gain weight from their treatment.
- An individual on CAPD must constantly function with fluid dwelling in his abdominal cavity.
- Potassium restriction in renal disease may be difficult but sometimes essential to prevent cardiac arrhythmias and potential heart failure.
- Sodium is restricted in renal disease primarily to help control thirst.
- It is medication, not sodium control, that controls high blood pressure.

12. Mrs. K has been told to restrict her sodium. "But I never add salt to anything," she tells you. "I don't need to do anything differently, do I?" Below is a typical daily diet.
- What suggestions would you make to help Mrs. K understand her sodium restriction?
- Should she make any changes in her diet? If so, what?
- Are there any foods she should ADD to her diet to help meet her basic nutrient needs?

24-hour recall for Mrs. K:
Breakfast:
3 links smoked sausage, broiled
Low-cholesterol egg substitute, on toast
Orange juice
Coffee with sugar
Lunch (In a Chinese restaurant with friends)
Sweet and sour soup
Fried rice
Chinese vegetables in sauces
Tea
Snack
Diet soda
3 Dill pickles
4 Crackers
Dinner
Broiled fish, lemon, and tartar sauce
Canned peas and corn
Regular margarine on vegetables
Baked potato with processed cheese

Store-bought pastry
Coffee with sugar
Snack:
1 Apple

REFERENCES

1. The Nutritional Origin of Cataracts. Nutr Rev 42(11):377–379, November 1984
2. Goodhart RE, Shils, ME: Modern Nutrition in Health and Disease, 6th ed, pp 389, 393. Philadelphia, Lea & Febiger, 1980
3. Thomas CL (ed): Taber's Cyclopedic Medical Dictionary, 13th ed, p E-8. Philadelphia, FA Davis, 1977
4. World Health Organization: The Management of Diarrhoea and Use of Oral Rehydration Therapy: A Joint WHO/UNICEF Statement. Geneva, Switzerland, 1983. (Copies available from WHO, 1211 Geneva 27, Switzerland)
5. Gracey M: Therapy for mild diarrhea. Med J Aust 140(6)L 348–349, March 17, 1984
6. Bouma SF, Dwyer JT: Glucose absorption and weight change in 18 months of continuous ambulatory peritoneal dialysis. J Am Diet Assoc 84(2):194–197, 1984
7. Burton BT, Hirschman HGH: Current concepts of nutritional therapy in chronic renal failure: An update. J Am Diet Assoc 82(4):359–363. 1983
8. Parrott–Garcia M, McCarron DA: Calcium and hypertension. Nutr Rev 42(6):205–213, 1984
9. Langford HG et al: Dietary therapy slows the return of hypertension after stopping prolonged medication. JAMA 253(5):657–664, February 1,1985
10. Sherman HC, Sinclair JE: The balance of acid-forming and base-forming elements in food. J Biol Chem 3:307, 1907
11. Dwyer J, Foulkes E, Evans M et al: Acid/alkaline ash diets: Time for assessment and change. J Am Diet Assoc 85(7):841, July 1985

Excellent resource material related to low-sodium diets is available from: U.S. Dept. of Health and Human Services, 5600 Fishers Lane, Rockville, MD 20857; U.S. Dept. of Agriculture; Health Education Associates, 211 S. Easton, Glenside, PA 19038, and from local heart associations, cooperative extension services, dietitians, and hospitals.

UNIT 4

Diet Therapy in Disease: Control of Mixed Factors

Anorexia: The Loss of Appetite

*A*norexia means "loss of appetite." It should not be confused with "anorexia nervosa," the self-starving syndrome seen in many young and teenage women, which will be discussed in Chapter 37. This chapter will discuss the poor appetite or simple anorexia, which is a common and often complicating *symptom* in many adult and childhood diseases.

A person may suddenly begin to eat less for many reasons. Anorexia may be a physical symptom, a direct result of some physical problem, such as a stroke, but it may also be a psychological response to illness or some other problem.

There are at least six common causes of ano-rexia: disease, drugs, depression, dysgeusia, anxiety, and aging.

DISEASE

The diseases that most commonly affect appetite are cancer, flu, neurologic disorders, gastrointestinal disorders, nephrotic syndrome (failing kidneys), and diseases that result from chronic alcoholism. But almost any disease may affect appetite in some way.

DEPRESSION AND FAMILY DISORDER

Many types of depression may affect appetite. In infancy, the syndrome called nonorganic *failure to thrive* (FTT) may cause a child to eat—and desire—less food than he needs for growth. The psychological effect of a disordered relationship may cause the child to stop growing and "fall off" the growth curve. Children with FTT need care that is immediate and aggressive. They may need to spend time as inpatients in the pediatric ward of a hospital while they are refed and the possible family or medical (organic) reasons for their FTT are evaluated. Some children diagnosed as "failure to thrive" may have stopped growing ("failed to thrive") because of some unknown physical problem. Close medical attention in the hospital can help uncover this condition. If a child eats well and begins to grow again after 10 days in the hospital, many physicians will suspect that the slowed growth is related to a family or relationship (nonorganic) problem, rather than a physical (organic) problem.[1] Children who suddenly drop below the 5th percentile of height-to-age or weight-to-height without any obvious reason may be at risk of FTT and need immediate attention and evaluation. A sudden change may be the sign that there is some unresolved problem needing attention to prevent long-term damage. If not caught soon enough, it is very difficult (and sometimes impossible) to catch up at a later date on that lost growth. Failure to thrive will be discussed in more detail in Chapter 33.

Older children, teens, and adults may also become anorexic as the result of some life tension that causes depression. Listed on page 260 are some common characteristics of what psy-chology calls a "major depressive episode."[2] Weight and appetite change is one of these symptoms. Resolving the cause of the depression may resolve the appetite problem; nutrition support alone is never sufficient.

DYSGEUSIA

Dysgeusia means an altered sense of taste. It is a physical problem that may be caused by

a. Disease, such as cancer, a flu, or hepatitis

b. A metabolic disorder or change; for example, pregnancy

c. A nutritional problem, such as a vitamin or

Table 29-1

Taste Distortions of Common Foods by Categories of Dysgeusia

Foods and Percentage Distortions Reported (by Group)	Category (and Definition)			
	I (Distortion of One Food in Any Group*)	II (Distortion of Several Foods But Not an Entire Food Group)	III (Distortion of All Foods in Any One Group)	IV (Distortion of All Foods and Beverages)
Meat & Meat Substitutes	No taste distortion reported		Poultry (29) Fish (38) Red meat (75)	(100) (100) (100)
Breads & Cereals	No taste distortion reported		Bread (25)	(100)
Fruits	No taste distortion reported	Fresh fruit (30) Citrus fruit (10)	(45) (25)	(100) (100)
Milk & Dairy	Dairy foods (12)	(20)	(33)	(100)
Miscellaneous (Beverages, condiments, chocolate)		Naturally sweetened carbonated beverages (20)	(38)	(100)
	Artificially sweetened beverages (14) Chocolate (12)	(10) (30) Coffee (50)	(21) (21) (33)	(100) (100) (100)
% Original body weight lost by first treatment	-0.4 ± 2.2	0.3 ± 1.4	-5.3 ± 2.2	noncancer group: -11.3 ± 2.4 cancer group: -13.6 ± 2.3

* Totals in these columns do not equal 100 because many other foods were reported with no consistent pattern and so were not included. (Adapted from Markley EJ, Mattes–Kulig, DA, Henkin RJ: A classification of dysgeusia. J Am Diet Assoc 83(5): 578–580, November 1983)

mineral deficiency (a zinc deficiency, for example)

d. A neurologic problem; for example, a head injury or brain surgery

e. Medications, either in treatment of a disease or in drug abuse.[3]

f. Aging.

A client with dysgeusia finds that foods taste "funny." Food may suddenly taste much more or less bitter, sweet, sour, or salty than usual. It may begin to taste metallic. The smell may be nauseating. Table 29-1 illustrates the common taste changes that happen in the various categories of dysgeusia. Depending on its cause, dysgeusia may progress from one category or degree to another. Or, taste changes may remain permanently at a certain level. And sometimes, fortunately, the person recovers and the tastes of food return to normal.

The major nutritional problem in this disorder is that when the taste of certain foods is suddenly different or undesirable, entire foods and food groups may be omitted from the diet. This can lead to weight loss and nutrient deficiencies. The problem may be temporary (as in pregnancy) or treatable (as in zinc deficiency or

Table 29-2

Ways to Add Nutrients and Concentrate Calories

Add Fat	*Add Protein*	*Add Carbohydrate*

Butter, margarine or oil to:
    Cooked vegetables
    Sandwiches
    Soups
    Casseroles
    All breads
	Dry milk to:
	    Soups
	    Whole milk
	    Pudding
	    Casseroles
	    Mashed potatoes
		Sugar
		
		Corn syrup
		
		Maple syrup
		
		Jams, jellies
		
		Pasta or cereals with added fat and protein
		
		Applesauce
		
		Fruit juice concentrate

Cream to:
    Soups
    Cereals
    Milk drinks
    Eggnogs
    Other beverages
	Yogurt
	Cheese (grated) to:
	    Eggs
	    Casseroles
	    Soups
	    Toast
	    Sandwiches	

Bacon to:
    Casseroles
    Sandwiches
    Soups
	Peanut butter to:
	    Soups
	    Milk drinks
	    Pancakes
	    Sauces
	    Baked goods	

Mayonnaise, cream cheese to:
    Salads
    Vegetables
    Potatoes
    Sandwiches
	Eggs in:
	    Custards
	    Eggnog (see recipe)	

Avocado (mashed) to:
    Salads
    Soups
    Casseroles
    Sandwiches
    Vegetables
	Ice cream in:
	    Frappes
	    All milk drinks	

Tahini (sesame butter) to:
    Casseroles
    Hot vegetables
    Sandwiches		

drug abuse) or it may be permanent and worsen, as in some types of cancer, neurologic disorders, and some drug treatments. Someone with dysgeusia needs to know which nutrients might become a problem (if any), considering the omitted foods, and then work with the medical team to acquire those missing nutrients in some other way.

Often the cause for the taste change includes an increased need for some nutrients and this may make treatment even more difficult. For example, a person with cancer may need more calories to fight the disease. A drug treatment may affect the absorption of other nutrients (see Chapter 36). A pregnant woman may be so nauseous that she cannot keep anything "down," yet the needs of her unborn child and her very state of pregnancy mean she needs more nutrients (Chapter 13). Dysgeusia is rarely a simple problem and requires as much ongoing support as possible. Support must be tailored to meet individual needs and to work with individual problems.

DRUGS

Many drugs affect appetite in some way. They may lead to taste changes, as discussed above, or they may make a person more or less hungry or thirsty. Treatment is difficult, because the medication is often essential for some disease that may be present.

Anorectic drugs ("diet pills") are used intentionally to help overweight clients lose weight. Usually these drugs have side effects that make them unsafe to use over long periods of time. They may raise blood pressure or cause the heart to beat irregularly. And they usually do not help an obese person learn lifestyle changes. They should be used only with a physician's approval and supervision and are, at best, a temporary help.

Sometimes a drug prescribed for some other medical problem may inadvertently cause anorexia. When this happens, the physician may try to find another, alternate drug, but drugs used for the same diseases may have similar side effects, and appetite change is a common side effect. Drug-nutrient interactions will be discussed in more detail in Chapter 36.

Drug abuse (including alcohol abuse) also affects appetite and is a much more complex problem. Treatment for anorexia of any kind means working with whatever is causing the anorexia. The person abusing alcohol or another drug needs to be willing to make changes and seek aggressive, long-term help before the situation can be expected to change. Anorexia may be the least of many medical and social problems.

ANXIETY ABOUT EATING

Sometimes a person loses his appetite because the pain or discomfort of eating outweighs the pleasure. The discomfort might be physical or psychological. It might occur for example,

a. In diseases such as gum disease, ulcers, or a gastrointestinal disorder that results in severe pain during or after eating;

b. After a conditioned aversion. For example, if a child chokes and nearly suffocates on a piece of meat, beans, or some other food, thoughts of that food may cause anxiety in the future. Or if a person becomes ill and vomits immediately after eating some food, the food may become associated with the vomiting, and be avoided

c. After tube feeding has been forced upon someone

d. As a result of psychiatric fears about food (for example, that it is poisonous or will cause some inevitable, unpleasant effect)

Persons anxious about eating for any of these or other reasons may avoid foods and lose weight or be at risk for deficiency. Or the anxiety may not influence health but may make it hard to enjoy certain social events. When these anxieties interfere with life, counseling sometimes is used to help a person learn to deal with the cause of the anxiety.

AGING

Taste sensations tend to dull with age. Taste buds die and the nervous system, which helps relay messages of hunger, may not work as efficiently as in younger years, so older people often complain that "food has lost its taste." Also, there may be less muscle action along the gastro-intestinal tract so that food remains longer in the tract, with a subsequent feeling of fullness. These are reasons aging itself may affect appetite.

Often, too, other factors may lead to anorexia in older persons, including those discussed above. Older persons often have more diseases than the young. They take more medications, experience more taste changes, and may also suffer from depression and anxiety.

DANGERS OF ANOREXIA

The most obvious danger is the effect that anorexia might have on the client's health and nutritional status. Avoiding whole food groups may cause deficiency syndromes. Any type of anorexia may cause weight loss.

Weight loss can be a health risk. Muscle may be lost as well as the ability to fight infection and disease. A person is at highest risk of problems resulting from underweight if

a. Weight is 20% (or more) below ideal body weight

b. There has been a *recent rapid* loss of 10% (or more) from normal weight

c. The person has been unable to eat anything for 10 days or more.[4]

TREATMENT

To treat anorexia effectively, the underlying problem first must be identified. If the problem is psychological, treatment must involve support and help in that area. Conditioned fears may need to be overcome. Anorexia that results from a disease may resolve when the disease is treated.

Unfortunately, though, sometimes the underlying disease cannot be easily cured. The nephrotic syndrome of kidney failure cannot be cured; it can only be treated and controlled. Many gastrointestinal diseases (see Chapter 33) also cannot be "cured", but diet may be controlled so the individual is more comfortable and may begin to enjoy eating. Drug therapies can sometimes be changed, but other drugs may cause other problems. Anorexia in pregnancy usually accompanies nausea and vomiting and was discussed in Chapter 13. Often, too, a person may be sick, not feel like eating, but actually may need those nutrients more than ever before to help fight the disease. It is not always safe or accurate to "let the body tell you what it needs" through subjective feelings. When systems go wrong that "inner clock" is off balance and the appetite may also become distorted. And "cravings," even in a very healthy individual, usually reflect desires, not actual physiological needs.

Anorexia is common in cancer. The disease itself often seems to lead quickly to anorexia, and chemical or radiation treatments may make it even more difficult to eat. Chapter 30 will discuss in greater detail ways to try and help increase the appetite and minimize the nutrition problems of the anorexic cancer patient.

Many general suggestions are available to help boost nutrients in a diet (Table 29-2 and opposite). These guidelines can be used in working with a person no matter what the cause of the anorexia. Some of these suggestions are listed below. The guidelines and recipes will help boost calories and nutrients; they will not necessarily solve the appetite problem, but they may make food more appealing.

A person who has lost his appetite may not *want* to eat anything, but may be *willing* to take something that someone else prepares. In this condition, there is little pleasure or satisfaction in eating. Since most people associate eating with pleasure, eating becomes much more difficult — and often completely undesirable — when the pleasure disappears.

This is why it is important to pack as *many* calories and other nutrients as possible into a *small* quantity of food for these clients. They may be wiling to take a small amount of food every few hours but be unwilling to eat a large tray of food, which may nauseate them. The secret of preventing malnutrition is to concentrate the nutrients in an acceptable form. The concentration is usually done in one or more of three ways:

1. By adding fat to the diet (at 9 Kcals per gram, fat is the most concentrated source of food energy available)

2. By adding protein to the diet (to help the

MEALTIME TIPS FOR ANOREXIA

1. *Eat often.* This may mean eight (or more) small snacks throughout the day and no large meals. Small meals and snacks are often more acceptable than a large amount of food. Keep snacks full of calories and protein. Keep them readily available. Keep offering them.

2. *Eat the foods that most appeal and that stay down.* This is especially true if nausea is a problem. This may mean only fruit and milk. It may mean only gingerale and toast. When nausea and vomiting are problems, foods that stay down are more nourishing ultimately than foods that don't. A sick adult may only want spaghetti with cheese and sauce four times a day for a week, or cucumbers, or the same type of sandwich. This is alright, to a point. If the illness continues, other ways of feeding necessary nutrients need to be considered.

3. *Keep mealtime stress at a minimum.* The anorexic person may become even more anorexic if his family constantly worries about him at mealtime.

4. *Try to understand fussy or angry eating behaviors,* especially in children. Some children express anger about their sickness or loss of control in some area by trying to control meals. Firmly offer specific foods or choices. Let a child make certain decisions about meals and snacks. Draw reasonable limits, as calmly as possible, to prevent food from becoming a battleground.

5. *Feed foods at whatever temperature is desired.* Heat and cold do not add or subtract calories. Many people who have a poor appetite prefer slightly warm or cool foods, rather than extremes.

6. *Make meals colorful.* Use foods that are attractive. Add colored napkins, flowers, fresh fruit, pleasing tablecloth or placemats and dishes. Add amusing or fun garnishes. Make eating as pleasurable as possible.

7. *Try again.* If a food does not appeal today, try it another day. Tastes may change.

8. *Don't force foods.* If weight loss is severe and feeding needs to be more aggressive, talk with the physician.

9. *Let someone else (not the anorexic individual) cook.* Some people lose their appetite by simply being around food.

10. *People with poor appetites sometimes complain that they get full fast.* This is called "early satiety." Some ways to prevent this include:
    - Small meals
    - Chew and eat as slowly as possible, so there is less food competing for stomach space at the same time
    - Avoid high fat foods. They trigger this feeling.
    - Make sure all liquids have calories. Never give only plain water.
    - Don't drink and eat at the same meal. This fills the stomach too quickly. Drink liquids 30–60 minutes before (or after) meals.

(From Sherman M: Feeding the Sick Child. National Cancer Institute, Department of Health, Education and Welfare Publication No. (NIH) 78–795, 1978 and National Cancer Institute: Eating Hints: Recipes and Tips for Better Nutrition during Cancer Treatment, National Institute of Health Publication No. 80–2079, August 1980)

CHARACTERISTICS OF A MAJOR DEPRESSIVE EPISODE

Exaggerated depressed mood. (In children under 6, a persistently sad facial expression.) Plus:

Four or more of the following symptoms lasting two or more weeks. (In children under 6, three of the first four):

Poor appetite and significant weight loss OR increased appetite and significant weight gain (in children under 6, failure to meet normal, expected weight gains)

Change in sleep pattern: not able to sleep or sleeping too much

Change in activity: energy level slows down or becomes unusually "hyper" (in children under 6, lack of energy)

Loss of interest in pleasures or usual activities (in children under 6, apathy)

Fatigue or loss of energy

Feelings of worthlessness, self-reproach, or excessive or inappropriate guilt

Complaints or evidence of diminished ability to think or concentrate

Recurrent thought of death or suicide, wishes to be dead, or suicide attempt.

(From Tishler CL: Depression in children and adolescents: Identification and intervention. Public Health Currents 24(5), October–December 1984. Columbus, Ohio, Ross Laboratories)

---

individual replace muscle mass and fight disease and infection)

3. By adding concentrated carbohydrates to the diet (to help meet basic energy needs)

The concentrated food must taste good and be medically safe. Remember osmolarity (Chapters 9,28): substances with a very high osmolarity or concentration of molecules may cause diarrhea. The nutritionist works with the patient to help with specific preferences, to check on actual intake, and to help encourage eating. She often keeps track of how much the patient is actually eating, and can alert the rest of the medical team to problems. When intake lowers to such an extent that the individual's health and weight are at risk, other methods of feeding, such as by tube or intravenous line, are often considered (see Chapter 38).

Listed on the opposite page are four recipes that may be incorporated into a diet to help concentrate nutrients, especially calories. Other resources for recipes and tips to help appetite are listed at the end of the chapter.[5,6]

The mechanisms that control appetite are very complex and not well understood. They seem to be controlled by certain areas of the brain with delicate sensors of balance. Unfortunately, as many overweight individuals know, the appetite center does not always act as an adequate "policeman". Persons eat or refrain from eating for many reasons that have little to do with appetite. Appetite sensors may not work well at all in many diseases and psychological disturbances. It is important to remember that:

"The wonder is not that there should be a great diversity of disturbances in the regulation of food intake, producing many different types of obesities and excessive thinness, but rather that in most animals and man, with feeding behaviour subject to so many influences, the mechanism of regulation of food intake works as extraordinarily well as it does."[7]

SOME RECIPES THAT BOOST CALORIES

Double Strength Milk

1 quart whole milk
1 cup nonfat dry milk

Mix the two. Let the mixture stand overnight for the best flavor.
Per cup: 286 Kcals, 15 g protein

Add to double-strength milk (options):

Scoop ice cream
2 tbsp chocolate, butterscotch, or other syrup
½ cup fresh or frozen fruit
2 tbsp frozen juice concentrate
Softened or melted peanut butter
Honey to taste
Flavoring extracts

Fruit Shake

1 cup double strength milk (above)
½ banana, not quite ripe
2 tbsp frozen orange juice concentrate
1 egg
1 tbsp sugar (optional)

Blend in blender: banana, egg, orange juice concentrate, and sugar. Slowly blend in milk. Serve cold and frothy. Per recipe: 517 Kcals, 22 g protein.

Peanut Butter Snack Spread

1 tbsp instant dry milk
1 tsp water
1 tsp vanilla
1 tbsp honey
3 heaping tbsp peanut butter

Combine dry milk, water, and vanilla, stirring to moisten. Add honey and peanut butter, stirring slowly until liquid begins to blend with peanut butter. Spread between graham crackers or milk crackers. Can also be formed into balls, chilled, and eaten as candy. Makes ⅓ cup. Per recipe: 440 Kcals, 17 g protein

Blender Eggnogs

Eggnogs are usually a popular food—but they can also be a source of trouble. Raw egg whites contain a substance, avidin, that interferes with the absorption of biotin. A more serious problem is that raw eggs can carry the salmonella organism that produces diarrhea and other problems of food poisoning. This is most serious if the person drinking the eggnog is already

(continued)

ill and less able to fight off infection. The solution? Cooked egg products. Since even commercial eggnog mixes may not be free of the salmonella organism, here is a recipe for an eggnog using a cooked egg.

1 cup cold fortified milk (use double-strength milk for extra protein and
    energy)
1½ tbsp sugar
½ tsp vanilla
1 fresh egg (make sure there are no cracks in the shell)

Put milk, sugar, and vanilla into the blender. In a small pan heat two inches of water to boiling. Rinse egg in warm running water for a few seconds and break egg into water. Cook for two to three minutes over medium heat until white is firm (do not boil since boiling will harden the egg). Scoop egg out of water and place directly into blender. Blend at high speed, covered, for about 15 seconds or until egg is well blended. Strain to take out any tiny particles. (Don't sniff the eggnog when you finish blending it; it will have the sulfur smell of a hot cooked egg for a few seconds).

You can serve the eggnog immediately for it will be at room temperature. You can make it in large batches and store it in the refrigerator or freezer. Try it with nutmeg, ice cream (or brandy if the doctor allows).

Calories: 423 (314 if you use a soy formula instead of milk)
Protein: 26 g (12 g with a soy formula)

(From National Cancer Institute: Eating Hints: Recipes and Tips for Better Nutrition during Cancer Treatment. National Institute of Health Publication No. 80–2079, August 1980)

STUDY QUESTIONS

1. Define:
  ● Anorexia
  ● Failure-to-thrive
  ● Dysgeusia

2. List and describe five possible causes of anorexia.

3. What is a "major depressive episode?" What role does nutrition play in such an episode?

4. What may cause dysgeusia?

5. Jane was six years old when she became violently ill right after eating chocolate cake at a birthday party. Now a senior in high school, Jane still avoids chocolate cake. Why?

6. Bill has an ulcer that feels worse whenever he eats or drinks anything except skim milk and white bread with butter. As a result, his daily diet right now is a half gallon of skim milk and a half loaf of bread with butter and sometimes sugar. He has lost 15 lb from his usual 160 lb frame in the three weeks since the ulcer began to bother him. He feels the weight loss is probably the result of stress from studying for finals, which are now over.
  ● In what way(s) are Jane's and Bill's problems similar?
  ● What is wrong with Bill's diet?
  ● What would you suggest to Bill?

7. How may anorexia be treated successfully?

8. Is "appetite" a reliable measure of what the body needs? Why or why not?

9. List and describe at least four suggestions for meals and mealtimes that may help an anorexic client acquire the nutrients he needs.

10. Drew is five and has just come down with the flu for the third time in two months. He has no appetite but his mother is able to feed him fluids. How can she help him get enough calories and enough protein?

REFERENCES

1. Bithoney W, Rathbun J: Failure to thrive. In Developmental Behavioral Pediatrics. Philadelphia, WB Saunders, 1983
2. Tishler CL: Depression in children and adolescents: Identification and intervention. Ross Laboratories, Public Health Currents 24(5)October–December 1984.
3. Markley EJ, Mattes–Kulig DA, Henkin RI: A classification of dysgeusia. J Am Diet Assoc 83(5): 578–580, November 1983
4. Butterworth CE, Weinsier RC: Malnutrition in hospital patients: Assessment and treatment. In Goodhart RE, Shils ME (eds): Modern Nutrition in Health and Disease, 6th ed, pp 667–684. Philadelphia, Lea & Febiger, 1980
5. Sherman M: Feeding the Sick Child. National Cancer Institute, Department of Health, Education, and Welfare Publication No. (NIH) 78–795, 1978
6. National Cancer Institute: Eating Hints: Recipes and Tips for Better Nutrition during Cancer Treatment. National Institute of Health Publication No. 80–2079, August 1980
7. Mayer J: Physiology of hunger and satiety. In Goodhart RE, Shils ME (eds): Modern Nutrition in Health and Disease, 6th ed, p 576. Philadelphia, Lea & Febiger, 1980

CHAPTER 30

Nutrition in Cancer

OBJECTIVES

1. To define cancer and related, common terms
2. To discuss possible causes and common responses to a diagnosis of cancer
3. To define and discuss common nutrition problems in cancer
   a. Weight loss
   b. Anorexia
   c. Cancer cachexia
4. To emphasize the importance of adequate nutritional status in the treatment of cancer
5. To define and discuss common nutrition-related side effects of
   a. Chemotherapy,
   b. Radiation therapy,
   c. Surgery for cancer
6. To outline appropriate responses to the common nutrition-related problems and side effects
7. To discuss several areas of nutrition commonly associated with the prevention and treatment of cancer
   a. Outlining, defining, and discussing the role and dangers of unconventional cancer treatments, laetrile, macrobiotic diet, and exclusive dependence on supplements
   b. Outlining the role of food: fats, antioxidants, fiber, and vegetables of the brassica family
8. To define and to discuss hospice care

The diagnosis of cancer brings a chill to many persons. Some still take it as a death warrant, even though many forms may be cured easily in their early stages. Others deny that anything is wrong, and may refuse treatment or choose unconventional alternatives. And many accept the diagnosis and the medical treatment that may prolong life and even cure them. Fortunately, more and more of the population is realizing that not everyone who develops cancer dies of that cancer.

TERMS

Cancer is the abnormal, uncontrolled growth of some lump or mass *(tumor)* of cells in the body. A growth may be *benign,* growing very slowly, and carry little or no risk; benign growth is not a cancer. A growth that is cancerous is *malignant,* that is, it grows quickly. It has potential to spread and cause great damage to the body in one, a few, or many areas.

A cancer that spreads is said to have "metastasized." *Metastases* are related tumors that appear in parts of the body other than that of the original tumor. For example, breast cancer may be found and removed; then, in the next year, metastases (the same type of cancerous cells) may be found in the liver or some other organ. A metastasis may be a sign that not all of the cancer was removed, or that it had already begun to spread before surgery. Malignant cancer is sometimes compared to a housefire. The earlier it is caught, the less damage it can do. And to keep the house from eventually burning down, *all* of the fire must be extinguished, wherever it is. When it spreads in some unseen, quiet way (for example, through the walls), it may break out again in stronger force in some unlikely place and soon be out of control. This is also the greatest danger of cancer.

Not all cancer is created equal. Cancer cells usually look very different from normal cells, but they also may look very different from other types of cancer cells. The same type of cancer cells may affect different areas of the body. Some grow and spread quickly; others hardly seem to grow at all.

CAUSES

How cancer actually begins is still not well understood. Most authorities believe it begins with a normal cell that somehow "goes wild." Many things can play a role in this process.

Substances that are more likely than others to induce or lead to the development of some type of cancer are called *carcinogens.* A carcinogen may be mild and likely to lead to cancerous growth only after a long-term, extensive exposure. Others are more powerful, more likely to lead to cancer quickly in more people. Some carcinogens are familiar substances: radiation (ultraviolet light from the sun may lead to skin cancer after long exposure), environmental chemicals (in mines, in cigarette smoke, in chemical waste products), viruses, some hormones, and even foods and food substances. Nitrosamines, which may be converted in the body from nitrites, from saffrole (a substance in sassafras and some other oils and spices), from aflotoxins (fungi) on peanuts and some affected grains, from cereals as well as from bracken fern and some substances in other plants, are all "natural" carcinogens.[1] In addition, some additives — now off the market — such as some food dyes are well known for their role in cancer.

Any food additive that has been clearly proved to cause cancer in any way may legally be taken off the market. Saccharin remains available, with a warning label, as the result of lobbyists who fought to keep it on the market: a special and perhaps temporary concession. However, it is often many years before the substances are found to be potential carcinogens

and during these years many people have been using them regularly.

Diet is not the only factor in the development of cancer. Environmental risks, such as working in a mine, smoking cigarettes, and excessive use of alcohol are also linked with cancers. Although there are some general dietary guidelines (discussed below) to help persons work to prevent cancer, especially diet-related cancers, no diet or lifestyle is guaranteed to completely protect anyone. In this way, cancer is like many other diseases.

ATTITUDES

The client diagnosed with cancer, or the client's family or friends, may still react to the diagnosis with fear, denial, depression, and a host of other responses that may be more severe because the diagnosis is "cancer." Some feel guilty and believe the disease is a type of punishment. Others know how unpredictable cancer can be, and are suddenly faced with the reality of death. One such patient saw it as a type of dragon and described her attitude vividly in a lecture she later gave to a group of physicians:

> "We will never kill the dragon. But each morning we confront him. Then we give our children breakfast, perhaps put a bit more mulch on the peas, and hope that we can convince the dragon to stay away for a while longer . . . Having cancer is an embodiment of the existential paradox that we all experience: we feel that we are immortal, yet we know that we will die."[2]

A client's attitude toward the cancer will affect the attitude toward treatment. Since nutrition is a key part of treatment for most types of cancer, a client's attitude may also affect the way he eats. To help him accept nutritional recommendations, the health professional must try to accept, understand, and work with the client's attitude.

Other health professionals on the team (see Chapter 21) are all deeply involved, as well, in individual and family support of the client with cancer, since this disease, more than many others, may require major short- or long-term lifestyle changes. The medical team often works together closely to help the client and family receive the medical, social, vocational, emotional, and spiritual support they will need.

While some persons may see nutrition as a minor issue in cancer, it is actually a critical one. Cancer changes the way the body uses nutrients. Several common nutrition problems, including serious malnutrition, often result from the disease itself, and several other nutrition problems are common side-effects of cancer treatments. A cancer client who stays well nourished, keeps a normal weight, and learns to control some of the treatment-related side-effects is very likely to come through treatment with some excess energy. This client will probably feel better than the malnourished client. He will probably be better able to resist later infections, and may be able to go home sooner, go back to work, or return to satisfying and productive hobbies with energy and enjoyment.

NUTRITION PROBLEMS: THE IMPACT OF THE DISEASE

There are three major, nutrition related problems that are often manifested in the client with cancer: weight loss, anorexia, and cancer cachexia.

Weight loss is probably the most common nutrition problem in cancer. Persons with cancer often lose large amounts of weight quickly, losing both muscle and fat. For some persons, weight loss is the first sign that something is wrong. And weight lost may be very hard to gain back again. As cancer progresses, the client may actually lose more weight, become weaker, and be less able to fight minor infections.

Weight loss is probably due in part to anorexia; many persons with cancer *do* lose their appetite, eat less, and notice taste changes. But weight loss often happens too quickly to be due only to a lower energy intake. It seems more likely that energy needs increase. The tumor may actually cause metabolism to increase to a much higher level. The tumor uses energy to grow, and the rest of the body is drawing on energy to fight this abnormal growth and to fight any damage being done. Both the tumor and the

"host" (normal tissue) may be "competing" for nutrients, including calories.

Then, "doesn't feeding the client also feed the cancer?", some ask. Indirectly, perhaps. But the client must be fed to stay alive. Food gives the individual the strength to go through therapy and to prepare to continue living. One physician sums up the value of good nutrition in cancer by saying he knew of no cases "in which feeding a cancer patient adequately . . . diminished the beneficial effects of therapy . . . and no merit from having the patient die from starvation".[3] In fact, starving the patient probably will not help starve the cancer at all; the tumor can adapt better to a starvation state than can the patient![4]

As weight is lost, so are many of the stores usually available to the body to fight back during treatment. Nitrogen stores are lost. Some types of cancer also lead to other nutrient imbalances (such as electrolytes, vitamins, or minerals).[5]

Weight loss in cancer is usually treated aggressively. A dietitian must calculate how many calories the client needs for weight gain.[6] In detailed counseling, she works with the client (if he is well enough) to decide *how* to work to meet these energy needs. Special high calorie recipes and liquid supplements and snacks are often used for the person who is treated as an outpatient, who is well enough to live at home during therapy. Some sources for these recipes can be found in the "Resources" section at the end of this chapter. Supplements are also used while the patient is in the hospital, if these supplements can be tolerated. Many individuals receive enteral or parenteral nutrition (feeding by tube or a vein, discussed in Chapter 38) to help prevent weight loss, especially if weight loss is already so severe that cancer cachexia (below) has developed, and the individual cannot gain the nutrients needed from a standard hospital diet.

Anorexia is common, though the reasons for it are not well understood. There is no clear evidence that any of the appetite control mechanisms in the brain or throughout the body are affected by the cancer.[7] The anorexia of cancer may be related partly to the depression and pain of the disease, as well as to the side effects of treatment.[8] Most likely, it is a persistent result of many factors in the disease process. The greatest problem is the weight loss that develops as a result, leading to the syndrome called cancer *cachexia.*

Cancer cachexia is a general term for a person with cancer who has become thin, weak, and wasted. The term "cachexia" comes from two Greek words and literally means "bad condition." A cachectic person is someone who is emaciated, weak, debilitated, and malnourished. Anyone who has been starved over a long period of time (as in famine or concentration camp victims) becomes cachectic. A person with cancer cachexia is at high risk of developing infections and not having the strength to resist them.

Cancer cachexia is different from simple starvation. In starvation the body metabolism "slows down." Lean muscle tissue is conserved to some extent and the "extra" fat becomes the main source of energy.

In cancer cachexia, however, metabolism does not slow down. There is little or no "safety mechanism" working to protect muscle mass from being wasted. Nitrogen is quickly used, either by the body or by the tumor. Basal metabolism goes up, not down. The body may become resistant to insulin and blood sugar rises.[9] Elsewhere on this page is a list of the major dangers that may result from the malnutrition that follows. In fact cancer cachexia is simply a physical response to a trauma (the disease, in this case, cancer). These physical responses are the same ones that follow other types of trauma, such as shock and sepsis, which will be discussed in more detail in Chapter 39. When this hypermetabolism is allowed to continue until the cachectic patient has lost 30% to 50% of original body weight, the individual is at serious medical risk and quite possibly may die.[10]

With the current and careful treatment available, cachexia can be reversed. Treatment usually includes "hyperalimentation," a term generally used to mean aggressive, high calorie refeeding, often by tube and/or an intravenous solution. Usually at this stage the cachectic person simply cannot eat enough to gain weight. Often body fluids need to be replaced as well.

Other nutrition-related problems may depend on the location or site of the cancer. If the tumor is in the stomach, it will affect eating. With pancreatic cancer, the client may lose the ability to produce insulin and diabetes may result. If cancer is in the throat, many foods become too difficult to swallow. So the way that the disease affects nutrition will depend partly on where the disease is located.

NUTRITION-RELATED SIDE-EFFECTS: THE IMPACT OF TREATMENT

While cancer affects nutrition, so may its treatment.

There are three basic medical treatment programs for cancer. An individual might be ad-

RISKS OF MALNUTRITION IN CANCER

- Muscles, enzymes, and other necessary protein tissues are lost.
- The immune system becomes less effective, the individual more susceptible to infection
- Wounds heal poorly and are more likely to reopen
- Persons may develop supersensitive, abnormal reactions to drugs and other treatments
- Expense, inconvenience, and increased risk of longer hospitalization

(Adapted from Daly JM, Ang SD: Profiles in Nutrition Management: The Oncology Patient. North Chicago, Abbott Laboratories, 1983)

vised to go through one or more of them. When the cancer is first diagnosed, the physician determines

1. The stage of the tumor (how big and extensive it is)
2. The grading of the tumor (which tells how fast it is growing; it is expressed in grades from I to IV)
3. The type of cells involved.

Recommended treatment depends both on stage and grade, and the actual type of the cancer. Treatment may include surgery, chemotherapy, radiation, or a combination of these.

Surgery

Surgery is performed to remove the tumor. If all of it is successfully removed and there are no metastases, surgery may be the only necessary treatment. The individual may be "cured."

Surgery that affects any part of the digestive system may in turn affect nutrition. Surgery itself is a type of "trauma" that increases nutrient needs temporarily, especially needs for extra energy and protein to encourage recovery and healing. The person who is well nourished before surgery is likely to recover more quickly than one who is malnourished.[11] This is discussed in more detail in Chapter 39.

Chemotherapy

Chemotherapy actually involves "poisoning" the tumor with the administration of toxic drugs. There are many different types and combinations of these drug treatments. Once they are in the blood and traveling through the body, the drugs work to stop the cancer cells from multiplying. Eventually the cancer cells will die. Because chemotherapy treatment involves the use of toxic drugs, it is done only for a few days at a time and is repeated only as often as a physician feels is truly necessary. Chemotherapy may be combined with surgery or radiation therapy.

Because the drugs are poisons, they also affect normal cells. Hair loss and reproductive changes may occur. Some digestive enzymes may be wiped out temporarily, causing diarrhea

or malabsorption. Nausea and vomiting often make it difficult to eat. Sometimes foods eaten just before treatment become associated with the treatment because they may be vomited immediately afterwards. This conditioned aversion may make many foods undesirable and the person may be nauseated at the sight of them for a long time after treatment. Taste changes are often common and may affect nutrition if a whole food group is avoided. This symptom, dysgeusia, has been discussed (Chapter 29). Nutrition treatment during chemotherapy may also include hyperalimentation, which can help keep the client well nourished throughout the treatment.[12]

Radiation Therapy

Radiation therapy is the third common treatment of cancer. It does not affect the entire body, as chemotherapy does, although it may be combined with either or both of the other two treatments. In radiation therapy (also known as therapeutic radiology or TR), the person comes to the clinic or hospital each day for a period of days or weeks to receive carefully specified doses of radiation to the cancerous areas of the body. The patient may receive TR in this way or cobalt implants on an in-patient basis. Also called X-ray or cobalt therapy, radiation destroys the ability of cells to grow. It too may affect healthy cells. The goal of TR is to make sure the tumor cells will not grow back; the healthy cells will usually grow back once treatments have ended. Radiation for these treatments may come from a large machine or from radioactive materials temporarily "implanted" in the cancerous areas of the body.

The nutrition-related side effects of TR depend on the type of cancer, the length of treatment, and the part of the body receiving radiation. Side effects of treatments for head and neck cancers include dental caries and tooth loss, taste changes, nausea and vomiting, sore throat, and discomfort experienced in chewing or swallowing. Common side effects of treatments for tumors in the abdominal area include nausea, and vomiting and diarrhea (called radiation enteritis).

The most common nutrition-related side-effects of treatments are discussed below, with general recommendations to help the client overcome them or work with them.

Anorexia is a common problem, discussed in Chapter 29. The general guidelines discussed there apply to all types of anorexia, including that of cancer. Dietitians who work on the medical team with cancer patients can help a client and his family apply these (and other) suggestions to the specific situation. Publications from the National Cancer Institute are available (see listings in the "Resources" section at the end of this chapter) and include many helpful hints and guidelines. Anorexia cannot always be resolved, but it may be minimized with an appealing, calorie- and protein-concentrated schedule of small meals and snacks.

Diarrhea (also called "radiation enteritis" or "steatorrhea" — fatty diarrhea —) is likely to be a problem when treatments irritate or damage the cells of the small intestine. Diet treatment involves limiting three groups of foods

1. Fatty foods, which may be poorly absorbed
2. Certain fiber foods, including fresh vegetables, some fresh fruit, and legumes that cause gas
3. Foods that may irritate sensitive tissue, such as hot spices, alcohol, and caffeine

Sometimes very hot or very cold foods also irritate the intestines; foods that are only warm or cool may be better accepted.

The best medicine is preventive medicine. A client who will be receiving treatment to this area that might cause diarrhea should talk with a dietitian about the specific diet changes needed to be made *before* problems develop. The irritation in the intestines often continues for a while after treatments end, while destroyed cells are given a chance to grow back, so diet restrictions should also continue until the client feels it is time to reintroduce certain foods once again.

Dry or sore mouth and problems with chewing or swallowing. Treatment to the head and neck area may temporarily destroy the glands that manufacture saliva. The cells in the mouth and throat then dry out and swallowing is often difficult. Common methods recommended to help keep the mouth moist and help keep discomfort to a minimum include the following:

1. Frequent liquids. If weight loss is a problem, choose liquids that contain calories, such as juices, gingerale, milk drinks, eggnogs, ices.
2. Throat lozenges or hard candies. These stimulate saliva and keep the area moist, *but* they may also do great damage to the teeth, as a result of constant, close exposure to sugar (see Chapter 41). For this reason many physicians may recommend "dietetic" hard candies, sweetened with sorbitol or artificial sweeteners that do not promote tooth decay.
3. Soft or pureed foods. Most foods, even meats, can be pureed in a blender by cutting the food into tiny pieces and blending it with some liquid. Cream soups can be prepared with double-strength milk (see Chapter 29) to help provide the needed protein and energy. Vegetables with cheese or cream sauce can be mashed or pureed. Hot, fortified cereals, topped with melted cheese, butter, milk, or sugar can be an appealing and filling source of nutrients. Some persons find baby foods acceptable and convenient; others prefer to spend time blending standard table foods or casseroles with bouillons or sauces to assure themselves that they are eating "regular" foods. Soft foods need not be boring; seasonings can be added as needed to achieve the required "tang" and flavors.
4. Use of a straw instead of a spoon. Sometimes it makes swallowing easier.
5. Avoiding seasonings or foods that irritate.

Dental problems may sometimes be severe. Normally, saliva helps to protect the teeth from bacteria. But when the mouth is dry and there is little saliva, teeth may become more susceptible than ever to rampant cavities. Some TR clinics teach clients who are receiving head and neck treatments various ways to help prevent cavities. Treatment may include

1. A substitute for saliva ("artificial saliva")
2. Frequent flossing and brushing
3. A diet low in foods that feed bacteria. (These

foods and the role of nutrition in dental health are discussed in detail in Chapter 41)

4. Some other method for keeping the mouth moist and clean

Nausea and vomiting may occur in any type of treatment. Guidelines are usually the same for clients with cancer as for the pregnant woman

1. Eating dry foods, such as crackers, toast, rice, or other grain products

2. Drinking beverages separate from meals

3. Letting someone else cook while nausea and vomiting continue

4. Serving foods cool instead of steaming hot

5. Avoiding foods that obviously aggravate the problem. These will depend on the individual

6. Eating small, frequent meals and snacks, even in the middle of the night if this is a wakeful time

7. Drinking replacement fluids, preferably fluids with calories, taken in very small sips.

Early satiety, described in Chapter 29, occurs when the person feels full very quickly. A small snack may feel like a three-course meal.

Sometimes the cause of early satiety is a sluggish intestinal tract. When peristalsis, the muscle movement that propels food through the intestines, slows down, foods stay in the stomach longer. There is no easy answer. Small meals need to be taken frequently to provide the body with enough calories, patiently refilling the stomach as it slowly empties.

An individual with cancer may feel better and help prevent the complications of malnutrition when he follows the suggestions listed here:

1. Chooses foods with enough calories, protein, and other nutrients to maintain normal weight

2. Lets others do the cooking

3. Gets needed rest

4. Uses alcohol only as advised by the physician

More detailed, personalized suggestions may be available from the medical team. Each person is unique; some suggestions work for some individuals and not for others. This is why anyone going through cancer treatment should be in close contact with the physician and his team. They can help individualize the diet to family preferences, treat side effects, and answer specific questions. They can help the individual work to meet unique and usually high energy needs.

WHAT ABOUT UNCONVENTIONAL TREATMENTS?

Unconventional treatments are methods that most well-qualified physicians will not use or recommend as the *principal* or *primary* treatment, because they are usually methods that have not been proven to be worthwhile. Three types are popular in cancer treatment: *laetrile,* special diets, and *megavitamin* therapy. None of these has proved to help treat cancer. Potentially, they may all be harmful, shortening a client's already short life. Most significant, they may prevent a client from receiving the sound medical treatment that may be able to reverse or cure the cancer if it is caught early enough. Any treatment or alternate therapy that encourages someone with cancer to *wait* before going to the doctor is a dangerous therapy indeed. Some cancers can grow and spread quite rapidly.

Laetrile

Laetrile or *amygdalin* is a substance that comes from powdered apricot pits. It has been called *vitamin B_{17}* although it is not a vitamin and is not needed by the human body in any way.[4] It has been used in Mexico on cancer patients and many North Americans have gone to Mexico for treatments. Laetrile treatment is illegal in the USA. Since apricot pits contain cyanide, cyanide poisoning is one of the most likely effects of these treatments. The Federal Food and Drug Administration has flatly stated that there is "no valid scientific evidence which indicates that laetrile has any potential value in cancer management."[13]

Special Diets

Often a client with cancer will begin to eat in a certain way after the diagnosis, believing it will somehow help to treat the disease. There is often no danger in this, as long as all major nutrients are supplied and there is no risk of vitamin or mineral overdose.

Some diets, though, may actually increase the client's nutritional risk. The *macrobiotic diet* proposed by some groups, is one of these. This is a vegan diet that has been suggested by several lay books and critically reviewed by the medical profession.[14]

The biggest problem with the macrobiotic diet is that it is not calorically dense. It is high in fiber and low in fat, meaning a person must eat a large quantity of food to acquire enough calories. This makes the diet particularly inappropriate for the cancer patient with a poor appetite who is probably going to lose weight on a regular diet, and for whom weight loss can cause or lead to serious cachexia. The diet is based on the Eastern philosophy of yin and yang, hot and cold forces that must be in balance or illness will result. (The yin/yang theory of food was discussed in Chapter 18). There is nothing in medical science that supports this philosophy of disease. Illness is caused by imbalances that often have little or no relevance to diet or spiritual forces. Even if followed completely, the diet does not provide all the nutrients a cancer patient needs.

The greatest danger of this type of unconventional treatment is its claim that diet alone can cure cancer, advising "patients with advanced cancer . . . that with a macrobiotic diet they are more likely to recover than if they received conventional treatment."[14] This encourages the cancer patient to ignore the physician, who may actually be able to rid the patient's body of cancer, in favor of another method that almost certainly cannot do so. Nutrition is a very important *support* for medical treatment of cancer, but it should not be used to replace it. The final choice for treatment lies with the patient himself, but he should certainly be properly informed and wisely advised, since no one else has more to lose.

Megavitamin Treatment

Vitamins A, C, and E have all been connected at different times with cancer treatments. Vitamin A seems to have some effect in topically treating certain types of skin tumors,[15] but not when it is ingested. Vitamin A can of, course, build up in the body and become toxic, with serious side-effects, eventually leading to convulsions, coma, and death from respiratory failure.

Some researchers believe carotene (the substance that makes carrots orange and that can be converted in the body to vitamin A) might be an important substance on its own for the treatment of cancer.[15] Research is currently testing this theory. Carotene does not have the dangerous side effects of vitamin A, although high levels may pigment the skin, especially the palms of the hands, to a yellow orange.

Vitamin C does help prevent the conversion of nitrites into nitrosamines[15] but this does not justify the use of supplements. High doses of vitamin C tablets seem to aggravate heartburn, nausea, vomiting, and edema in cancer patients and even seem to lead to a larger tumor.[15] It simply may be enough to drink a large glass of orange juice, eat some nitrite-containing bacon, and avoid supplements altogether!

Vitamin E is an *antioxidant,* that is, a substance that helps protect cells from the destruction and changes that oxygen may cause. Some people believe antioxidants may help protect cells from environmental pollutants and may retard aging, but this has yet to be proved. E is still not completely understood, but it does not seem as toxic as the other fat-soluble vitamins. Very high doses (over 300 IU per day[15]) may, however, affect the way the liver handles vitamins A and K. There is little or no definite evidence to prove any role vitamin E may have in the therapies associated with cancer.

HOSPICE CARE

Hospice is a type of medical care that provides support and encouragement to the terminally ill. The idea, an old one with roots in the convents of the Middle Ages, was renewed in this century by Dr. Cicely M. Saunders who founded St. Christopher's Hospice in England in the

1960's. In the USA, most hospice care is provided to terminally ill persons by visiting nurses, doctors, and dietitians whose services are reimbursed by federal funds and by some private insurance companies. Hospice care is for anyone suffering a terminal illness, not simply cancer alone. In hospice care, a person is treated with dignity and allowed to die with as much support, pain relief, maintenance nutrition, and encouragement as possible during the last period of life. Hospice care usually depends on medical support and volunteers.

The goal of good nutrition support in hospice care is comfort. Food may help a patient or client feel as well as possible for as long as possible. Feeding should include whatever is most acceptable to the client and to the family. Sometimes tube feeding is accepted and preferred because it can help the person retain some strength to make the most of each day without having to worry about eating a sufficient quantity of food. Sometimes soft foods or liquids are preferred.

In hospice, life is supported by natural or comfortable means until it goes of its own accord. Sensible, appropriate nutrition is a very important part of that support. (Some hospice resources are listed at the end of this chapter.)

CANCER PREVENTION

In 1983 the National Academy of Science issued a "Diet, Nutrition, and Cancer Report." [16] Based on current research, the academy made three policy statements and suggested six dietary guidelines that may help prevent cancer. They concluded that no special diet will help cure cancer, that certain dietary changes may play a role in prevention, and that herbal teas, laetrile, and megadoses of nutrients are ineffective in cancer treatment. The dietary guidelines are listed below.

One year later, early in 1984, the American Cancer Society issued seven dietary guidelines to help the general public prevent diet-related cancers. These included all of the NAS recommendations plus the added advice to eat less and stay trim.

NUTRITION-RELATED CANCER PREVENTION GUIDELINES

1. Limit fats to 30% of total calories. For example, a 1500 calorie diet should acquire slightly less than 500 calories from fats in all foods.

2. Include foods high in fiber, carotene, vitamin C, and include cruciferous vegetables (cabbage, kohlrabi, broccoli, brussel sprouts, and cauliflower) in the diet daily.

3. Avoid foods that have been smoked or pickled. They may contain nitrosamines. These foods include sausages, smoked fish and ham, bacon, hot dogs, bologna, and other luncheon meats.

4. Monitor food additives and toxicants.

5. Drink alcohol in moderation and do not smoke. Stomach and lung cancer are more likely when alcohol intake is high, especially when the drinker also smokes.

6. Vitamin supplements are unnecessary, unless they have been medically advised.

7. Maintain normal weight for height.

(Adapted from American Cancer Society: Nutrition and cancer: Cause and prevention; an American Cancer Society special report. CA-A Cancer Journal for Clinicians 34(2), 1984)

Cancer is one of the leading causes of death in the USA.[17] Dietary changes in some populations have seemed to change the incidence of cancer for that group of people.[18] Once an individual has cancer, he may encounter many nutrition-related problems and need careful, ongoing support. But it may also be possible to lower the risk of developing cancer at all by making a few, generally simple, lifelong dietary changes.

STUDY QUESTIONS

1. How is a "malignant" tumor different from a "benign" tumor? Are both cancerous? Why or why not?

2. List at least five substances that may cause cancer.

3. How is nutrition important in the treatment of cancer?

4. Why may cancer patients lose weight quickly? Explain the risks of this weight loss.

5. How does cancer affect
   - Metabolism?
   - Appetite?
   - Taste sensations

6. List the three common treatments in cancer therapy and at least three side effects that may be associated with any type of treatment.

7. Mr. P. is a 58-year-old school teacher who has all three of the side effects you have listed in the above question. What can he do about them?

8. What is laetrile? Is it safe to use in cancer treatment? Why or why not?

9. What other unconventional treatments (described in the text or encountered in your own experience) are sometimes used to "treat" cancer? What are the potential risks?

10. What is a hospice?

11. List at least five recommendations that may help prevent cancer. Which of these are already part of your lifestyle? What can you do to incorporate the rest into your life?

REFERENCES

1. Miller JA, Miller EC: Carcinogens occurring naturally in foods. Fed Proc 35(6): 1316–1321, May 1, 1976

2. Stewart-Trillin A: Of Dragons and Garden Peas. N Engl J Med 304(12): 699–701, March 19, 1981

3. Gori GB: Summation: Conference on nutrition and cancer therapy. Cancer Res 37: 2469–2471, July 1977

4. Goodhart RE, Shils ME: Modern Nutrition in Health and Disease, 6th ed, pp 449, 1159. Philadelphia, Lea & Febiger, 1980

5. Blackburn GL et al: The effect of cancer on nitrogen, electrolyte and mineral metabolism. Cancer Res 37: 2348–2353, July 1977

6. Bozzetti F: Determination of the caloric requirement of patients with cancer. Surg Gynecol Obstet 149: 667–670, November 1979

7. DeWys WD: Anorexia in cancer patients. Cancer Res 37: 2354–2358, July 1977

8. Holland JCB et al: Psychological aspects of anorexia in cancer patients. Cancer Res 37: 2425–2428, July 1977

9. Daly JM, Ang SD: Profiles in Nutrition Management: The Oncology Patient. North Chicago, IL, Abbott Laboratories, 1983

10. Brennan MF: Uncomplicated starvation vs. cancer cachexia. Cancer Res 37: 2359–2364, July 1977

11. Shils ME, Randall HT: Diet and nutrition in the care of the surgical patient. In Goodhart RE, Shils ME (eds): Modern Nutrition in Health and Disease, 6th ed, pp 1082–1124. Philadelphia, Lea & Febiger, 1980

12. Copeland EM: Intravenous hyperalimentation and chemotherapy: An update. J Parenter Enter Nutr 6(3): 236–239, May–June 1982

13. Federal Food and Drug Administration: Drug Bulletin 7:2, 1977

14. Stare FJ: Book Review: The cancer prevention diet: Michio Kushi's nutritional blueprint for the relief and prevention of disease. N Engl J Med 309: 677, September 15, 1983

15. Huber A: The Effects of Megadoses of Vitamins and Minerals. Presented at Conference on Controversial Issues Confronting the Cancer Patient. Boston, March 8, 1984

16. American Cancer Society: Nutrition and cancer: Cause and prevention; An American Cancer So-

ciety special report. CA: A Cancer Journal for Clinicians 34(2), 1984

17. US Department of Health and Human Services, Office of Health Research, Statistics and Technology: Facts from the National Center for Health Statistics, Department of Health and Human Services Publication No. (PHS) 81–1002

18. Van Eys J: Nutrition and neoplasia. Nutr Rev 40(12): 353–359, December 1982

RESOURCES

Many government publications devoted to cancer and its treatment are available for the client and his family. Three excellent resources on diet and cancer are:

National Institutes of Health: Eating Hints: Recipes and Tips for Better Nutrition during Cancer Treatment. National Institutes of Health Publication No. 80–2079, 1980

National Institutes of Health: Diet and Nutrition: A Resource for the Parents of Children with Cancer. National Institutes of Health Publication No. 81–2038, June 1981

Sherman M: Feeding the Sick Child. Department of Health, Education, and Welfare Publication No. (NIH) 78–795, 1978

(All the above available from the Office of Cancer Communications, National Cancer Institute, Bethesda, MD 20205)

Some hospice resources and related publications include the following:

Hamilton MP, Reid HF: A Hospice Handbook. Grand Rapids, MI, Wm B. Eerdman, 1980

Zorza V, Zorza R: A Way To Die. Westminster, MD, Alfred Knopf, 1980

(Many states are forming or have formed local hospice organizations that are listed in the telephone directory)

CHAPTER 31

Diabetes Mellitus

OBJECTIVES

1. To introduce and define the major terms commonly used in the diagnosis and treatment of diabetes mellitus

2. To outline the history, disorder, symptoms, and potential complications of this disease in both insulin-dependent and noninsulin-dependent diabetics

3. To explain the interrelated role of diet, activity, and insulin, and the importance of monitoring blood sugar for disease control

4. To list and explain the factors that may make "tight" control difficult
   a. Disease
   b. Stress
   c. Lack of knowledge or understanding
   d. Use of alcohol
   e. Attitude toward the disease that leads to noncompliance
   f. Pregnancy
   g. Medications

5. To discuss and illustrate the diet therapy of diabetes mellitus, explaining
   a. Goals of diet therapy for insulin and noninsulin dependent diabetics
   b. Role of the exchange system
   c. Why and how to space meals
   d. Preparation for emergencies
   e. Need for fiber and other carbohydrates that may help maintain stable blood sugars

f. Ways to be an informed consumer regarding
   "Dietetic" foods
   Convenience foods
   Eating out
   Sugar substitutes

6. To emphasize the importance of the diabetic taking the fullest responsibility possible for the control of his disease

7. To provide additional, detailed resources for the diabetic, the diabetic's family, and the health care provider

Around 10 AD, the Greek, Celsus, first described what is now known as diabetes. Another Greek, Aretaeus, gave the disease its name. *Diabetes* means "to siphon" or "run through." Centuries later, in 1679, a scientist noticed the sweetness of a diabetic's urine; thus the term "mellitus," meaning honey. Yet through all those centuries, although there was a name for the disease, most persons afflicted with it died within a few years of its onset. Not until 1921, when Banting and Best discovered insulin, could a diabetic hope to live more than a few years.

BLOOD SUGAR LEVELS

Normally the beta cells in the pancreas manufacture insulin, a hormone that helps govern the body's narrow, "tight" control of blood sugar

(BS) levels. When blood sugar rises, mechanisms normally trigger the pancreas to manufacture insulin. The hormone travels into the blood and helps to carry away the extra glucose or sugar from the blood into the cells where it is needed most (see Fig. 31-1). When this process lowers BS to normal once again, insulin production slows down. When BS becomes too low, the hormone balance sends messages that cause cells to break down and manufacture glucose. These hormone balances may also trigger hunger. Food supplies additional glucose (see Chapters 1, 2 and 4). In the healthy body, when insulin production is normal, blood sugar nor-

mally ranges between 80 mg and 120 mg per deciliter (mg/dl or mg %). It may rise after a meal to 150 mg and perhaps to 160 mg, but rarely goes higher, and is back to its normal range within several hours. Sometimes normal BS may drop to a level as low as 60 mg, but rarely lower.

Diabetes mellitus begins when the natural insulin produced by the body becomes ineffective or less plentiful. When insulin balance is upset, tight blood sugar control is lost. Blood sugar rises, and keeps rising, as it builds up in the blood but is unable to link up with insulin to reach the cell. This usually happens because

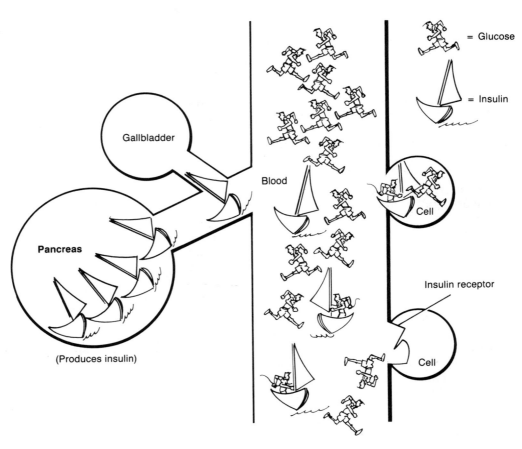

Figure 31-1
The role of insulin in controlling blood sugar.

there is not enough insulin available. In some diabetics, there is plenty of insulin but it cannot work properly. These individuals are called "insulin-resistant" and are usually overweight.

When blood sugar rises over 160 mg to 180 mg/dl, the kidneys are not able to conserve this large quantity of sugar. The extra sugar is lost, carried to the bladder where it is emptied in the urine. The presence of sugar in the urine is a sign that something is wrong.

This critical limit of the kidneys is called the "renal threshold." It can be compared to the water in a flood, which rises higher than the walls built against it (see Fig. 31-2). When blood sugar tops this threshold and glucose "spills" into the urine, urine tests become positive (+) for sugar. Since the urine can only carry so much sugar at a time it cannot rid itself of all the excess, so blood sugar levels may continue rising. This condition of high blood sugar is called *hyperglycemia.* A person may have high blood sugar but not spill sugar into the urine; the renal threshold tends to rise with age.

Diabetics on insulin sometimes experience another problem: low blood sugar or *hypoglycemia.* Insulin works so well that blood sugar may plummet below 60 mg to 80 mg/dl; this usually happens when there is too much insulin for the available glucose.

INSULIN-DEPENDENT DIABETES (IDDM)

There are two major types of diabetes mellitus: one that is insulin-dependent (IDDM), which is sometimes called type I or juvenile-onset, and one that is not necessarily insulin-dependent (called noninsulin-dependent diabetes— NIDDM—also known as type II or adult onset). The differences between these two types are outlined on the following page. Only about 10% of all diabetics belong to the first group. These individuals have no natural insulin production, and need insulin injections daily. The normal pancreatic production of the hormone has, for some reason, shut down completely. The causes vary.

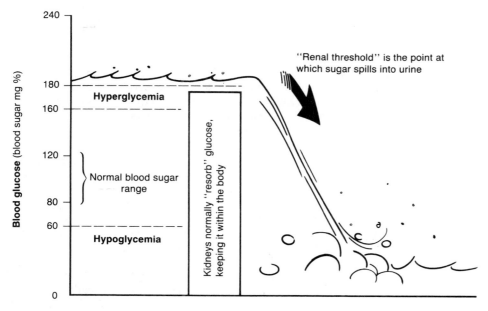

Figure 31-2
The renal threshold.

INSULIN- vs. NONINSULIN-DEPENDENT DIABETES: A COMPARISON

	IDDM	NIDDM
Onset	• Usually onset in childhood or as young adult	• Usually after age 40 or during pregnancy
Treatment	• Lifelong insulin injections and a diet controlling carbohydrate, protein, and fat	• Weight loss • Sometimes insulin or oral hypoglycemic agents may be treated by weight loss alone • Diet controlling carbohydrate, protein, fat
Importance of diet	• Critical for blood sugar control • Meals, snacks, and food quantities must be planned around insulin dose to prevent hypoglycemia	• Critical for weight loss • Rigid timing of meals and snacks not important unless on insulin
Importance of exercise	• Stimulates circulation • Helps body use insulin	• Makes body more sensitive to its own insulin • Uses energy to help weight loss
Hypoglycemia	• May occur; diabetic must carry emergency sugar source at all times	• Not a problem unless individual also on insulin or oral hypoglycemic agents
Hyperglycemia	• Common when diabetes control is poor	• Common when diabetes control is poor
Cause	• Pancreas "shuts down;" unable to manufacture insulin	• Pancreas may continue to produce insulin, but cells insensitive to it
Outcome	• No known cure • Treatment is lifelong • Potential risk of complications leading to vision problems (retinopathy), cardiovascular disease, neurologic problems (neuropathy), and renal disease	• Symptoms may resolve with weight loss • If uncontrolled, potential long-term complications may be same as IDDM

The tendency to develop diabetes, or impaired glucose tolerance, may be inherited. However, persons with this tendency may still need some stressor or precipitating factor before they actually develop the disease. Some factors that increase the risk for disease in persons with the tendency toward diabetes include obesity, pregnancy, disease, infections, and some drugs; certain types of drugs (discussed below) may lead to high blood sugar levels.

The actual causes of diabetes are still not well understood. Current thought seems to indicate that diabetes may be a type of autoimmune disease, in which something in the body interprets the beta cells as "foreign" and forms antibodies against them, destroying them.[1] This theory is currently the subject of much research. In some individuals, antibodies have been detected long before the onset of the disease. In the meantime, there is no cure for the disease; all treatment is intended simply to control blood sugar and minimize the risks of complications.

IDDM may also develop when severe malnutrition, starvation, and disease cause the pancreas to shut down.[2] The insulin-dependent diabetic will probably never again be able to manufacture insulin.

This type of diabetic is usually underweight (or of normal weight), and is still in childhood or early adulthood when diabetes suddenly develops. Weight loss is a common early symptom because the human body cannot use food properly without insulin. Other indications of the disease include polyuria (excess urination), polydipsia (excess thirst), polyphagia (excess hunger), a sweet, fruity breath (due to ketone by-products of fat breakdown in the blood, urine, and lungs) and, ultimately, unconsciousness and diabetic coma. The body has lost its balance completely; blood and urine are full of sugar and other abnormal substances, and the cells are starving.

Once the disease is diagnosed, it takes several weeks or months finally to stabilize a person on a particular level of insulin and on a particular diet. Often one reason this adjustment takes so long is a phenomenon called a "honeymoon period." After injections of insulin for a few days (or less, or more), the pancreas may actually "revive" once again to pump a small amount of natural insulin. The diabetic needs less insulin through injection, and may wonder if the diagnosis were correct. Sometimes the body continues to pump its own insulin for weeks and even months, before it finally fades and shuts down for the last time. This in-between time is often a helpful time for the diabetic to begin to adjust to the disease and begin to adapt his lifestyle to include regular exercise, regular injections, and a predictable diet.

NONINSULIN DEPENDENT DIABETES (NIDDM)

The second type of diabetes mellitus is quite different. Adult-onset diabetics may be over 35 before they notice any symptoms. They can, and probably will, continue to produce insulin. Their pancreatic islet cells still function, but inadequately. Somewhere there is a "communica-

tion breakdown" between the needs of the cells and the action of the insulin. The pancreas may not produce a sufficient quantity. The cells may "resist" the insulin that is produced. Blood sugar rises and the cells may begin to develop imbalances.

Overweight is the most common precursor of insulin-resistant NIDDM. Population studies have shown a definite relationship between obesity and NIDDM. In fact, if two similar groups of people are compared, and the only difference between them is that one group has an average weight that is 20% higher than its peers, the heavier group is TWICE as likely to develop diabetes than is the thinner group.[3] Typical diets of the two population groups do not seem to matter; the factor that most influences the potential for type II diabetes is the percent of ideal body weight. This may be why NIDDM is more common in wealthier than in poor nations.

The overweight diabetic may not have the same early symptoms of diabetes as his younger, thinner counterpart. High blood sugar, detected at a routine physical, may be the first sign of NIDDM. The new diabetic may have no weight loss, and may feel fine. Sometimes he may experience the same or similar symptoms (thirst, excess urination, and so forth) as the insulin-dependent diabetic. Or he may have other complaints: frequent infections, blurred or altered vision, pains or cramps in legs, feet, or fingers, slow wound healing, intense itching and/or drowsiness.[4]

TREATMENT

Treatment for the two types may differ. But both share the same goals: to normalize blood sugar and postpone or prevent disease complications. IDDM is treated with insulin, diet, and recommended regular exercise. Insulin-dependent diabetics usually do not need to lose weight. NIDDM is treated primarily with diet. Exercise is also strongly recommended and should be taken as seriously as diet. Regular diet and exercise are designed to help a person maintain blood sugar within normal range and begin to lose weight.

Sometimes overweight, adult-onset diabetics are so resistant to their own insulin that they do need injections of the hormone until they are able to lose weight.* Many adults are not comfortable giving themselves injections. Others may need to take *oral hypoglycemic agents,* drugs that stimulate the body to respond to its own insulin. The pills (which do not contain insulin) often have risks and side-effects of their own. As it loses fat, the body becomes more and more sensitive to its own insulin, and the injections—or pills—are often no longer necessary. Weight loss does *not cure* diabetes, but it is the prescribed, *lifelong treatment* for control. A person with NIDDM who successfully loses weight, and then maintains the desired weight with balanced diet and exercise may truly enjoy life, free of diabetes-related hospital crises, insulin injections and complications. There is much evidence that diabetics who lose weight can protect themselves from the dangers and health risks of both diabetes and obesity.[5] Some of these health risks are discussed below.

GESTATIONAL DIABETES

A third, common type of diabetes is *gestational diabetes,* or the diabetes of pregnancy. Some women seem able to produce and use insulin well until the body is stressed with the added demands of pregnancy. Then blood sugar shoots up. This hyperglycemia may be caused by a limited production of insulin, an altered ability to use it, or some other poorly understood function.

The woman who "spills" sugar into her urine during each pregnancy should follow carefully the diet advice of a dietitian and physician during her pregnancy, and take insulin if it is necessary. There is the 50% possibility that she may someday "stay" diabetic, even after the baby is born, if her gestational diabetes is not properly controlled.[6] Most women with gestational diabetes do not require insulin and can control the symptoms by adjusting their diet. Women who develop gestational diabetes may increase their infant's medical risks as well as their own; good control protects the infant as well as the mother.

Overweight women with gestational diabetes should *not lose* weight during their pregnancy, since this also may be a risk for the infant. Weight loss may be recommended after delivery, though, and may help prevent the women from developing gestational diabetes during her next pregnancy.

Women who are already diabetic and then become pregnant face the risk of miscarriage, birth defects and the range of health problems of uncontrolled diabetes. However, with close monitoring and control, a healthy pregnancy is possible for a diabetic woman; the better her blood sugar control, the more likely that she will have a safe and healthy pregnancy.[7,8]

LONG-TERM COMPLICATIONS

Most of the complications of diabetes are related to blood circulation or neuropathy. Tiny blood vessels tend to break, clog, or change in some way, causing poor circulation over many years. These changes may be caused by chronic, abnormal blood sugar levels or by some other unknown disease factor. When the blood vessels break or become clogged, problems develop in the cells affected by that blood flow. When this occurs in the eye, for example, the condition is called retinopathy and can cause blindness. Diabetes is one of the leading causes of blindness in the USA. Vascular changes may also develop in the tiny filtering nephrons of the kidneys and may lead to renal failure.

Larger blood vessels may also become clogged with fatty deposits and lead to cardiovascular complications. Diabetics are at a higher risk of developing atherosclerosis earlier than nondiabetics.[4] There are probably many reasons for this. When diabetes is out of control, fat breaks down to produce energy. Since insulin is not necessary to move the energy from fat into the cells, the blood may contain more fat, including cholesterol and triglycerides, than normal. High blood levels of these fats increase the risk of heart attack and stroke.

Neuropathy or nerve damage is the other common complication. A diabetic may have neuropathy in the peripheral areas, that is, in the fingers, toes, legs, and hands. As a result of this peripheral neuropathy, the person may not feel

---

* This is often a "Catch-22" situation, since dependence on insulin may make weight loss difficult.

as sharply the pain of a sunburn, of stepping on glass, even a stubbed toe or scraped finger. The wound may not receive the prompt attention it needs. And since circulation may also be poor in these areas, it will take longer for the wound to heal. Infection and even gangrene may develop. When these problems become serious, some diabetics may eventually need to have fingers or toes surgically removed.

Many authorities believe that careful blood sugar control may help to postpone the development of at least some of these complications. Without natural insulin it is very difficult to adequately control blood sugar.

Persons who work hard for many years to keep their diabetes well controlled do frequently still develop certain complications. Renal disease seems to be inevitable for a small percentage of diabetics.[9] To some degree retinopathy may also simply be part of the disease. Blood sugar control, through diet and exercise, may help prevent neuropathies and certainly helps to prevent the weariness, thirst, frequent urination, hunger, and vision problems of hyperglycemia. Triglycerides, a type of fat in the blood, may also be kept to a minimum with improved blood sugar control and the cardiovascular risks of diabetes may also be minimized with a diet low in fat, especially saturated fats and cholesterol.

While professionals agree that diabetic control is important, there are many opinions regarding just how "tight" that control should be. What is the safest, narrowest, range of blood sugar that a diabetic can most easily maintain? This issue is the object of much ongoing research and several different schools of thought. Some advocate close monitoring, strict diet, and very tight insulin control that allows for occasional hypoglycemia. Others try to prevent hypoglycemia by allowing a slightly more liberal diet, and slightly different insulin therapy. It is not the purpose of this text to discuss these theories in detail; each has its benefits and drawbacks. Whatever method a diabetic learns for his own control, blood sugar must be regulated in some way and to some degree. The closer the blood sugar level stays in the normal range, the more likely it seems that the body will be able to function normally and well for many years.

CONTROLLING BLOOD SUGAR

Normal fasting blood contains 80 mg to 120 mg of glucose per deciliter. After a meal, the level rises. In the diabetic, blood sugar may start high and go higher.

While the uncontrolled diabetic's blood sugar level is very high, the cells are starving, so fat cells break down for needed energy. Even though the energy (like money in a bank account) is there, it does not reach the cells, so they begin to draw on their own reserves. This results in the emergency state of ketosis or ketoacidosis (ketones or acetones as well as sugar are in the urine) and the individual may lapse into coma.

The symptoms, causes, and treatment of diabetic hyperglycemia are listed in Figure 31-3.

Insulin injections allow the blood sugar to finally enter and feed the cells. Fat breakdown stops and the diabetic begins to recover, using blood sugar properly, for energy.

Hypoglycemia (discussed in detail in Chapter 24) is almost never a problem for a diabetic who does not use insulin. But when the insulin dose is too high (as mentioned above), the blood sugar level may drop too low. And, unlike reactive hypoglycemia, which can often correct itself, the results may be very serious. Severe, untreated hypoglycemia can also lead to coma, as well as cell damage (including brain cells), and death. When detected early and treated properly, however, hypoglycemia can be quickly corrected. The symptoms, causes, and treatment of diabetic hypoglycemia are also listed in Figure 31-3. The insulin-dependent diabetic is constantly living in and maintaining a balance between the two extremes. The *hypo*glycemic reaction is called an "insulin reaction." While *hyper*glycemia is corrected through diet and medication or insulin, insulin reactions can be quickly corrected by giving the diabetic a source of sugar. Some emergency sugar sources are listed on page 283. Diabetics, especially those on insulin, should always carry some source of sugar (glucose is best) in a pocket, purse, jacket, string around the neck, or pinned somewhere on the body. Diabetic drivers should *always* keep some sugar source in the car. They may also want to keep other foods in the car in case of a breakdown or traffic jam. Foods such as crackers,

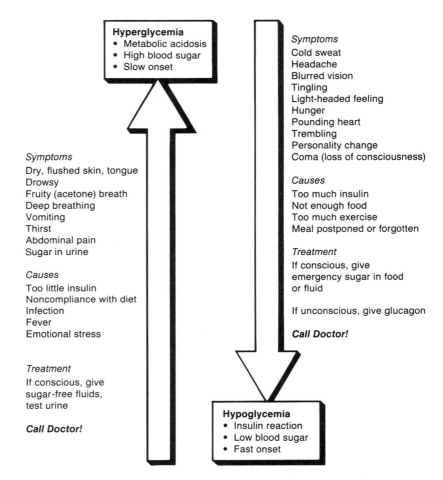

Figure 31-3
When blood sugar goes out of control.

peanut butter, and some canned or bottled beverages store well in most temperatures.

In summary, blood sugar in the healthy diabetic is controlled by three factors: diet, activity, and insulin. These must be kept in balance in health and in disease and must be monitored carefully at all times. Many different factors can affect their control, as illustrated in Figure 31-4.

Insulin

In IDDM, injections of insulin are given once or several times each day to replace that missing natural hormone.

There are many different types of insulin. Some types act quickly while others reach their "peak" or full activity level more slowly. Many persons take a combination of several types of insulin in order to have insulin available all day, since even after its peak activity, all insulin stays in the blood for several hours. Table 31-1 lists the types of insulin and their different levels of activity.

Mealtimes must be balanced with the times a diabetic takes insulin. If food is not available to break down into glucose for the insulin available, insulin reactions can develop quickly. A diabetic must plan regular meals and snacks

EMERGENCY SUGAR SOURCES

Each of the items below provides 10 grams of fast-acting carbohydrate:

Juice, equivalent to 1 fruit exchange (*e.g.,* ½ cup orange juice)

½ cup (4 oz) Regular soda

5 Small sugar cubes (2 packets)

2½ tsp Sugar

¼ cup Regular jello

6 Lifesavers (chewed quickly)

½ Regular popsicle

6 Jelly beans

10 Gumdrops

2 tsp Karo or Coke syrup or honey

Commercial glucose alternatives available in most pharmacies include:

2 Glucose Tablets®

⅓ of an 80-g bottle of Glutose® concentrated sugar liquid

10-g pkt of Monogel®

Note: NEVER give "dietetic" or "diet" candy or jello or whole fruit to help treat an insulin reaction. It will not work!

---

around the times when insulin is most active in the body. Since the person usually takes the same dose of insulin at the same time(s) each day, the health team can work together with the diabetic to help determine the best timing for meals and snacks.

Drugs

As mentioned above, oral hypoglycemic agents (OHA's) are sometimes used to stimulate the body to use its own insulin. These drugs are not recommended in pregnancy and do not work if a diabetic is unable to produce insulin. Some of these drugs include Diabinese, Tolinase, Orinase, Diabeta and Glyburide. While a pill is usually more appealing than an injection, these pills also may carry risks. Individuals on the pills may have an increased risk of heart attack and other cardiovascular complications, which are

already a risk for the overweight diabetic. Any diabetic on an oral agent should be aware of the potential side-effects and complications. Often weight loss and exercise alone will bring BS down toward normal so OHA's can be discontinued.

Activity

Activity or exercise helps control blood sugar. Regular aerobic exercise such as walking, jogging, swimming, tennis, or some other consistent sport makes the cells of the body more sensitive to insulin. The overweight adult diabetic may be able to control blood sugar because exercise has decreased insulin resistance. The insulin-dependent diabetic who exercises may need less insulin. Since exercise promotes blood flow, it may also prevent cardiovascular complications and help a diabetic stay healthy.

Despite all these advantages of planned, regular exercise, the insulin-dependent diabetic who exercises also needs to guard against insulin reactions. Exercise may lower blood sugar so effectively that hypoglycemia develops. The physician and dietitian can help a diabetic plan exercise, balancing it around meals and insulin. All insulin-dependent diabetics who exercise MUST carry some sugar source *even* while they are exercising. When a diabetic on insulin loses weight, the insulin dose may need to be changed in proportion to the new weight or, again, insulin reactions may occur.

Self Monitoring

The diabetic who is trying to control blood sugar — by diet or insulin and diet — needs to be sure that the control methods are working. This is why diabetics must check their urine and often their blood sugar regularly. Urine tests are usually done in the morning, but may be done several times each day. Test tapes are available that tell whether the urine contains sugar and/or ketones. Urine testing tells whether the sugar level is high enough to spill into urine, but urine testing cannot determine exact blood sugar levels. Blood tests alone will do that. The best

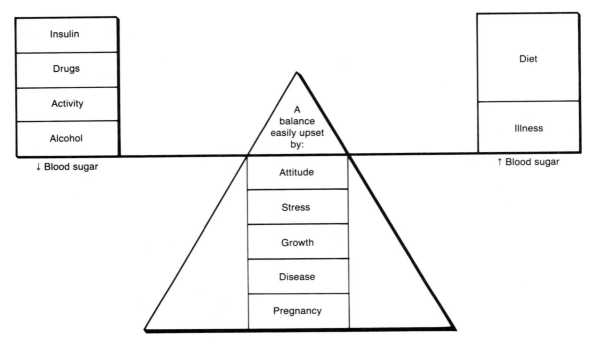

Figure 31-4
Factors that influence blood sugar balance.

control of blood glucose involves monitoring it. In the past few years, fingersticks and test tapes for blood sugar (such as Diascan® and Chemstrip-BG®) have become more available and more commonly used. A diabetic may test blood sugar by himself at any time, and then adjust diet and activity accordingly. Diet control is discussed elsewhere in this chapter.

Confounding Factors

A confounding factor is an element or situation that interferes or causes confusion. There are

Table 31-1

Common Insulin Preparations

Preparation	Onset (hr)	Peak (hr)	Duration (hr)
Rapid-acting			
Regular	½–1	2–5	6–8
Prompt Insulin Zinc Suspension	½–1½	5–10	12–16
Intermediate-acting			
NPH	1–1½	8–12	24
Lente	1–2½	7–15	24
Long-acting			
PZI (Protein-zinc insulin suspension)	4–8	14–20	36
Ultralente	4–8	10–30	over 36

(Scherer JC: Lippincott Nurses' Drug Manual, p 583. Philadelphia, JB Lippincott, 1985)

several factors (listed in Figure 31-4) that sometimes interfere with control of normal blood sugar in the diabetic.

Illness

Illness increases the energy need for healing and usually decreases the energy need for activity. An insulin-dependent diabetic who is ill needs the same amount of energy as usual, and at least the same amount of insulin (unless the physician recommends more). Control in illness is difficult because, although insulin needs do not decrease with flu, fever, and other infections, appetite usually drops. Blood sugar often rises in illness (see Fig. 31-5) yet the diabetic is at risk of an insulin–energy imbalance if calorie intake is not as close to normal as possible.

When "sick days" come, food energy is usually most acceptable in the form of small, frequent meals. Liquids may be better accepted than solids; for example, an eggnog might be more appealing than a scrambled egg and milk. Soups, juices, custards, and even ice cream and

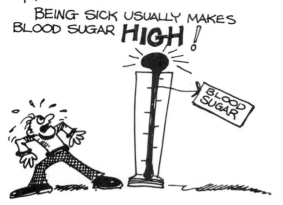

Figure 31-5
An important reminder. (From Notes for Diabetics: What to Do if You Are Sick. Boston, Joslin Diabetes Foundation, 1976)

sherbet may be worked into the "sick day" diet. Any insulin-dependent diabetic should be prepared with a list of "sick day" foods and their exchange values. The days should begin by notifying the physician of the illness, in case special needs develop.

Stress

Emotional or physical stress will change blood sugar balance. It may decrease the need for insulin and lead to insulin reactions, or it may have the opposite effect. A diabetic who is under frequent stress should discuss the condition with the physician.

Growth

The insulin needs of the diabetic diagnosed in childhood will change as the child grows. And this is often complicated because growth is never steady. A child who is going through a "growth spurt" may at first appear to be totally out of diabetic control. Parents need to be aware of this, and to work with the child to learn gradually to adjust insulin and diet to promote the best possible growth. The biggest growth spurt for most diabetics is puberty. This may affect the insulin needs of girls quite suddenly, shortly after age ten, and of boys later and more slowly.[10] Since teens may continue growing for almost ten years, their insulin and diet will need close medical follow-up during these years.

Poor Compliance: The Human Factor

Unfortunately adolescence is the period when poor *compliance* is most common. A teen may consider diabetes as part of his childhood, part of dependence, and try to rebel against it, to the great concern of many parents who may also be struggling with this loss of childhood and dependence. Adolescence is not the only time when compliance may be poor; a diabetic of any age may have problems accepting the responsibility and the lifelong reality of the disease. Children diagnosed early may learn their attitude from their parents. Adults diagnosed later in life may not understand the freedom they would gain with weight loss and control, or they may simply reject the concept that they are "weak" enough to have diabetes. As a result of their poor control, they may do yet more damage. Some persons reject the idea of placing any limits on their diet.

No man, including a diabetic, is an island. Attitudes and belief systems are shaped and reinforced by family, friends, and other influences. Meals and activities are usually shared. Because diabetes will affect someone for life, the other persons in the diabetic's life should be involved. An adolescent may want to be in control of his own insulin and diet and this independence should be encouraged. But the family needs to know it and talk about it. Persons who prepare meals must understand the reasons for the diabetic's diet and lifestyle. The mothers of a diabetic child's friends need to know.

Poor compliance may result from a negative attitude or from lack of knowledge. It may happen as the result of not receiving sufficient diet instruction; not being able to adapt the diet to cultural preferences; disagreement with the doctor; distrust of the medical staff; lack of family or other support; resentment about being told what to do, or belief that the diet is too expensive or causes hunger or dizziness.[11] Whatever the reason, it should be considered, discussed and, whenever possible, prevented by clear, effective, early counseling and planning. But it *must* be discussed. The diabetic is the one who must live with the disease and seek to control it. No one else can do it for him. Sometimes a child may feel alone and different and welcome the support of a summer camp for diabetic children, or some other contact with diabetic peers who can remind each other that they are not alone, and they are not freaks.

Alcohol

Alcohol has an acute effect on blood sugar balance. It does NOT act like sugar; instead it temporarily competes with the liver's ability to produce an emergency supply of glucose; as a result blood sugar may drop to a dangerously low level while alcohol is being metabolized. A diabetic who has a few drinks on an empty stomach may pass out in a hypoglycemic state and may even die after being mistaken for drunk.

Alcohol *can* be a part of the diabetic diet, but usually only with or immediately after a large meal and only as advised by a physician. Food in the stomach slows the time it takes for alcohol to get into the blood. Liqueurs or mixed drinks that contain sugar are usually not recommended; wine, beer, and occasional hard liquor may be acceptable.

Alcohol's calories count. They may be calculated by the equation

$$0.8 \times proof \times ounces^{12}$$

This will result in calories from alcohol, not from sugar or any other substance in the drink. Table 31-2 lists common wines that are low in sugar and may be allowed. Any diabetic should check with the physician and/or a nutritionist for ways to fit specific drinks into his diet.

Diabetics who take oral hypoglycemic agents, discussed above, usually should not drink. This is only because the alcohol may interact with the medication, causing nausea, dizziness, flushing, or other unpleasant side effects.

Pregnancy

Pregnancy causes serious stress in the diabetic. Pregnant diabetics often have a good deal of difficulty maintaining blood sugar and insulin balance because the needs of the fetus are constantly increasing. A woman may also have trouble maintaining the pregnancy, and there is a greater risk of the infant being miscarried or born with some abnormality.[7,8] Pregnancy also increases the woman's risk of developing complications of diabetes. With much medical support and diabetic control, though, a healthy pregnancy is possible. Infants born to diabetic mothers may be larger than other infants as the result of extra fat the baby manufactures from the high sugar levels in the mother's blood.

These women need close medical care and diet counseling throughout their pregnancy. Often they are encouraged and taught to check their own blood sugar levels several times each day and to adjust diet accordingly. This may help improve control, and lower the risk for both mother and infant.[8]

Drugs

Drugs may also affect blood sugar control. Steroids, beta-blockers, and diuretics may all

Table 31-2

Low-carbohydrate Wines (a selection)

Red	White	Other
Burgundy	Chablis	Dry Rosé
Cabernet Sauvignon	Chardonnay	Dry Champagne
Claret	Dry Chenin Blanc	Dry Sherry
Gamay Beaujolais	French Colombard	
Merlot	Dry Gewurztraminer	
Petite Sirah	Dry Riesling	
Pinot Noir	Dry Sauterne	
Zinfandel	Dry Sauvignon Blanc	
	White Burgundy	

(McDonald J: Alcohol and diabetes. Diabetes Care 3(5):634, September–October 1980)

impair glucose tolerance, leading to hyperglycemia, making diabetes control difficult. A diabetic on these drugs should discuss this with his physician.

THE DIET

Diet is the cornerstone treatment of diabetes. Meals must be coordinated with insulin and exercise to keep blood sugar stable. The insulin-dependent diabetic usually follows a diet that is divided into three meals and two snacks daily. The adult-onset, overweight diabetic has a diet that promotes weight loss, with timing not critical and snacks optional. Both types of diabetics usually follow a diet based on the exchange system introduced in Chapter 22.

Personalized Exchange Diet

The exchange system is printed in Appendix 2 at the end of this text. It may take time to learn, especially for someone who has never before grouped or measured food. Usually a diabetic must meet with a dietitian regularly over several weeks or months to learn how to adopt the diet to cultural preferences and how to adapt "family recipes" and favorite foods to the diet. If the diabetic is on insulin, mealtimes are scheduled around the actions of the insulin.

Be Prepared for Emergencies

The diabetic must learn the symptoms of an "insulin reaction" and begin to carry an emergency sugar source at all times. A physician may also want the client to have glucagon available. Glucagon is a substance that raises blood sugar rapidly and can be injected if the diabetic loses consciousness.

Choose Carbohydrate Wisely

Emergency sugar sources are usually the only simple sugar source allowed in the diet. Other uses of these sugars that cause a fast rise in blood glucose are usually limited. However, the research that developed the "glycemic index" described in Chapter 24 proved that many other types of carbohydrates, alone, also cause a rapid rise in blood sugar. As a result of this research, the American Diabetes Association has recommended that "more emphasis should be placed on those carbohydrate-containing foods that produce the smallest rise in blood glucose, and less emphasis on those that are associated with higher glycemic responses."[13]

There has also been much recent research on the role of fiber in diabetes and blood sugar control.[14–17] Fiber seems to help keep blood sugar from rising quickly and may become an important part of dietary control. A diabetic who fills bread, fruit, and vegetable exchanges with high fiber selections may eventually require less insulin and find weight loss easier. Some researchers recommend and others provide guidelines for planning a high carbohydrate, high fiber diet as treatment for both types of diabetes. Often, in such diets, the bread exchange list is further divided into bread, starchy vegetables, dry cooked beans, and bran.[18-19]

"WHAT ABOUT . . ."?

Dietetic Foods? A food that is called "dietetic" makes some diet claim. It may have nothing to do with a diabetic diet. Dietetic is not the same as diabetic. If a person wants to fit certain "dietetic" foods into the diet, he should first check with a physician or nutritionist.

Convenience Foods? An exchange diet requires that mixed foods be calculated according to the meat, milk, fruit, vegetable, bread, or fat exchanges they contain. It may be hard to calculate a convenience food unless it is labelled in terms of diabetic exchanges. Some diet products, for example "lean" or "diet" or "Weight Watchers®" frozen dinners, may have diabetic exchanges listed on them. A dietitian may be able to advise on other foods that might not be labelled.

Eating Out? Yes, diabetics can eat out, but they need to know what they can order and how many exchanges each food represents. Many restaurants serve known portion sizes of individual foods; fast food chains may have exchange lists available from the parent company, if not from the individual store. Without these lists, it is difficult to guess exchanges in mixed dishes and casseroles. Diabetics often find it easiest to order simple foods, eat only what is necessary for the diet, and *plan meals ahead,* often with the counsel of a dietitian.

Sugar Substitutes? Nonnutritive sweeteners (for example, saccharin and aspartame) are usually permitted on the diabetic diet. Other types of sugar may include fructose and sorbitol. Fructose and sorbitol both have the same energy content as glucose: 4 calories per gram, but unlike glucose or table sugar, they do not cause a rapid blood sugar rise. "Dietetic" candies are often sweetened with sorbitol. Fructose is used less frequently, but is often available in grocery stores; it is expensive. The calories from these and all other sugars must be counted in the diet. The use of honey and other syrups is usually discouraged because they contain high concentrations of glucose.

INSULIN PUMPS

One recently developed method of diabetic control is the insulin pump. This pump is a small machine worn at all times that provides continuous subcutaneous insulin infusion (CSII). Insulin enters the blood at a continuous rate through an injected needle that remains in the body. Before each meal, a diabetic on CSII can inject a larger dose of insulin than usual. Blood sugar, which is checked several times a day, can be adjusted immediately by a snack or by added insulin. Care is simple, but it is crucial that the site of the needle stay absolutely clean at all times, or infection may develop.

The advantages of the pumps are obvious: constant insulin is supplied, copying the normal pancreatic function better than any other type of insulin control. Diet is still as important as ever, since the disease is still present. But controlled, scheduled meals are not as important. The diabetic on a pump should still carry an emergency sugar source at all times. Maintenance of the pump requires diabetics with a high degree of interest and commitment. The pump may eventually become a safe, ideal choice for eligible, pregnant diabetics. And because it provides constantly available insulin, the pump may prevent whatever blood changes might result from abnormal blood sugar; there is some evidence that this may significantly lower the blood cholesterol, VLDL, and triglycerides that often are dangerously high in diabetes.[20]

There are disadvantages to pumps. They require meticulous care. They might be appropriate for a responsible adolescent but probably not for a child. They introduce a risk of infection at the site of the infusion. Wearing a machine may make exercise awkward for some persons, and they tempt the diabetic to abandon a carefully balanced diet. In this way they may lead to weight gain.[21] They have also been known to malfunction, releasing too much or too little insulin. For some individuals, however, the benefits may outweigh the costs.

In summary, the diabetic is simply a person whose available insulin is inadequate. Diabetes is a disease with specific disadvantages, complications, and no known cure. Overweight diabetics may be able to control the disease symptoms by weight loss, preventing many of the complications. But the child and the person of normal weight who is insulin-dependent has no "easy out." Controlling diabetes is a lifelong process, a constant balancing act. And ultimately the balance is the responsbility of one person: the diabetic. A child who learns this, and begins to take gradual responsibility for his own care early in life may find it easier to live with diabetes than the child who is always controlled by others.

With almost six million diabetics in the USA alone, there are many support resources available.[21,22] Some of these are listed at the end of this chapter. There are clubs, journals, diabetes centers, cookbooks, and many, many educational materials available. Since the disease may occur among the semiliterate as well as the literate, the nonEnglish speaker as well as the English-speaking population, multilingual and pictorial teaching materials are available and listed with other resources.

STUDY QUESTIONS

1. Define the following:
   - Polydipsia
   - Ketone
   - Compliance
   - Polyuria
   - Renal threshold
   - Gestational diabetes
   - Insulin reaction
   - Insulin pump
   - Mellitus

2. What are the two major types of diabetes mellitus? How do they differ?

3. Is either of the two types curable? Explain your answer.

4. List and describe at least three possible complications of diabetes.

5. Why do some women develop diabetes in pregnancy?

6. What are the three major factors in the control of diabetes mellitus?

7. List and explain at least four things that might lead to poor control of blood sugar.

8. What type of diabetes requires the diabetic to carry an emergency sugar source at all times? Why?

9. Where could this sugar source be stored so that it is immediately available?

10. How does diet help control blood sugar?

11. Why should protein and fat be controlled in the diabetic diet?

12. Can diabetics drink alcohol? Explain your answer.

13. What organizations are available to help diabetics learn to live with and control their disease? What are their addresses and phone numbers in your area?

REFERENCES

1. Eisenbarth GS: Type I diabetes mellitus: A chronic autoimmune disease. N Engl J Med 314(21): 1360–1368, May 22, 1986
2. Abu-Bakare A, Gill GV et al: Tropical or malnutrition-related diabetes: A real syndrome? Lancet 1 (8490), pp 1135–1138, May 17, 1986
3. Goodhart RE, Shils ME: Modern Nutrition in Health and Disease, 6th ed, p 984. Philadelphia, Lea & Febiger, 1980
4. Krall LP (ed): Joslin Diabetes Manual, 11th ed, pp 33–34. Philadelphia, Lea & Febiger, 1978
5. Arky R, Wylie–Rosett J, El–Beheri B: Examination of current dietary recommendations for individuals with diabetes mellitus. Diabetes Care 5(1):59–63, January–February 1982

6. Butman M (ed): Prenatal Nutrition: A Clinical Manual, p 97. Boston, Massachusetts Department of Public Health, 1983
7. Folkman J, Hollerorth H: A Guide for Women with Diabetes Who Are Pregnant . . . or Plan To Be, 1985. Available from Joslin Diabetes Center, One Joslin Pl., Boston, MA 02215
8. Faiman G et al: Dietary adjustment during self-blood-glucose monitoring in pregnant women with insulin-dependent diabetes mellitus. J Am Diet Assoc 84(7): 816–817, July 1984
9. Rimmer J: Is the Natural History of Diabetic Renal Disease Changing? Presented at the Fifth Annual Aline Coffey Nutrition Symposium, Burlington, VT, April 5, 1986
10. Jackson RC: The child with diabetes. Nutrition Today, pp 2–9, March–April 1971
11. Broussard BA, Bass MA, Jackson MY: Reasons for diabetic diet noncompliance among Cherokee indians. J Nutr Ed 14(2): 56–57, June 1982
12. McDonald J: Alcohol and diabetes. Diabetes Care 3(5): 629–637, September–October 1980
13. American Diabetes Association Council on Nutrition: Policy statement: Glycemic effect of carbohydrates. Diabetes Care 7(6): 607–608, November–December 1984
14. Simpson HCR et al: A high carbohydrate leguminous fibre diet improves all aspects of diabetic control. Lancet 1(1): 1981
15. Anderson JW, Ward K: High carbohydrate, high fiber diets for insulin-treated men with diabetes mellitus. Am J Clin Nutr 32:2312, 1979
16. Mann JJ: Letter to the Editor: Fiber and diabetes. Diabetes Care 8: 192–193, 1985
17. Munoz JM: Fiber and diabetes. Diabetes Care 7:297–300, 1984
18. Suitor CW, Suitor RE, Adelman MO: Planning high-carbohydrate, high-fiber diets with a microcomputer. J Am Diet Assoc 82(3): 279–282, 1983
19. Anderson JW: HCF Exchanges—A Sensible Plan for Healthy Living and User's guide to HCF Diets. (Both available from HCF Diabetes Foundation P.O. Box 22124, Lexington, KY 40522)
20. Pietri AO et al: The effect of continuous subcutaneous insulin infusion on very-low-density lipoprotein triglyceride metabolism in type I diabetes mellitus. Diabetes 32: 75–81, January 1983
21. Capper AF, Headen SW, Bergenstal RM: Dietary practices of persons with diabetes during insulin pump therapy. J Am Diet Assoc 85(4) 445–449, 1985
22. Prater B: Educational guidelines for self-care living with diabetes. J Am Diet Assoc 82(3): 283–286, 1983

OTHER RESOURCES AND LAY INFORMATION CONCERNING DIABETES

Organizations

- American Diabetes Association
  1660 Duke St.
  Alexandria, VA 22314
  (800)-ADA-DISC
  (Many resources and publications available)

- Canadian Diabetic Association
  123 Edward St., Suite 601
  Toronto, Ontario M5G-1EZ
      or
  4480 Main St.
  Vancouver, British Columbia V5V-3R3
  (Multilingual material available)

- National Diabetes Information Clearinghouse
  Westwood Bldg., Room 603
  Bethesda, MD 20205

- Juvenile Diabetes Association
  23 E. 26th St., Suite 1014
  New York, NY 10010

- New York Association for the Blind
  111 E. 59th St.
  New York, NY 10022

Food Models to Teach Exchanges

- National Dairy Council (cardboard models)
  Rosemont, IL 60018

- Nasco (life-like rubber models)
  Fort Atkinson, WI 53538

- "The Diabetic Picture" by Fry and Wetterlin is a 67-page manual designed to teach diabetes to those who are illiterate, read slowly, or are visually impaired. It is available from Donna Wetterlin, RD Nutrition Services Department, Kettering Medical Center, Southern Boulevard, Kettering, OH 45429.

Cookbooks

- *Family Cookbook,* co-authored by the American Diabetes and Dietetic Associations, published by Prentice-Hall, Vol I (1980) and Vol II (1984). Available from the American Diabetes Association.

- *The Calculating Cook* (1978) by Jeanne Jones is available from the Diabetes Association of Delaware Valley, 919 Walnut St., Philadelphia, PA 19107.

CHAPTER 32

Obesity

OBJECTIVES

1. To define the complex physical and psychological disorder of obesity

2. To discuss briefly the difficulty in determining safe versus "ideal" weight

3. To identify the common problems inherent in obesity:
   a. The serious health risks
   b. The social disadvantages

4. To define and discuss what causes obesity, including the role of
   a. Genetics and fat cells
   b. Excess energy intake
   c. Activity
   d. False beliefs and pressures
   e. Improper and psychological "use" of food
   f. Apathy
   g. Habits begun in childhood

5. To emphasize, from the above discussion, the absolute "law" of all obesity: energy input exceeds energy output.

6. To discuss common unhealthful weight loss techniques:
   a. Crash diets
   b. Diet pills

7. To explain successful, healthful dieting techniques
   a. Emphasizing attitudes:
      the ultimate responsibility of the dieter for control
      the need for changed, lifelong habits

   b. Discussing
      Dieting alone
      Role of a counselor or partner
      Role of a group
   c. Providing specific guidelines for modifying
      Diet
      Exercise
      Other food-related behavior

Obesity is a psychological disorder.[1] That is, its underlying cause is in the mind, in the personal attitude toward food that leads to overeating. Attitude alone does not place excess fat on the body. It is a physical energy imbalance that leads to obesity; energy output is less than energy input. But the essence of this behavior is usually an attitude and a mindset.

Obesity is defined as the condition of being 20% over ideal body weight. It refers to excess fat, rather than to large, heavy bones, or a large, muscular body. Yet, what is "too fat" and what is "too thin?" What is "ideal?" Cultures and subcultures vary in their definitions of these standards, linking them to a desirable appearance, but rarely to health. Yet both excess and inadequate fat can be health risks.

Most of the research done on weight and health seems to agree that weight ranging between 10% below and 10% above standard weight charts is not a health risk. Within this 20% range, where weight does not seem to affect health, what a person weighs really depends on personal preference. There is still a great deal of debate, though, about what weights are desirable or ideal.[2] This was discussed briefly in Chapter 12. The current weight tables (1983 Metropolitan Life Tables) do not list "ideal" weights. They simply state average weights of men and women of different heights and frames who carry life insurance. For decades, life insurance tables have been the common USA standards.

Most groups measure "ideal" weight by appearance and make appearance far more important than health. The results are some very mixed messages. The media is filled with mixed messages about weight, especially for women. Women's magazines alternate pages of thin models with pages of fattening foods. Most grocery stores sell booklets encouraging crash diets, all placed in racks near the candy counter. Few women are a "perfect" size anything. The extreme pressure of weight appears to be less of an appearance problem for men, although it is equally a health factor. Being 10%–20% overweight is socially more acceptable for men than women. Perhaps because of this extreme social pressure, women often feel they must be even thinner than men would prefer.[3] Few personal issues are more sensitive to a woman than her weight.

THE RISKS OF OBESITY

Yet overweight is a real problem both for men and for women. In fact, obesity is probably the most common form of "malnutrition" (a term that simply means "bad nutrition") in the United States.[4] It may play a role in the development of many diseases, including heart diseases, diabetes mellitus, hyperlipoproteinemia, respiratory problems, liver and gallbladder disease, toxemia in pregnancy, arthritis in the weight-bearing joints, uterine and gallbladder cancers.[2,5,6] Overweight persons are more likely to have accidents and more risks in surgery (since more tissue is involved and surgery may take longer). Every excess pound requires one mile of extra blood vessels to keep the cells healthy.[7] An overweight condition may limit activity because activity is exhausting or embarrassing. This restrictive, sedentary lifestyle can lead to still more

physical, emotional, and relational problems — and more weight. Although overweight is a real health risk for many, its prevalence (15%–50% of adults and 25% of children[6]) often makes it seem acceptable. Very frequently, the habits leading to obesity are learned and reinforced from childhood. These deeply rooted habits make treatment and long-term success very, very difficult.

Yet obesity is also a social stigma. The obese may be teased, paid less, and assumed to have poor self-discipline. Their "ungainly" appearance may be a subtle discriminatory factor working against them in interviews for certain professional positions. Attractive, well-fitting clothes are often hard to find.

THE CAUSES OF OBESITY

All overweight is caused at some point by consuming more food energy than the body can use. The excess is stored as fat. If stores are not used and the diet continues to be higher in energy than necessary, more and more fat is stored, and obesity results. This is true for infants; it is true for children; it is even true for those rare persons with hormonal imbalances. Hypothyroid persons have a very slow metabolism. If they eat more than their body's basic needs (which are lower than average), they gain body fat. While some drugs do cause the body to hold more water, true obesity is caused by overfat. All fat comes from excess stored calories. Very few persons actually have a genetically "low thyroid;" instead, they may maintain a low metabolism by being very inactive (though regular exercise may raise metabolism). The tendency to be obese does seem to be inherited[8] but the actual fat comes from more food energy than the body needs.

Obesity is not necessarily caused by a "bad" diet. It is often simply caused by too much food. A young child may become obese by eating as much as his mother. A woman may become obese by eating as much as her husband. A "sensible" diet may cause obesity if it contains more calories than a person needs.

Obesity is also related to socioeconomic status. Between infancy and adolescence, children of wealthy parents tend to weigh more than children of poor parents. For adult women, the tendency reverses, and poor women are more likely than wealthy women to be overweight.[9] Close to 60% of all low-income women may be obese.

Although excess caloric intake is the only reason for excess fat, there are many reasons that some persons gain weight easily. Some of these may include

Not enough activity

A body made up largely of fat, which requires less energy to maintain than does muscle tissue

An individual may believe he needs more energy than is actually necessary

Yielding to pressures from other persons to eat more than is necessary

Using food inappropriately, that is, eating simply as a result of depression, anger, or boredom

Any successful treatment of obesity must address the reasons for overeating.

ACTIVITY

As outlined in Chapters 2 and 22, even the inactive body needs energy to function at a basic level. This "basal metabolism" has been compared to the gas needed to keep a car idling. Whenever the activity level rises, so does the energy requirement of both the car and the body. The amount of extra energy used depends on how strenuous the activity—and how long it continues. It also depends on how much weight the body carries through this activity. Lighter people require less energy than heavier people to perform the same exercises.

Activity can make an enormous difference in energy requirements. Figure 32-1 illustrates this for a sample student who is moderately active. Because he is involved in running and horseback riding, he is able to eat almost 600 more kcals each day than his inactive counterpart, without gaining any weight. Because he is active, his body may have a larger proportion of lean tissue that requires more energy to stay healthy. Not only is he healthier, he can also afford to eat more food because his body will use

it. There is some evidence that increasing *general* activity in every possible part of daily life (e.g., taking the stairs, "fidgeting," tapping one's foot) may help weight loss *more* than aerobic exercise two to three times per week, although the latter is important for general health.[10]

Exercise does not just use up energy. It may also change the proportions of the body to include more muscle and less fat. Because of this difference, a person may actually be able to raise basal metabolism by a regular diet and exercise routine that replaces fat with muscle.

FALSE BELIEFS AND PRESSURES

Some persons hold false beliefs about calories and weight loss. They follow crash diet after crash diet without understanding the basic principles of energy balance. When the body is subject to these principles, weight is lost regardless of the person's beliefs about weight loss. Sometimes, however, persons may be unable to lose weight because they act on false beliefs that do not help them lose fat. For example, a diet of grapefruit alone may work simply because it is difficult to obtain enough food energy (each grapefruit contains about 120 calories), not because of any special "fat-burning" substance in the grapefruit. On the other hand a person on a low carbohydrate diet may continue to eat so much of the "allowed" foods (meats, salad dressings, butter, cream, all very high in fat and energy) that only a small amount of water weight is lost. "Water weight" usually comes back quickly as soon as the diet is changed.

A person may also choose to overeat in response to outside pressure. Relatives (especially female relatives) often feel love is best given by food. If food is accepted, love is accepted. If food is left or rejected, then so, they seem to believe, is love. This pressure may be clearly stated or it may be subtle. Sometimes outside pressure is not clearly linked to any one person but to social pressures. No one is forced, but many choose to yield to these influences.

"USING" FOOD INAPPROPRIATELY

Many learn early in life that food is more than a warm, healthy, strengthening substance. Food is

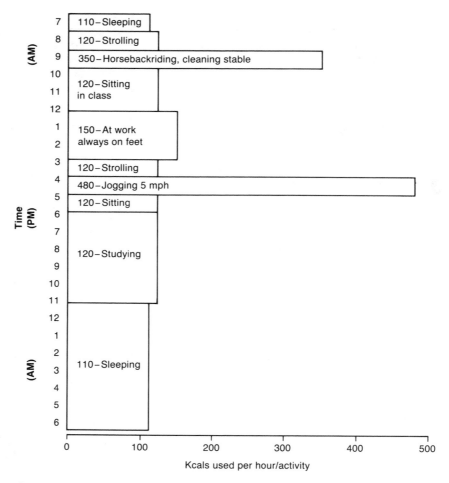

Figure 32-1
Activity/energy expenditure of a 19-year-old man. (Total calorie output: 3480 Kcals)

also a reward, a great pleasure. It is often used to help relieve tension, to express grief, sometimes it is an activity that expresses frustration. These psychological lessons about food begin at birth. An infant feels her mother's warmth and hears her emotions as she is fed. As the infant grows, meals and snack times may equate with certain emotional messages. For example, the infant learns her parents' attitude toward food and the feelings connected with it. If parents commonly use food as an outlet for anger or boredom, the child may learn to use the same outlet in the same way. These associations may eventually lead to obesity.

Many weight loss diets ignore these associations or assume they can be changed easily. Habits that have been learned over many years may also take years to *unlearn* or to adapt in order to help control weight.

DISINTEREST IN DIETING

Many persons overeat simply because they enjoy eating. Food is a great pleasure and obesity is a cost they are willing to pay. Sadly, they are sometimes even willing to pay the price of their health — and even their life — for this instant gratification. This is a psychological dependence on food that may become as dangerous as an alcohol or drug dependence. In all these situations, education and knowledge are not sufficient. Change will only occur when the person is motivated and willing to take responsibility for the problem and begin to initiate changes.

THEORIES OF OBESITY

Once a person begins to overeat, gains weight, and becomes obese, there are many theories about why it may be "harder to 'cure' than cancer." [6] Certainly learned habits make change difficult. The instant pleasure of food makes it hard to control and hard to exchange for a reward (better health and appearance) that is less instant and less tangible. But some researchers also believe that there are physical reasons weight loss is difficult once a person becomes overweight.

Fat stores itself in "fat cells," not in muscle or bone or other tissue. Fat cells deposit themselves in many different areas of the body: in the liver, heart, blood vessels and, largely, under the skin. The "fat cell theory," common in discussions of obesity, hypothesizes that infants are born with a certain number of fat cells that may multiply at certain points in the growth process. Once the number of fat cells is finally established, cells either become bigger or smaller as persons gain or lose weight, but the fat cells no longer multiply. Some researchers believe that diet may influence how many fat cells are produced at critical times and that persons with more fat cells are more likely to stay obese than people with a normal or very small number of fat cells.[6] The theory suggests that if the fat in fat cells drops to a certain level, the body receives "messages" that make further weight loss difficult. Once the fat cell number is established, it cannot be depleted; weight loss will empty the cell of fat but will never destroy the cell itself. The person may experience hunger and a "physiological desire" to refill the cells with fat. This theory certainly appeals to many, but it has never been clearly proven.

Other theorists believe that each body has a biologically "ideal" weight and resists weight loss below a certain point. This theory is not an explanation for obesity, however, because chronic obesity is never ideal for the organism. But this (also unproved) "setpoint theory" may explain why many persons find it almost impossible to maintain weight below a certain point.

OBESITY IN CHILDHOOD

Obesity in childhood is a serious problem for health reasons but especially because of the damage it may cause to a child's self-image. Fat children are often ridiculed, teased, and ostracized. If this is their first lesson about their place in their society, it may affect them for life. They may grow up and eventually lose weight but still view themselves as inferior.

Many obese children remain obese for life. "Baby fat," which is usually gone by the end of the first year, becomes toddler fat, and habits continue that carry overweight into adulthood.

Childhood obesity often involves the habits of an entire family. Thus, families need to be involved in treatment in some way and must be willing to make changes that will affect the family and not just the child in treatment. Often overweight children have overweight parents who may need to relearn eating habits themselves. The parents also need to learn what quantities of food their child really needs and they must also be convinced that a thinner child will really be a healthier child. Since treatment becomes more difficult the longer a person is obese, childhood is an ideal time to diagnose and aggressively begin to prevent further obesity. The importance of peers can sometimes be used to advantage by involving overweight children in groups for counseling and exercise. Depending on the child's age, the parents may be counseled together or separate from a nutritionist's session with the child. Counseling often needs to be long-term (weekly or bimonthly over a period of months). It must also be practical for the parents, interesting to the child and encouraging for all.

WEIGHT LOSS

Basic Math of Dieting

Dieting is rarely fun. It takes motivation, hard work, and a willingness to control behavior over a long period of time. Every gram of fat that is stored stands for almost 9 Kcals that must be lost. Since there are 454 grams in a pound, a pound of fat represents a "savings" account" of 3500 Kcals to use. (This is a little less than 454×9 because fat cells are made up of some protein and water, not just fat alone.) To lose a pound of fat, one must eat 3500 Kcals less than necessary. To lose one pound per week, each day's energy intake must be 500 Kcals less than maintenance requirements ($500 \times 7 = 3500$). To lose two pounds, it is necessary to deduct 1000 Kcals per day from requirements. Thus a woman who needs 2100 Kcals to maintain her weight must either (1) go on a diet of 1600 Kcals per day or (2) begin an exercise that uses up 500 extra Kcals each day to lose one pound per week. If she chooses both diet and exercise, her net loss is 1000 Kcals per day and she will probably lose 2 pounds per week.

This is the "basic math" of weight loss. The scale often seems to tell a different story and this is usually caused by water balance. The body retains different amounts of water under different conditions. Each pint (2 cups or ½ liter) of water weighs 1 pound. Many people "diurese" or lose several pounds of water at the beginning of a diet. But energy balance does not affect water balance in the long run. And no one can gain permanent weight by simply drinking large amounts of water. The healthy body retains the water it needs and excretes the rest.

Crash Diets

Many diets, especially "crash" and "fad" diets, try to ignore the basic math of weight loss and the need for changing lifelong habits. These diets are often unsafe, severe semistarvation diets that are not adequate in any nutrients and should not become lifetime patterns.[11,12] Weight loss does occur but with fat loss comes muscle loss and water loss, as well. If a person follows these diets for a long period of time, she may become weak, with poor endurance and with emotional changes. Essential nutrients are often missing. Eventually the diet may become too frustrating and old eating habits return. When old habits come back, so does old weight. Virtually nothing has really changed. The person returns to "fat" clothes and begins to look for another diet. Continued weight loss and the rebound of weight gain is called the "yo-yo" effect. Recent research suggests that there is more harm in "yo-yo" dieting than in not dieting at all. Each attempt at dieting will be more difficult than the last. With these frequent weight fluctuations, the body adapts and uses calories more efficiently.

Diet pills are another technique commonly used when trying to lose weight. Both prescription and over-the-counter diet pills are easy to acquire. They often work in several ways: (1) by lowering appetite; (2) by increasing energy output, since they are often amphetamines or stimulants (and many over-the-counter pills contain caffeine, also a stimulant), or (3) by a diuretic effect; water is excreted.

Diet pills work for many people — while the prescription or supply lasts. Just as with any medication, though, they have side-effects. Often they become less effective as the body adapts to them. Sometimes they cause anxiety, insomnia, palpitations, and mental changes. They should never be used without a physician's supervision. And often they are treated like another "easy, instant" answer. They rarely help the obese person learn to make lifelong habit changes. When the pills are gone or become ineffective, the old habits return, and the cycle begins again.

Successful Diet Techniques

The only secret ingredient in a successful diet is a truly motivated dieter. There are many sensible diet programs, tips, and support groups to help this person act on his motivation, but absolutely nothing can replace willingness and personal commitment to make changes. The responsibility for the choices lies with the dieter. Because people are different, different approaches work well for different individuals. Yes, the counselor must be competent, able to communicate, supportive, and honest. But when failure occurs, it is ultimately the responsibility of the dieter. It is he who makes the final food and activity choices. The dieter makes day by day, moment by moment decisions to succeed or to fail. If he succeeds, it is his own ultimate success. If he fails, he, not the counselor, loses. Any successful diet demands this honesty and willingness to take responsibility for the choices. It is the dieter who must choose and make the gradual, lifelong changes.

Chapter 2 discussed the basic principles of energy balance and Chapter 22 outlined basic energy-controlled diets. Some type of energy control must be a part of any diet that is going to work. But energy control is more than just food math. In order to begin to control food intake, food intake must be understood. Why eat? What kind of individual pressures make a person choose excess food? The dieter must learn to understand what "triggers" eating before beginning to control or to respond properly to those triggers. The dieter must also understand energy balance so he can decide how to control it. Thus, in summary, the successful dieter requires (a) self-awareness, (b) honesty, (c) a diet-activity balance that encourages weight loss and health, (d) modified behaviors that help lower food and energy intake, (e) support during the diet, and (f) support and help for life, relationships, and eating behaviors as a new, thin person.

There are three ways persons choose to diet. They may choose to diet (a) alone, (b) with the support of a private counselor, ideally a registered dietitian, or (c) with the support of a group setting, led by a qualified professional and promoting sound nutrition principles.

Going It Alone
Dieting alone is hard. It is most successful when only a few pounds and a few habits need be lost. It is not wise to go on a long-term crash diet alone, since some of these diets may lead to serious side-effects that might be ignored. A person who feels strongly about dieting alone should at least check with her physician regularly.

Individual Counseling
Most persons benefit from the support of one other person when dieting, whether it is a private counselor or another dieting friend they can trust. Two people can help each other with ideas, draw each other away from temptation, and force each other to be accountable. Programs such as Overeaters Anonymous® and others involve both private counseling and pairing of two dieters to help one another.

Many hospital outpatient facilities and diet centers involve private counseling sessions with a qualified nutritionist (a registered dietitian or qualified person with a graduate degree in nutrition).[13,14] Client and counselor meet regularly for a period of weeks or months until the client's goals are met. Personal diet counseling has many advantages. Trust can be established. Weight loss techniques can be tailored to the individual's lifestyle and preferences. Problems can be addressed readily and privately. However, individual counseling (which varies widely in techniques and details) is often expensive and may not be covered by health insurance if the weight loss is not directly related to another health problem.

Groups
Many obese persons choose to join a group program. Weight Watchers International® and TOPS (Take Off Pounds Sensibly)® are two examples. Some colleges may even offer diet and exercise classes for credit.[1] Dieters meet on a regular basis and are weighed. Group sessions cover many different aspects of weight loss. Details of these group programs may vary widely.

Weight loss groups may also be expensive, but many persons feel more committed to something for which they have paid. Group programs are ideal for those persons who feel most comfortable in a group setting; the struggle of other dieters often helps motivate them to continue.

However, groups may not be able to address individual problems. Anyone who is considering a weight loss program should first check with his physician for approval and for any particular diet advice that may be relevant to personal health or health problems. Leaders of diet groups frequently are not health professionals but simply successful fellow-dieters who have completed the program. They may have an incomplete understanding of nutrition and so may not always present accurate nutrition information.

Any of these programs works with the client to help modify two behaviors: (1) food intake and (2) other food- and energy-related behavior patterns.

Presented below are some basic tips that may be used to help lower total energy intake. They are tips that can help control weight for the person who may not be on a specific diet. They are tips that can become lifelong behaviors.

Exercise

The benefits of exercise have been discussed. The most effective exercises for weight loss are

EATING TIPS FOR DIETERS*

1. Eat before you go to the grocery store. It is easier to shop with self-control on a full stomach!

2. Eat several meals each day, and regular snacks as well, if it helps. Self-control at mealtime is easier if you are not starving.

3. Weigh and measure foods. To the hungry eye, all portions seem small. Measuring helps you obtain every calorie you're able to have — and then stop!

4. Drink beverages with meals. This includes water, juices, coffee, tea, or hot soup. Fluids help slow down eating and add a sense of fullness.

5. Try to make the first serving last 20 minutes or more. It takes this long for your stomach to signal your brain that it is filling up. If you make the portion last as long as possible, you may not want as much.

6. Trim as many calories as possible from all meals and snacks. Since fat is the most concentrated source of energy, cutting fat is the most effective way to cut calories. Some ways to do this include:
   - Choose low fat milk and milk products; ice milk instead of ice cream.
   - Choose low fat meats; poultry and fish are lower than beef, pork, and lamb. Cut off any visible fat (including the skin) and throw it away or give it away.
   - Cook foods in water, meat juice, lemon juice, wine, any liquid except fat (the alcohol calories in the wine will boil off). Never fry or cook in oil. If you like to sautée foods, coat the pan with a nonstick spray instead of oil or use a pan with a nonstick surface. Or stir-fry foods in a wok in ½ teaspoon of oil with soy sauce and water.
   - Choose low fat toppings. Instead of regular mayonnaise or margarine try the "lite" or "diet" types (and use the same amount as usual, not more!). Instead of sour cream, try plain yogurt with herbs, spices, or lemon juice. If you like "creamy" salad dressings, make your own, substituting yogurt for mayonnaise. Instead of butter or margarine on vegetables try grated, farmer's, or ricotta cheese.

7. Know food well. Many otherwise "healthful" foods are full of hidden fat calories. Avocados, olives, and nuts are very high in fat. Many "natural" ice creams contain far more fat than other, more common varieties and are sometimes sweetened with honey, which is a more concentrated source of calories than sugar. Frozen yogurt and sherbert, while usually low in fat, are often high in sugar.

8. Let yourself "splurge" when it is really important. If a diet is really going to fit into your lifestyle, there must be room for controlled freedom.

9. Alcohol counts at 7 calories per gram (that's almost 200 Kcals per ounce of pure alcohol!) but if it is used in cooking, the calories (from the alcohol) will evaporate.

10. Plan ahead to guard against "weak" times. If you "simply must" eat as soon as you get into the house an hour before

aerobic exercises, or those that increase the muscle action of the heart and increase the need for oxygen. Aerobic exercises include walking, running, biking, swimming, dancing, and most exercises that involve moving the whole body from one place to another in a way that raises heartbeat above a certain level for 20 minutes or more. These exercises use up energy. *Isometric* exercises, those that involve flexing and stretching muscles while remaining in the same position, are less effective for weight loss. They tone muscles but do not necessarily help burn fat.

Exercise only works when it is enjoyable and easy enough to do regularly. An overweight person can lose weight by exercise alone IF energy

---

dinner (or while you prepare the meal), plan a number of low calorie, nutritious snacks and set them up attractively just for that time. Some ideas include: a bowl of fresh fruit; a "frappe" of low fat yogurt; frozen juice cubes or concentrate and frozen fruit; a plate of chopped raw vegetables, or a bowl of plain, air-popped popcorn.

11. At parties, talk — or listen — to others. Choose the foods you are allowed and keep them on your plate; eat as slowly as possible. Stay away from the buffet table. If you are staying away from alcoholic beverages, try club soda with lemon or lime. Eat before you go if it will help you resist temptation. Ask if you can bring food, then bring lowfat, low calorie choices. Before you eat, decide what you will eat, in total, and limit yourself to that intake. If there is no one at the party you want to talk with, go home.

12. At mealtimes, serve portions onto each plate rather than "family style." If nibbling on leftovers is a problem, put leftovers away before the meal or put someone else in charge of cleanup. If you cannot use the crumbs and fragments for a future meal, throw them away. You help no one by adding crumbs to your own fat stores.

13. If you keep sweets in the house for the family or for emergencies, choose foods you don't like. Or give children money for snacks instead of buying them yourself. If you bake for the family, bake foods that would least appeal to you.

14. In restaurants, ask for baked or broiled meat, not fried, breaded, au gratin, or meat swimming in melted butter, cream sauce, or gravy. Cut off the visible fat or skin and leave it on the plate. Ask for salad with dressing "on the side;" this way, you can control the amount you want. Use milk or lemon instead of cream in tea or coffee. Skip dessert or have fruit or fruit cocktail (or save your appetizer or salad to eat while your companions have dessert). Or get one dessert for two or three people and split it. Feel comfortable asking for a doggie bag.

15. If you "break" your diet, stop as soon as you can. Many dieters who eat something they wanted to resist feel they have "gone off the wagon" and go on to eat more. "I had one — I might as well eat the whole thing now." This is a deception. The closer you are to the "wagon" when you fall off, the easier it is to get back "on the wagon." The body will count every extra calorie as a little more fat. And if you can limit your intake of these forbidden foods, even when you slip, you are learning how to limit them later on, when you have lost all that fat, and can begin to have those foods again in limited amounts.

---

* (These suggestions, as well as suggestions for exercise and behavior changes are adapted from the following sources: Brody J: Jane Brody's Nutrition Book. New York, Bantam Books, 1981; Mahoney MJ, Mahoney K: Fight fat with behavior control. Psychology Today, May 1976; Kearney P: The Jack Sprat Program for Behavior Modification. Boston, Tufts-New England Medical Center, Frances Stern Nutrition Center, July 1977; Nutrition Action Ideas for Weight Control [Food Life Series] from New England Dairy and Food Council 1980)

intake stays at the same low level. For example, a 250-pound woman who can maintain her weight on an 1800 to 2000 Kcal diet because she is very inactive may be willing to continue her normal diet (being careful to limit foods that might push her over this limit) and begin a regular exercise program, for example, 30 minutes daily on a stationary rowing machine. She may lose weight quickly. If she reaches 140 pounds in this way and feels so good that she wants to continue the exercise but does not want to lose more weight, she will be able to ADD several hundred Kcals to her diet, keep on exercising, *and* remain thin. This is the benefit of exercise. Below are listed some other ways to use fat or food energy.

EXERCISE TIPS

1. Whenever possible, use stairs instead of elevators or escalators. If you work or live on the fourth floor, you can start by walking up several flights and then taking the elevator the rest of the way or riding up and walking down.

2. Park further away from your destination than necessary.

3. Get off the bus or train a stop or two before your usual stop and walk the rest of the way.

4. If you rarely have time in the morning to allow for this extra exercise, do it at lunch or on the way home.

5. If you have somewhere to hang out your laundry to dry in the sun, use it. You get exercise, you save money on the drier, and the wash usually smells better.

6. If you need to go somewhere within walking distance (½ to 2 miles — you decide your limit), walk or bike instead of driving. Get a knapsack, cart, or other tool for comfortably carrying parcels, bags, children, whatever you need to carry.

7. Involve children in exercise when possible. Mothers of toddlers sometimes use children as an excuse NOT to exercise. Yet the exercise, within their limits, is healthy for them too.

8. Make exercise fun, even if this is hard to do. Listen to music tapes (or language or a lecture tape — whatever interests you) as you walk. Join an exercise group with a friend. Choose the most enjoyable, scenic area of your neighborhood in which to run or walk. Buy exercise clothes that you really like and allow yourself to wear them only when you are doing particular exercises. Make a chart to keep track of your progress and plan specific rewards at certain points (*e.g.*, "Walked 25 miles, attended exercise classes 10 times without missing," etc.)

9. Walk as fast as you can — everywhere. If you walk twice as fast as usual, you may use twice as many calories.

10. Use coffee breaks to walk instead of eat.

11. Think of exercise in terms of food calories. A cheeseburger may equal a 90-minute walk. A candy bar may take 30 minutes of a vigorous swim or tennis game to burn it off. If you are tempted to splurge, decide how much exercise you are willing to do to burn it off. Then, do the exercise *first*.

12. Do housework more often than usual.

13. Exercising 1 to 3 hours *after eating* helps burn more calories than exercise on an empty stomach. This is because fasting metabolism is slightly lower than the body's metabolism after a meal, so energy is conserved even during exercise.*

---

* (David Levitsky, M.D., professor of nutrition sciences at Cornell University, as quoted in Mademoiselle, p 220, November 1983)

Behavior Modification

The term "behavior modification" in dieting gained popularity in the mid 1970s.[15,16,17] It usually refers to techniques that can help change eating patterns. Many of these steps have already been discussed briefly.

The first step in behavior modification is awareness. A client keeps a record of all meals and snacks and the "cues" around them: (a) time; (b) place; (c) presence or absence of other persons and who they are; (d) the reason for eating; (e) feelings experienced before or during eating, and (f) exactly how much of what foods are eaten. Table 32-1 illustrates a sample behavior modification chart. This record is continued for a week or more *before* any changes begin. It helps the person understand his own psychological food associations and when (and maybe why) he overeats. Then the counselor works with the dieter to begin gradually changing cues or responses. They discuss what can be changed,

how it may be changed, and what cannot be changed. Behavior is modified slowly, with support from a counselor or a group, over a long period of time until the client begins to gain more and more control over his eating patterns. Some common, basic eating behaviors and ways they may be modified to help cut down on energy intake are outlined on page 302.

Diet groups that address behavior and self-image rather than diet do exist. Some of these programs work well for some persons. Obesity (like other eating disorders) relates as closely to psychology as it does to nutrition. Many special, intense counseling and diet options exist for the morbidly, or dangerously, obese person.

However, any group only works insofar as it leads members to a net negative energy balance: energy/food input is less than energy/exercise output. Diet groups that do not formally address this issue must ultimately lead to the same goal or they will not work. The principle holds, and

Table 32-1

Sample Baseline Food Record

Time	Place	With Whom	Position	Feelings	Hunger	Food	Exercise
7 a.m.	Kitchen table	Alone	Sitting	Tired	Very hungry	1 Fried egg 2 Strips bacon 8 oz orange juice Coffee with cream/sugar	At 8 walked to bus stop one block away
10:30 am	At work	Coworkers	Standing by coffee machine	Frustrated	None	3 Donuts 1 Cup coffee	At 12 walked 1½ miles instead of eating in cafeteria
12:15	Outdoors	Alone	Walking	Peaceful	None	1 apple	
2:30	At work	Alone	At desk	Angry	Slight	1 Candy bar	
							At 5 walked ½ mile to bus
5:30	Home	Spouse	Sitting	Hurried, tired	Very	½ of 16" Pizza Diet soda 1 Fresh, peeled orange	
9	School parking lot	Friend	Walking to car	Exhausted	None	Piece gum	
10:30	Living room	Spouse	Sitting	Content	Slight	1 Beer ½ Bag pretzels	

BASIC BEHAVIOR MODIFICATION TECHNIQUES

1. For one week, keep a record of everything you eat and drink (that contains calories). For each meal or snack, record time, where you were, who you were with, your position, how you felt, your hunger, what you ate, and include any exercise you have done (see Table 32-1).

2. At the end of the week, using this record, analyze some of the key times and reasons you eat more than you want, or foods you would rather avoid. Eating habits can only really change after you understand why they exist.

3. Choose new habits that can replace the old ones. If, for example, you always eat when you feel sad, plan ahead what you will do *first* (before eating) next time you are sad. Plan something that can (or will) not be combined with eating, for example, listening to favorite music, taking a walk, doing calisthenics, knitting, etc.

4. Change the environment to make eating less of a constant temptation. Some common suggestions include
  - Stay out of the kitchen as much as possible, since this room is an immediate reminder of food
  - Limit the places in the house where you will eat. Eat all meals and snacks *only* in those places
  - Design a full table setting for all meals and snacks. Eat only at this setting, even if you don't need to use the utensils. This often means you must sit down to eat or drink anything

  - Separate eating from all other activities. Concentrate on enjoying only one activity at a time. When you eat, just eat. Appreciate the taste and smell of your food (even if you eat fast). Don't read, listen to the radio or stereo, or watch TV while you eat. If some sound is "on" when you want to eat, turn it off. This gradually helps to break the mind's association of eating with other activities that have always unconsciously told you to "eat!" Decide what you will disassociate with eating. Decide what (if any) foods you will allow to be associated with what activities (*e.g.,* "When I watch football games I will eat only celery and plain popcorn and drink only diet soda.")
  - Keep foods out of sight. Put tempting foods in opaque containers or in the freezer. If you like attractive centerpieces, buy fake or wax fruit, candles or fresh or silk flowers—or anything—except candy, nuts, and fresh fruit.
  - Put away leftovers immediately

5. Plan meal and snack times to prevent ravenous hunger.

6. Decorate your kitchen in pale pastels instead of bright colors. Bright colors stimulate the appetite and may cause you to eat more.

7. You may not be able to modify the behaviors (or attitudes) of your friends and family, but you *can* modify your own response to them. *You* are in control of what passes your lips. Repeat "no, thank you" as often as necessary. Modify it. Be creative. Be funny. Smile a lot. But be in control, the guardian of your body. You know what is best for you.

---

will work, even when it is not the primary focus of therapy.

A Note about Surgery
Surgery has become an alternative weight loss technique for a select few persons whose health is endangered because of their weight (*i.e.,* morbidly obese persons). Several techniques have been used; the most common is one that closes off part of the stomach. Because this results in a smaller stomach size (30 to 50 cc), less energy and nutrients can be taken in at one time. A

person is forced to eat less and as a result, loses weight. This gastric bypass or gastric partition is less drastic than the earlier methods of intestinal bypass, which removed a large section of the small intestine.

Because this method worked by promoting malabsorption, vitamins, minerals, and electrolytes were also lost. Diarrhea, a symptom of malabsorption, was common and at first was quite severe. The surgery is a risk and some persons die. Surgery itself is a risk factor for anyone, and more so for the severely overweight.

After surgery, eating must resume, but very gradually or severe vomiting and gastric damage may result.[18] Unfortunately, the effects may not last for life. Yet surgeries, performed selectively by highly trained specialists, have helped many persons add years to their lives. But like all the other techniques that treat obesity, they are not the "ticket to a free lunch." The cheapest, safest way to treat obesity is to prevent it, and to begin to do so early in life.

STUDY QUESTIONS

1. Is obesity a health risk? Explain your answer.
2. What imbalance causes obesity? What factors in a person's society or environment lead to this imbalance?
3. Is it true that "a fat child is a healthy child?" Why or why not?
4. Below are five "excuses" for obesity. For each excuse, what are some real reasons the person may be overweight? What would you discuss with him to help him lose weight? Be specific.
   1. "Everyone in my family is fat. It is in my genes."
   2. "I have a low thyroid."
   3. "When I started having back problems, I had to stop exercising. That's when I put on this weight. I guess I can't do anything about it now."
   4. "My sister has anorexia nervosa. Everytime I go on a diet, my mother forces me to stop because she's afraid I'll become like my sister. I really don't want to upset my mother."
   5. "I eat because I hate my job."
5. Discuss
   • The fat cell theory of obesity
   • The setpoint theory of weight
6. What are the disadvantages of
   • Crash diets
   • Diet pills
7. What is "behavior modification"? How can it help an obese person lose weight?
8. Examine the behaviors and eating habits of the person described in Table 32-1.
   • What changes would you suggest?
   • What positive behavior would you continue to encourage?

REFERENCES

1. Hudiburgh NHK: A multidisciplinary approach to weight control. J Am Diet Assoc 84(4): 447–450, 1984
2. Keys A: Overweight, obesity, coronary heart disease and mortality. Nutr Rev 38(9): 297–307, 1980
3. Goleman D: Dislike of own body found common among women. New York Times, March 19, 1985
4. Levy RI: Obesity—an overview. Health Learning Systems' Dialogues in Nutrition 3(1), 1978
5. CME Communications: Clinical Impact of Overweight: Positive Management Techniques. New York, CME Communications, 1980
6. Brownell KD: The psychology and physiology of obesity: Implications for screening and treatment. J Am Diet Assoc 84(4): 406–414, 1984
7. Brody J: Jane Brody's Nutrition Book, pp 277–328. New York, Bantam Books, 1981
8. Stunkard AJ et al: An adoption study of human obesity. N Engl J Med 314(4): 193–198, January 23, 1986
9. Garn SM: Socioeconomic aspects of obesity. Contemp Nutr 6(7), 1981
10. Bogardus C: Exercise and Diabetes. Presented at Fifth Annual Aline Coffey Nutrition Symposium, Burlington, VT, April 5, 1986
11. Morgan BLG: The nutritional truth about popular diets. Nutrition and Health 6(3). New York, Columbia University, 1984
12. Fisher MC, Lachance PA: Nutrition evaluation of published weight-reducing diets. J Am Diet Assoc 85(4): 450–454, 1985

13. Atkinson RL, Russ CS et al: A comprehensive approach to outpatient obesity management. J Am Diet Assoc 84(4): 439–444, 1984

14. Russ CS, Ciavarella PA, Atkinson RL: A comprehensive outpatient weight reduction program: Dietary patterns, psychological considerations and treatment principles. J Am Diet Assoc 84(4): 444–446, 1984

15. Ferguson JM: Learning to Eat: Behavior Modification for Weight Control. Palo Alto, CA, Bull Publishing Co., 1975

16. Ferguson JM: Habits, not Diets: The Real Way to Weight Control. Palo Alto, CA, Bull Publishing, 1976

17. Mahoney MJ, Mahoney K: Fight fat with behavior control. Psychology Today, pp 39ff, May 1976

18. Bukoff-Priddy ML: Gastric reduction surgery: A dietitian's experience and perspective. J Am Diet Assoc 85(4): 455–459, 1985

CHAPTER 33

Gastrointestinal Disorders

OBJECTIVES

1. To review the basic parts of the gastrointestinal tract
2. To describe common causes and consequences of gastrointestinal disorders
3. To discuss the cause, symptoms, and nutrition implications of treatment for several common GI disorders
   a. Esophagitis
   b. Hiatus hernia
   c. Peptic ulcers
   d. Gallbladder and pancreatic disease
   e. Diarrhea
   f. GI bowel resections and side-effects
   g. Diverticular disease
   h. The major inflammatory bowel diseases:
      Crohn's ileitis
      Ulcerative colitis
   i. Irritable bowel syndrome

The gastrointestinal (GI) tract was described in detail in Chapter 1. It is a tubelike passageway that runs through the body from the mouth to the rectum and is technically considered to be "outside" the body. Food is propelled through the tract, broken down by the force of muscles and the many substances released into the different areas of the tract. Once the food is broken down completely, it can cross the membranes and get "inside" the body to nourish it. When problems or illnesses develop in the GI tract, they will usually affect the way food reaches the cells.

GI disorders may develop anywhere along the GI tract. Figure 33-1 lists the major disorders to be discussed in this chapter.

Disorders may cause damage to any or all of the layers of the cell wall. Figure 33-2 shows the basic design of the cell wall. It is composed of several layers of muscle, nerve, blood, and epithelial (surface) cells. The innermost layer may look slightly different in each part of the tract, but the basic structure is the same. Food is absorbed within the first few inside layers. These are the same layers that will be damaged quickly by a GI disorder.

GI disorders may have many causes. Some of these include

1. Another organ disease. For example, some diseases cause the release of too much gastric acid, which then eats away at the cell wall
2. Muscle changes. Muscles may weaken with age. When the muscles in the GI tract slow down, it will take longer for food to pass through and be digested
3. Chronic irritation from vomiting, laxative abuse, smoking, drug use, or an allergic or sensitive reaction to some substance in the GI tract
4. A foreign substance such as bacteria or parasites

5. Previous damage, for example from surgery or disease

6. Missing enzyme(s)

7. An emotional or psychosomatic disorder

8. An unknown cause

Below is a discussion of some of the major GI problems that affect nutrition. Problems that affect chewing and swallowing are discussed in Chapter 35.

THE ESOPHAGUS

Esophagitis

Esophagitis, a sensitive, painful esophagus, is the result of irritation caused by something, usually gastric juice, forced *up* into the esophagus from the stomach. The opening between the esophagus and the stomach is usually kept closed by a muscle called the esophageal sphincter. When gastric juice backs up and is forced through the sphincter into the esophagus, this action is called *gastric reflux.* The stomach wall is designed to hold a very acidic liquid, but the esophagus is not protected against this acid by any mechanism except the normal protection of the closed sphincter. Acid that is forced up "eats away" at the cells on the tissue wall, causing painful swallowing. Serious damage can result, since constant exposure to the stomach acid may "burn" a hole through the wall of this "tube."

Treatment depends on the cause. Sometimes the stomach fills quickly and "backs up" into the esophagus. Very small, frequent meals will

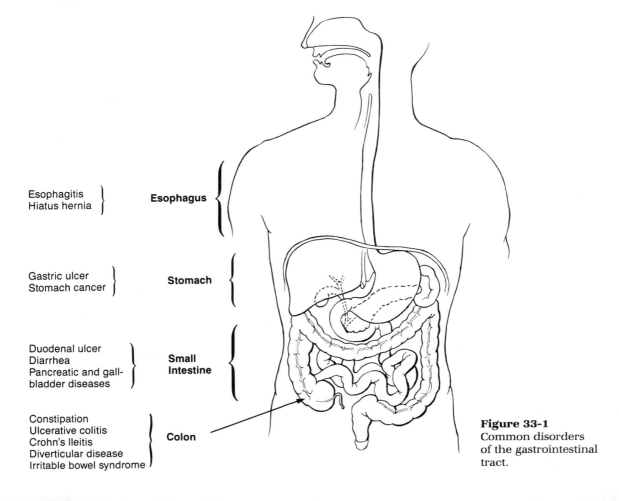

Esophagitis
Hiatus hernia
Esophagus

Gastric ulcer
Stomach cancer
Stomach

Duodenal ulcer
Diarrhea
Pancreatic and gall-
bladder diseases
Small Intestine

Constipation
Ulcerative colitis
Crohn's Ileitis
Diverticular disease
Irritable bowel syndrome
Colon

Figure 33-1
Common disorders of the gastrointestinal tract.

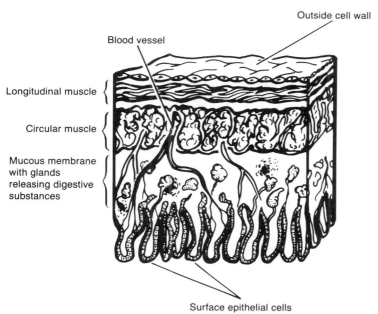

Outside cell wall

Blood vessel

Longitudinal muscle

Circular muscle

Mucous membrane
with glands
releasing digestive
substances

Surface epithelial cells

Figure 33-2
Typical cell wall along the digestive tract.

help prevent this from occurring. Chronic vomiting from disease or bulimia can cause the same damage; the esophagus will heal only when the vomiting stops.

Hiatal Hernia

Sometimes a hiatus hernia causes esophagitis. The area containing the esophagus and the lungs is separated from the lower abdomen by the diaphragm, a large muscle that holds the esophagus in place. (The diaphragm is the muscle that helps the lungs expand and contract in the breathing process.)

A hiatus hernia occurs when a part of the stomach is pushed up through the muscle of the diaphragm where it does not belong. When this happens, the esophagus cannot empty "down;" its contents must first flow sideways, through the hernia, to reach the stomach. As a result, there are many problems and discomforts. Gastric reflux may occur, causing heartburn and damaging the esophagus. Often discomfort is a greater problem than pain. Food "comes back up" often, and people with hiatal hernias complain of indigestion or heartburn that may last for hours. At first, some sufferers come to the physician thinking they have the symptoms of a heart attack. They feel worse when they bend over, lie down after meals, eat large meals, or drink highly acidic beverages.

Persons with a hiatus hernia are often overweight; weight loss helps the hernia to resolve and the symptoms to disappear. Sometimes weight loss is the only treatment necessary, but sometimes medication or surgery become necessary.

Diet is very important in the treatment of the symptoms of the hernia. The following suggestions are often recommended to minimize the discomfort:

1. Many small meals are better than two or three large meals, so the stomach is never so full that it is forced "up"

2. Drink fluids between meals. Include little or no fluids at mealtimes. This, too, prevents an overly full stomach

3. Avoid eating or drinking anything two to three hours before bedtime. When the body is prone (lying flat), any food still in the stomach may "flow" back up and cause discomfort

4. If recommended, lose weight

5. Avoid whatever aggravates the symptoms

6. Adjust bed so the entire head and chest are slightly elevated while sleeping. Pillows only elevate the head; the entire mattress must be raised at the head end. Usually gravity (and the esophageal sphincter) help keep food in the lower part of the GI tract and out of the esophagus. The angle of the stomach in a hiatus hernia makes this more difficult. These suggestions help prevent stomach acid from damaging the esophagus while the physician and client can talk about other treatments.

STOMACH AND SMALL INTESTINE

Ulcer

Of the several disorders that may occur in the stomach and small intestine, ulcers are the best known. An *ulcer* is an area in the wall of the GI tract that may be destroyed or eaten away by gastric acid. When this happens, a "crater" develops in part of the cell wall. Nerves are exposed to the acid, causing pain. The ulcer may bleed. If it bleeds over a long period of time, the individual may become anemic.

Fifteen percent of all ulcers develop in the stomach.[1] These are called gastric ulcers and may sometimes be related to a stomach cancer that is causing an overproduction of acid.

Most ulcers, however, are *duodenal* ulcers; that is, they develop in the duodenum, the first 25 to 30 centimeters of the small intestine. Often the ulcer develops in the portion of the duodenum near the stomach.

Ulcers may be caused by other diseases or by emotional and psychological pressure and stress. Medication and diet therapy can promote healing but the ulcer may recur if the basic cause is not treated. People at highest risk for ulcers include relatives of individuals with ulcers and people with blood type O.[2]

For many years ulcers were treated with a bland diet that included large amounts of milk and cream. Sufferers were told to avoid fiber, acid, alcohol, caffeine, and spicy foods. They were told to take frequent sips of milk because milk was believed to "coat" the ulcers. These diets were called *sippy diets.*

As research continued and new drugs developed, it became clear that the ulcer diet does not need to be this restricted except, perhaps, in the very beginning of treatment. In fact, milk and other proteins, which do slow down acid production temporarily, ultimately lead to an "acid rebound." While the milk is in the stomach, little acid is released. But after the milk is digested into the duodenum and jejunum, the stomach produces more acid than when it was first empty. Many individuals with ulcers can actually enjoy very spicy foods and even high fiber foods without pain. As a result, most ulcer patients are now told to eat whatever foods they can enjoy. Acid production is now controlled by medications, not milk, although milk and dairy products are still important for general nutrition.

Some beverages are still restricted in ulcer treatment, however. Alcohol may irritate an ulcer, since it stimulates gastric acid secretion. Coffee — both regular and decaffeinated — also stimulates gastric acid so it is not usually recommended. Soda may bother some people. It may also be wise to avoid other acidic liquids such as vinegar, lemon juice, grapefruit, pineapple, orange, tomato, and cranberry juices, *if* they irritate. A diet that is too strict may lead to a nutrient deficiency. Borderline ascorbic acid deficiency has developed when the diet has tightly restricted fresh fruits and vegetables.[2]

When the empty stomach produces gastric acid, it has a *p*H (acidity level) of 0.9–2.0.[3] An environment becomes more acidic as the *p*H drops. Food in the stomach causes the *p*H to rise, and almost all foods, including the liquids listed above, have a higher *p*H than that of the empty stomach. The higher the *p*H, the LESS acidic the stomach, and the more *basic* it becomes. Food and liquid in the stomach *buffer* the stomach so the juices are less acidic and can do less damage to the ulcer. This is why persons with ulcers may be told to eat small meals and to eat often. Frequent feeding helps relieve the pain.

Fats also buffer the stomach. Less acid is produced when a meal contains fat. But too much fat may not be recommended for other reasons. A person whose ulcers seem related to stress may also, because of stress, be at risk for cardiovascular disease. Because of this risk, a physician may suggest using low fat milk and vegetable oils instead of whole milk, eggs, cream, and butter.

Gallbladder and Pancreatic Diseases

The gallbladder and pancreas share the common bile duct. Through this duct they release digestive enzymes and other substances into the small intestine. When something goes wrong with these organs, digestion is affected.

The gallbladder normally stores bile produced by the liver. It works together with the liver to produce hormones and to empty stored bile into the small intestine. Bile helps break down and emulsify dietary fat so it can be digested and absorbed.

The most common disorder of the gallbladder is the production of gallstones. These stones are made of cholesterol that has combined with calcium or oxalate and become solid. Problems occur when these stones obstruct or block the flow of bile. The result, acute cholecystitis, is extremely painful and may also result in infection in the area of the blockage. The stones may be dissolved with medication, removed surgically, or the gallbladder itself may be removed (cholecystectomy).

Diet probably plays a very small part in this disorder. Between diagnosis and treatment a low-fat diet may be prescribed; this helps keep bile secretion to a minimum and avoids aggravating the area. After treatment, no special diet is necessary; as long as the liver functions normally, bile will still be available.

Pancreatic diseases have a more serious and long-term effect on nutrition. The pancreas releases pancreatic juice, an alkaline substance that helps raise the pH of the chyme coming from the stomach. Enzymes need this alkaline environment to survive and function. The pancreas also produces and secretes major enzymes involved in digestion: trypsin, chymotrypsin and carboxypeptidase, which all work to break down proteins; pancreatic amylase, which breaks down dextrins (starches) into disaccharides; and pancreatic lipase, which breaks down fat (triglycerides) into fatty acids and glycerol. In addition, the pancreas produces insulin and glucagon, which are essential for blood sugar control.

Common diseases that damage the ability of the pancreas to produce and release these enzymes include:

1. Pancreatitis
2. Cystic fibrosis (CF)
3. Pancreatic cancer
4. Protein-energy malnutrition
5. Diabetes mellitus

Pancreatitis or inflammation of the pancreas, is usually the result of alcohol abuse. Consequently, individuals with pancreatitis may be malnourished as a result of many other factors involved in alcoholism. Pancreatitis is extremely painful. Eating stimulates action of the pancreas; therefore patients are usually not encouraged to eat and may instead be put on total parenteral nutrition (see Chapter 38).

The person with CF, pancreatic cancer, or malnutrition is usually eating and encouraged to eat. However the pancreatic enzymes have either been destroyed or they are not working properly. Other enzymes and functions along the digestive tract are able to compensate and digest the proteins plus carbohydrates, but fat digestion and absorption is seriously diminished. The results may lead to fatty diarrhea, malnutrition, and rapid weight loss. Without pancreatic lipase, the person loses all fat calories and essential fatty acids, and fat-soluble vitamins are also inadequately absorbed. These individuals need special treatment to replace

a. Pancreatic function
b. Calories from fat
c. Essential fatty acids
d. Fat-soluble vitamins

Pancreatic enzymes may be given orally in the form of enteric-coated pancreatic extracts.

These are large pills that must be taken with each meal; they do not work as well as natural endogenous pancreases. Medium-chain triglyceride oil is often used to add calories and keep diarrhea to a minimum; however MCTs do not contain the essential fatty acids. It may be necessary to give EFAs parenterally (directly into the blood). Fat-soluble vitamins may be given in a water-soluble form.

Diabetes mellitus is discussed in detail in Chapter 31.

In summary, pancreatic diseases are quite serious. Nutrition support must be aggressive and often involves major adjustments in the diet, especially as related to the fats. Appropriate dietary changes are important to help a person function as normally and in as healthy a fashion as possible.

Diarrhea

Diarrhea is a GI symptom, not a disease. It may be a symptom of many things, including maldigestion and malabsorption. Malabsorption may develop when

1. The gallbladder does not release enough bile to break down fat
2. The pancreas does not release needed enzymes for adequate digestion
3. The surface of the GI tract is abnormal and unable to absorb properly
4. Abnormal bacteria or parasites are present
5. The intestines have been surgically shortened ("short bowel syndrome")
6. There is some other cause[1]

Treatment, including diet treatment, depends on the cause. Diarrhea is always a sign of some type of malabsorption, which is probably not serious if the diarrhea is temporary. If it continues for many days or weeks, as in some GI diseases (below), the client may develop one or several nutrient deficiencies. The client probably will also lose weight, which may, at first, be a more serious problem. The medical team must work together to help determine what nutrients are being lost and how, practically, they can be restored.

Bowel Resection

Surgery on the colon or the small intestines often leads to diarrhea or "short bowel syndrome." Dangerously obese individuals sometimes have this type of surgery as a last resort in order to lose weight. Others who suffer from various types of inflammatory bowel disease (such as Crohn's or ulcerative colitis) or bowel cancer may have part or all of their colon surgically removed.

A quick look back at Figure 1-2 shows where various nutrients are usually absorbed from the intestine into the blood. If a particular section of the intestine is removed, a deficiency in the nutrient usually absorbed in that area may eventually develop. A person who cannot absorb fat may, over a long period of time, become deficient in one or more of the fat-soluble vitamins. The body may eventually adapt and absorb nutrients at other sites, but not as effectively. Sometimes supplements are prescribed in a form the body will absorb.

When parts of the stomach are removed, some persons eat less. They may feel full more quickly or they may be afraid to eat. This, too, may lead to nutrient deficiencies and the person may benefit from nutrition counseling.

The anemias and calcium deficiency are the most common nutrition problems in persons who have had gastric surgery or GI diseases. These deficiencies are usually caused by malabsorption and treated with supplements rather than diet. Because malabsorption is a major problem, nutrient adequacy of the diet is more important than ever for these individuals.

THE COLON

Diverticular Disease

Diverticular disease was discussed in some detail in Chapter 24. It has two phases. The first is diverticulitis, in which the colon is raw, swollen, and irritated by the infected diverticuli or pockets that have pierced its walls. The second stage, diverticulosis, is the general presence of diverticuli, but they are no longer inflamed. People with diverticular disease are at risk for bowel cancer. Treatment usually includes a low fiber diet when the colon is irritated and high fiber diet at other times to help prevent food residues from building up and exerting increased pressure against the colon walls.

INFLAMMATORY BOWEL DISEASES

Inflammatory bowel diseases (IBD) have many names. Within this group are several distinct syndromes that share the irritating characteristics of

No known, distinct cause

No known cure

Sporadic "flare up," causing great pain and distress, and often hospitalization, followed by

A period of rest without symptoms or problems.

The two most common IBD's are *Crohn's ileitis* (also called Crohn's disease, ileitis, or regional enteritis) and *ulcerative colitis* (sometimes simply called *colitis*).

The basic difference between these two is the degree of damage they can do to the GI tract. Colitis is the inflammation of the colon and rectum. It usually affects only the outermost layer of the cell wall. Ileitis may also cause an inflamed colon, but it can also inflame any other area of the GI tract from the mouth to the rectum. It also may penetrate the outermost layer of the wall and cause deeper damage to the layers beneath.

A flare-up of either of these diseases is extremely painful and distressing. The individual usually experiences abdominal cramps, bloody diarrhea, and sometimes anorexia, weight loss, nausea, and vomiting. The GI tract is sensitive to any irritation and often parts of the cell walls are worn away. It bleeds easily and appears to be covered with blisters.[1] Clients with IBDs are at a higher-than-normal risk of developing colon cancer.[4]

These diseases have a profound effect on the absorption of nutrients. Fluids and electrolytes are lost in diarrhea. Protein may be lost in bleeding, while malabsorption may cause the loss of many other nutrients. Lactose intolerance is common because the lactase enzymes have been destroyed with the surface cell layer.[1] In an acute attack, it may not be possible to eat or use the digestive tract at all; parenteral nutrition may supply the nutrients needed while the person receives medication and the gut is given a chance to "rest." Usually TPN must continue for at least 2 weeks and is the only way to prevent serious malnutrition.[4] If the disease is treated with surgery, malabsorption can eventually develop. When ileitis or colitis appears in childhood, the anorexia and discomfort that cause the child to eat poorly may also lead to nutrient inadequacies that impair growth. As in all disease, adequate nutrients are very important to withstand treatment and help healing. But because eating is the most effective way to obtain nutrients, and eating causes great discomfort, individuals with IBDs, especially Crohn's disease, may appear chronically underweight, anemic, and may benefit from ongoing nutrition support.[5,6]

There is no special diet for these diseases. Each person is unique and can tolerate a different range of foods. Foods may cause problems at some times but not at others. The diet should be as close to normal as possible. Most physicians recommend a low fiber diet during "flare-ups," since fiber stimulates the muscles of the GI tract to contract and may cause irritation and aggravate bleeding.[1,4,7] Also, there is increased risk of obstruction as a result of an inflamed, swollen inner lining and, as a result, a narrower intestine. Some recommend bran or another bulk-forming fiber to help treat diarrhea, which is common when the disease is mild.[4,8] Others discourage it.[1] The diet should include enough fluid to replace the fluid lost in diarrhea, and the person with IBD might enjoy small, frequent meals rather than large ones. Sometimes medium-chain triglycerides (MCTs) are used to help reduce calories lost in malabsorption. If the lactase enzyme is missing, regular milk should be avoided and low-lactose dairy products and lactase-treated milk should be chosen instead.

These persons may develop very restricted diets that could potentially cause as many nutrition problems as the diseases themselves. This is why periodic counseling and evaluation with a dietitian is very important.

Irritable Bowel Syndrome

Irritable bowel syndromes are different from IBDs, probably in their cause. Also called "functional bowel diseases," these syndromes seem to be brought on more by emotional stress than any physical cause. They are painful but rarely result in the physiological damage of the IBDs.

An individual with IBS suffers from periodic bouts of severe gastrointestinal discomfort. This may involve abdominal pain or cramps, diarrhea and/or constipation. Pain in the colon may be the result of high pressure there and a disordered motility (muscle contractions). Symptoms are aggravated by social and psychologic stress, and often certain foods.

A high-fiber diet is often recommended. Fiber tends to enlarge the colon and decrease colonic pressure. Certain fiber foods also help increase the bulk and form of the stool, which in turn can work to minimize constipation and diarrhea. A high-fiber diet should always involve a high fluid intake; otherwise the fiber (especially wheat bran fiber) could actually cause blockage and more discomfort! Diet counseling should include an evaluation of the current diet to identify what foods an individual is avoiding. An extremely minimal diet increases the risk of deficiencies.

The key treatment for IBS, however involves learning to cope, not learning how to eat. Since these syndromes seem stress-related, long-term cure and treatment must involve identifying and dealing with the psychological and social elements of the disease.

STUDY QUESTIONS

1. List the basic areas of the GI tract. List at least one disorder that may occur in each area.

2. For each disorder listed above, describe the role of nutrition in treatment.

3. What might cause gastric disorders?

4. Define the following:
   - Gastric reflux
   - Diaphragm
   - Duodenal ulcer
   - Acid rebound
   - Irritable bowel syndrome

5. What are some of the vitamins and minerals that may be malabsorbed or lost in IBDs?

6. What are some of the foods recommended and avoided in some types of IBD?

7. What nutrition-related problems may occur as a result of pancreatic insufficiency in cystic fibrosis? Why?

8. What does the gallbladder do? How should someone change his diet after his gallbladder is removed?

REFERENCES

1. Fishman MC, Hoffman AR, Klausner RD et al: Medicine, 1st ed, pp 245–280. Philadelphia, JB Lippincott, 1981
2. Fein HD: Nutrition in diseases of the gastrointestinal tract. In Goodhart RE, Shills ME (eds): Modern Nutrition in Health and Disease, 6th ed, pp 901–911. Philadelphia, Lea & Febiger, 1980
3. McClintic JR: Basic Anatomy and Physiology of the Human Body, p 457. New York, John Wiley and Sons, 1975
4. Kodner IJ, Fry RD: Clinical symposia: Inflammatory bowel disease 34(1). Summit, NJ, CIBA, 1982
5. Hodges P et al: Vitamin and iron intake in patients with Crohn's disease. J Am Diet Assoc 84(1): 52–58, 1984
6. Hodges P et al: Protein energy intake and malnutrition in Crohn's disease. J Am Diet Assoc 84(12): 1460–1464, 1984
7. Questions and Answers about Diet and Nutrition in Ileitis and Colitis. New York, National Foundation for Ileitis and Colitis, 1981
8. Brauer PM et al: Diet of women with Crohn's and other gastrointestinal diseases. J Am Diet Assoc 82(6): 659–664, 1983

CHAPTER 34

Inborn Errors of Metabolism

OBJECTIVES

1. To introduce/review the role of genetics in metabolism

2. To define the general effects of inborn errors of metabolism on the metabolic processes

3. To discuss the compensation versus "cure" of inborn errors, describing briefly several errors for which control is possible

4. To define six common inborn errors of metabolism:
   a. Lactose intolerance
   b. Phenylketonuria
   c. Maple syrup urine disease
   d. Glycogen storage disease, especially type I
   e. Homocystinuria
   f. Galactosemia

5. For each of the above (a) through (f), to explain
   a. The defect
   b. Damage caused when untreated
   c. Dietary and other common treatment
   d. Importance of individual, regular medical, and dietary follow-up

Persons inherit their genes from their biological parents. These "genes," containing messages with information about every physical aspect of the new person, are passed on in the *chromosomes.* Chromosomes are present in pairs in every cell of the body (except the reproductive cells). They resemble small threads that have been bound together in the middle. There are 46 chromosomes (i.e., 23 pairs) in every nonreproductive cell. The reproductive cells each contain one chromosome from each of the 23 pairs, or half the usual number. When sperm and egg join, the newly formed embryo receives 23 chromosomes from the egg and 23 from the sperm, or 23 unique pairs. In these chromosomes are all the necessary genes or messages for the inherited characteristics that form a new person.

Genes are not always perfect messages. Mutations or changes in genes can disrupt the "message," leading to an abnormal characteristic. Mutant genes can be the results of damage from drugs or other environmental "mutagens," causing severe problems. Some mutant genes are harmless and may be passed through many generations. For example, an albino, with white hair, pale skin, and eyes, is someone who has a mutant gene that deprives his body of pigmentation. Other inherited mutant genes involve deficiencies that are more serious: The inherited *inborn errors of metabolism* are genetic disorders caused by inherited mutant genes. These result in serious digestive or metabolic problems and will be the focus of this chapter.

There are at least 79 genetic disorders that relate in some way to nutrition and metabolism.[1] The error may include the deficiency of some minor substance or of some essential enzyme or protein. The enzyme is missing or the protein is defective and this prevents one (or more) substance(s) from converging to the next substance in the metabolic process. When these steps are disrupted, substances build up and may damage the cell. Disruptions may, for example, affect

The digestive tract

Nutrients normally carried across the intestinal wall

Excretion through the kidneys

Transport from one part of the cell or body to another

Breakdown of carbohydrate, fat, or the amino acids

The resulting problems may be mild. The person may still have some of the necessary functions. Or the problems may be severe and require a lifelong special treatment or diet. For example persons with Down's syndrome (which is not metabolic) are mentally retarded due to a defective chromosome, but with continued training and sheltered care they may live productive lives. On the other hand, the problems may be so serious that they are incompatible with life and the infant dies *in utero* or in early infancy.

It is usually impossible to replace what is missing in genetic disorders, including the inborn errors of metabolism. Proteins, including enzymes fed into the digestive tract, are usually destroyed, deactivated, and broken down by digestion. They rarely reach the intestinal lining intact and if, somehow, they do, there is no guarantee that they will cross the intestinal wall and work where they are needed. Nor can they usually be injected safely. Enzymes work within the cells, not in the circular (blood) system. They can cause serious damage if they are active in an area of the body where they do not belong. Indiscriminate administration might cause imbalances as severe as the defect itself. These are some of the reasons inborn errors are often difficult and usually impossible to cure.

Instead, treatment involves compensation. The diet must be changed to compensate or adapt, if possible, to the deficiency in order to prevent the harmful effects that can occur. A

few inborn errors can be treated with large (pharmacologic) doses of vitamins or other nutrients. In a few defects (among dozens) these treatments have been beneficial but each disorder is different and megavitamins are more a drug than a dietary therapy.

Sometimes nothing can compensate for these defects; they are fatal. Sometimes they are fatal *in utero;* at other times the child may be born and then die soon afterwards. For example:

1. Tay-Sachs disease, caused by an abnormal enzyme, in which afflicted infants are mentally retarded, develop blindness, and usually die by age 3.[2]

2. Niemann-Pick disease, caused by the deficiency of an enzyme and also leading to severe mental retardation, an enlarged liver and spleen, and death by age 2.

3. Anderson's disease, in which a defective enzyme produces amylopectin, an abnormal type of glycogen. Cirrhosis and enlarged liver and spleen usually lead to death by age 3.

Of the many other, more treatable types of inborn errors of metabolism, six are relatively common. They will be the focus of the remaining portion of this chapter. All of them include diet as a key treatment. None is fatal or seriously damaging if diet therapy is begun early in life. These six are (1) lactase deficiency; (2) phenylketonuria (PKU); (3) maple syrup urine disease (MSUD); (4) Glycogen storage disease; (5) homocystinuria, and (6) galactosemia.

LACTASE DEFICIENCY

This intolerance to milk sugar has already been discussed in detail in Chapter 24. It is different from a milk allergy where the offending substance is protein rather than sugar. A lactase deficiency may be primary (that is, genetic), or it may be secondary (caused by a viral or bacterial illness that destroys the enzyme from the small intestine). Treatment includes a diet low in or free of lactose. Many persons produce some lactase and are able to enjoy milk and other lactose-containing foods in small quantities. Lactase deficiency is a relatively harmless example of a genetic metabolic deficit.

PHENYLKETONURIA (PKU)

PKU has also been previously discussed, in Chapter 23. Caused by a deficiency of the enzyme phenylalanine hydroxylase, PKU leads to severe mental retardation caused by excess phenylalanine levels in the brain, and to fair skin and light hair caused by lack of the pigment melanin if it is not treated. Treatment involves a diet strictly controlling phenylalanine intake. This unusual diet can prevent brain damage and allow for a relatively normal life.

MAPLE SYRUP URINE DISEASE (MSUD)

Like PKU, MSUD is caused by a missing enzyme. Untreated, it also leads to irreversible brain and neural damage and mental retardation. It is called *maple syrup urine disease* because the urine and sweat of these infants has a maple syrup-like odor. The disease is also called branched-chain ketoaciduria because the three branched-chain amino acids (valine, leucine, and isoleucine) cannot be properly broken down. They build up, spill into the urine, and cause the serious tissue damage. Untreated, the infant will die young.

MSUD can be treated by omitting all protein from the diet and replacing it with a special commercial formula that has all the essential amino acids except the three branched-chain amino acids (BCAAs). These three must be added separately, according to individual needs as the child grows. As in PKU, the special formula is the major part of the child's diet. Regular blood tests, medical checkups and the involvement of a dietitian are also critical parts of treatment. The dietitian may teach the family how to incorporate the diet, as closely as possible, into their own lifestyle. Educational materials are available to help parents and other family members.* Often more than one family member has MSUD. Control is difficult because specific needs change with growth, disease, injury, and other physical stress, and formula mixtures are very expensive.

The pathways of these amino acids and the defects of PKU and MSUD are diagrammed in Figure 34-1.

GLYCOGEN STORAGE DISEASE, TYPE 1

Glycogen is a polysaccharide, the form of energy that is stored in the liver and muscle. Normally glycogen is converted to glucose whenever blood glucose levels drop and other sources (*e.g.,* from food) are not immediately available. The liver stores sufficient glycogen to provide 800 to 1200 calories. When glycogen stores are gone, the body begins to break down fat and muscle.

At least nine different metabolic errors can occur in the metabolic pathway of glycogen. These are called the *glycogen storage diseases.* The most common is Type 1 or von Gierke's disease.

In Glycogen Storage Disease, type I, the missing enzyme is glucose-6-phosphatase, which normally converts glucose-6-phosphate, a breakdown product of glycogen (see Figure 34-2) to glucose. These individuals cannot produce glucose from glycogen, although they can absorb glucose from foods. Dietary glucose is usually completely digested several hours after a meal. For the child with this inborn error of metabolism, it is at this point that glucose is suddenly no longer available, and he becomes hypoglycemic. Insulin production slows down as well. As a result, this chronic problem can also lead to slowed growth. When the disorder is uncontrolled, muscle — and some fat — breaks down to provide glucose to compensate for the hypoglycemia. Glycogen builds up because it cannot convert to glucose. Too much glycogen in the liver leads to a fatty, enlarged liver and other fatty deposits. Unless the defect is detected early and treated, the child may die.

Diet treatment includes small, frequent feedings. Most children also receive an enteral formula throughout the night delivered by a continuous drip through a feeding tube.[3,4] The remaining necessary energy and nutrients are divided into frequent meals and snacks

---

* One such guide is A Parent's Guide to the Child with Maple Syrup Urine Disease by Dr. Phyllis B. Acosta and Louise Bell, available from Florida State University, Center for Family Services, 103 Sandels Bldg., Tallahassee, FL 32306.

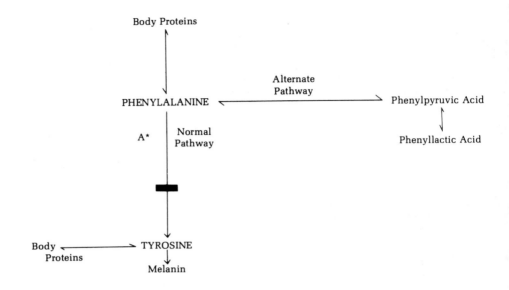

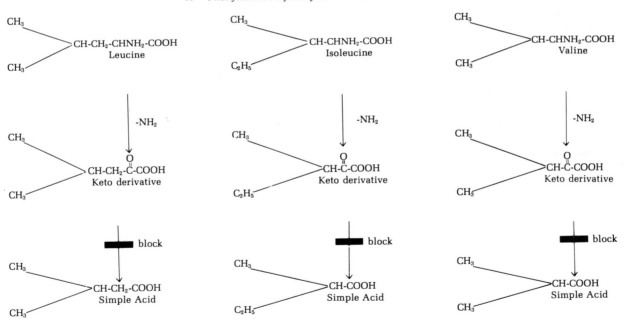

Figure 34-1
Enzyme deficiencies in phenylketonuria and maple syrup urine disease.

throughout the day. Parents sometimes learn to plan children's menus by a type of exchange diet specifically designed for the disease.[3] Fructose (in honey and many fruits) and milk products with lactose are usually not permitted because the same (missing) enzyme is required to break them down into glucose. Sucrose or table sugar is usually limited because half its composition is

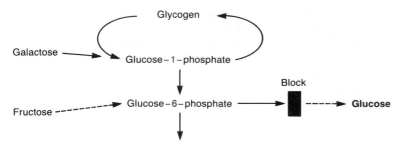

Figure 34-2
Diagram of glycogen storage disease type 1–deficiency.

fructose. Most of the carbohydrate permitted in the diet is in the form of glucose or starches.

Children with von Gierke's disease must usually stay on this careful diet therapy until at least their late teens and twenties.[3,4] Nocturnal feedings may be discontinued but frequent snacks are usually still necessary.

HOMOCYSTINURIA

Like PKU, *homocystinuria* involves a defect in the metabolism of an amino acid, in this case methionine. Methionine is one of the essential amino acids, necessary for protein metabolism to work properly. The defect, diagrammed in Figure 34-3, prevents methionine and its product, homocystine, from converting further to the next steps necessary for protein metabolism. As a result, excess methionine and homocystine build up in the body and spill into the urine. This buildup in the system leads to mental retardation, seizure disorders, liver disease, and poor growth.

Some children are treated with large doses of vitamin B_6; others begin a diet similar to that for the child with PKU, but with methionine, rather than phenylalanine, being restricted. Protein is provided from a special commercial formula. Three currently used include Methionaid, Product 3200-K and Low-methionine Isomil.[5] Soy products and other foods naturally low in methionine are usually incorporated into the diet as well.

GALACTOSEMIA

In *galactosemia*, the missing enzyme is galactose-1-phosphate uridyl transferase. This enzyme normally works to convert galactose into glucose. Galactose comes from the breakdown of lactose. It is also present in organ meats (liver, brain, pancreas), and can be produced naturally from glucose in the body. The dangerous galactose levels that can build up in the blood and spill into the urine within several days after birth can lead to vomiting, growth failure, cataracts, liver dysfunction, ascites, and mental retardation.

Treatment involves a galactose-restricted diet. Parents may need to

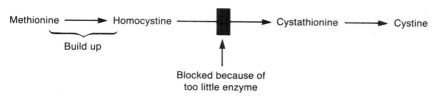

Figure 34-3
Enzyme deficiency in homocystinuria.

Omit all lactose products including all forms of milk, soy formulas if they contain any lactose, and all foods made with any milk or added milk solids

Omit less obvious sources of galactose. This involves careful planning with a dietitian, since galactose may be in certain fruits, vegetables, and grain products.[6]

The restricted diet is essential for infants. Later in life, though, it may be possible to reintroduce some galactose without further problems, since in some persons, the body seems to be able to bypass the defect and break down the carbohydrate by another pathway.

There are many other inborn errors that require diet or nutrient adjustments; the ones presented here are only a few of the most common. Since each person has a unique set of genes, the same general defect may be slightly different in individual children. As a result, treatment is also individualized and medical and nutrition follow-up and counseling must be tailored to the individual child and family.

Until the middle of the twentieth century, there was no hope of survival for most infants with these metabolic defects. Early death and/or mental retardation were inevitable and for the most part the cause was unknown. Much of the research in this field is recent and there are still many unknown areas. But for many children a normal life, if not quite a normal diet, is now possible; this is, at least, a beginning.

STUDY QUESTIONS

1. What is a chromosome?

2. What happens when a child, at conception, receives a mutant gene?

3. What systems in the body may be affected by an inborn error of metabolism?

4. If a child is born without an essential enzyme, can it be cured by giving the child supplemental enzymes of the same type from a health food store? Why or why not?

5. List the six inborn errors of metabolism discussed in this chapter. For each of them briefly describe the type of diet changes used in treatment.

6. Match the following:
  a. Lactase
  b. Deficiency of glucose-6-phosphatase
  c. Galactose
  d. Branched-chain ketoaciduria
  e. Melanin
  ___ Sweat smells like maple syrup
  ___ Enzyme that breaks down milk sugar
  ___ Pigment missing in phenylketonuria
  ___ Requires tube feeding during the night
  ___ Must avoid milk products, organ meats that contain this substance

REFERENCES

1. Holtzman NA, Batshaw ML, Valle DL: Genetic aspects of human nutrition. In Goodhart RE, Shils ME (eds): Modern Nutrition in Health and Disease, 6th ed, pp 1193–1219. Philadelphia, Lea & Febiger, 1980
2. Thiele VF: Clinical Nutrition, pp 160–181. St. Louis, CV Mosby, 1976
3. Folk CC, Greene HL: Dietary management of type I glycogen storage disease. J Am Diet Assoc 84(3): 293–301, 1984
4. Daeschel IE et al: Diet and growth of children with glycogen storage diseases types I and III. J Am Diet Assoc 83(2): 135–141, August 1983
5. American Academy of Pediatrics, Committee on Nutrition: Special diets for infants with inborn errors of amino acid metabolism. Pediatrics 57: 783–792, 1976
6. Mitchell HS et al: Nutrition in Health and Disease, 16th ed, p 499. Philadelphia, JB Lippincott, 1976

CHAPTER 35

Mechanical Feeding Problems

OBJECTIVES

1. To describe situations in which diet may need to compensate for a mechanical feeding problem.
2. To describe and define different types of mechanical feeding problems and their treatment:
   a. Preparing or grasping food
   b. Coordination
   c. Chewing
   d. Swallowing (dysphagia)
3. To discuss the nutritional risk of a mechanical feeding problem
4. To discuss the different causes of dysphagia and the three areas of treatment:
   a. Correcting the disorder
   b. Compensating
   c. Alternative feeding methods
5. To define and describe in detail texture-controlled diets that may be used in mechanical feeding disorders:
   a. Mechanical soft or ground
   b. Puree
   c. Full liquid
   d. Clear liquid
6. To outline briefly three common problems of a texture-modified diet that may be prevented:
   a. Tooth decay and gum disease
   b. Constipation
   c. Weight loss and malnutrition

A mechanical feeding problem exists when a person finds it physically difficult to obtain the necessary amounts of the necessary nutrients from a prepared meal because there is some impairment in handling, biting, chewing, or swallowing. Some physiologic interference makes it difficult to eat.

Many situations may cause feeding problems. A physiologic deficit such as blindness, lack of teeth, or a disabled or amputated limb may make mealtimes awkward. An infant born with cleft palate has a hole in the roof of his mouth that connects it to the nasal cavity and makes normal sucking almost impossible. The problem may also be caused by muscular or neural (nerve) damage. This may include genetic defects such as cerebral palsy, mental retardation, and diseases such as arthritis and multiple sclerosis. Paralysis and stroke as well as mental illness and neurologic diseases such as Parkinson's disease also involve mental and neural impairments that make it difficult to prepare meals, chew, and swallow. Mouth, tongue, and throat cancers often lead to mechanical feeding problems: because the diseased tissue is sensitive, tastes change, and eating may become unpleasant. Radiation treatment for these cancers may also irritate and further damage the mouth and throat. Radiation enteritis in which the tissue becomes raw, dry, and inflamed may develop. Saliva production is affected and may cease entirely. Eating may become a serious problem.

Drugs may also affect eating. Many drugs include "dry mouth" and "taste changes" in their list of side-effects. Swallowing requires the use of throat muscles; any drug that affects the muscular system may affect swallowing.

In addition, persons with any of these problems may become depressed about their disease or about the accompanying discomfort. This can lead to anorexia and make the nutritional problems even worse.

Mechanical feeding problems may be divided into five major categories:

1. Problems preparing or grasping food
2. Coordination problems
3. Biting
4. Chewing
5. Problems with swallowing (dysphagia), or with drooling

Many persons with mechanical feeding problems are at some risk for malnutrition simply because they might not obtain enough of the right nutrients for health. They may enjoy all the "right" foods. They may be able to afford them, able to cook them well, but simply find it too difficult to eat them. When eating is slow, embarrassing, or painful, most persons choose the foods that are easiest to eat. These foods may not provide enough calories, vitamins, or minerals. Nutritional problems may then make the disease worse and infection or weakness more likely. If this handicap or dependence is a recent result of disease, it may be hard to accept and may result in depression, denial, and an unwillingness to learn to cope. This usually involves counseling and family support and may take some time. To prevent nutritional problems that can result from a mechanical handicap, the patient must learn to compensate for or adapt to the problem. This is done with therapy, by changing the environment—and the diet—to make adequate eating easier. It also takes time. The compensation depends on which of the above five categories is the problem.

PROBLEMS PREPARING OR GRASPING FOOD

Persons who cannot grasp food well enough to prepare or cook it or who cannot grasp utensils well enough to feed themselves are sometimes fed by others. Often, though, they want the independence of self-feeding.

There are many ways to adapt utensils to help compensate for this difficulty. Spoons and fork handles can often be bent so they can be grasped more easily. Straws can help with most liquids. Plates with compartments help separate and confine food. Rubber disks between the plate and the table help to keep the plate in place.

Blindness is a common problem. Serving dark foods on a white plate or vice versa may help a partially blind person find food on the plate and thus be able to feed himself.

Compartmentalized plates with the same types of food in the same location help promote independent eating. Special plates, utensils, kitchen gear, and even cookbooks are also available from companies that make supplies for the handicapped (see Figure 35-1). Some such resources are listed at the end of this chapter. Often dietitians, occupational therapists, or members of a feeding team in a rehabilitation center will have information about further local resources.

COORDINATION PROBLEMS

Self-feeding is usually learned so early in life that it seems easy but actually it requires at least seven different skills, illustrated in Figure 35-2. These include the ability to (1) suck, (2) sit with head balanced, (3) bring hand to mouth, (4) grasp cup and utensil, (5) drink from cup, (6) take food from spoon, and (7) bite, chew, and swallow. Each of these skills requires muscle coordination. If one of these skills is missing, self-feeding skills are limited.

Treatment usually involves long-term physical therapy by a feeding specialist. Utensils and food are adapted to help encourage self-feeding. When self-feeding is clearly impossible, the person is fed but encouraged to use whatever skills are available. If the client can bite and chew, he should be offered normal table food. If these muscle skills are absent, diet is adapted so that only sucking and swallowing are needed. If these are impaired, tube feeding of some kind may be the best alternative. Whatever the problem, eating is an important part of rehabilitative therapy and should be as enjoyable as possible.

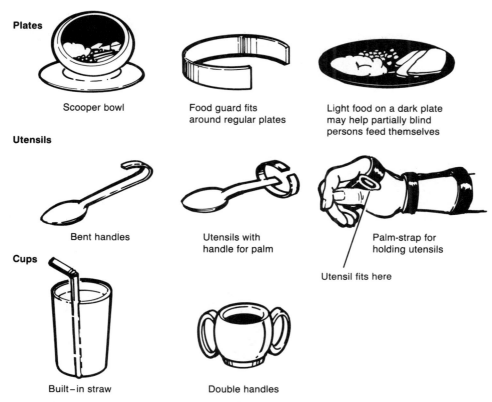

Plates

Scooper bowl

Food guard fits around regular plates

Light food on a dark plate may help partially blind persons feed themselves

Utensils

Bent handles

Utensils with handle for palm

Palm-strap for holding utensils

Utensil fits here

Cups

Built–in straw

Double handles

Figure 35-1
Examples of feeding aids and adaptations.

BITING PROBLEMS

Biting requires natural or false teeth and the strength to grip and bite. When, for some reason, teeth are missing, the diet needs to be soft enough to be gummed. This type of diet is sometimes called *mechanical soft* or ground and will be discussed below. Texture is often minimal. To maintain the interest and pleasure of eating, meals and snacks need to vary in color, acceptable softened textures (*e.g.,* cooked broccoli vs. mashed potato, and baked fish vs. fried clams), temperature, flavor, including sweet, sour, bitter, and salty foods, and seasonings. Table 35-1 provides a detailed list of foods appropriate in various texture-controlled diets.

CHEWING PROBLEMS

Chewing involves teeth, saliva, and tongue control. A person who cannot coordinate teeth and tongue needs a diet that is essentially liquid and easily swallowed. Most well-cooked foods can be blenderized with added liquid and fed by spoon, cup, or straw — whichever works best for the individual.

This type of diet is much more restrictive than the soft or ground diet. The consistency of food is that of baby food and often commercial baby foods are used. It is more monotonous and may be less acceptable. As a result, there is more risk of undernutrition, both from disinterest and from inadequate food choices. Many adults

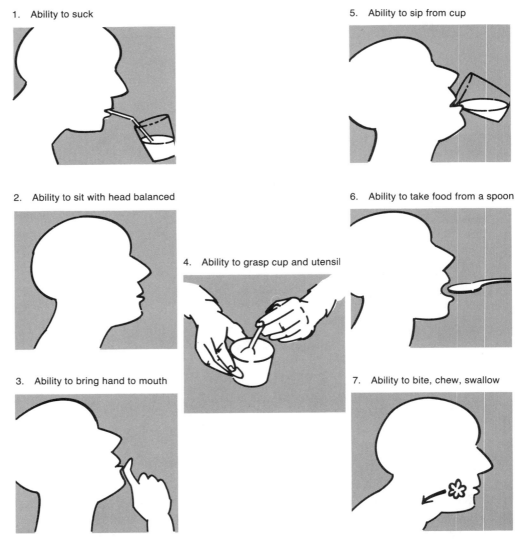

1. Ability to suck

5. Ability to sip from cup

2. Ability to sit with head balanced

6. Ability to take food from a spoon

4. Ability to grasp cup and utensil

3. Ability to bring hand to mouth

7. Ability to bite, chew, swallow

Figure 35-2
Basic abilities necessary for self-feeding.

object to "baby food." Consequently, table foods that have been blenderized may be psychologically more acceptable, even though baby foods are just as nutritionally adequate, easy and adaptable. Table 35-1 includes guidelines for this type of diet. As much texture as possible should be allowed.

SWALLOWING PROBLEMS

Difficulty in swallowing is called *dysphagia.* There are many different types of swallowing disorders, depending on what part of the swallowing process is affected, how severe the disorder is, and how permanent it is.

Swallowing is complex, with three phases: (1)

Table 35-1

Texture-Controlled Diets

Food Group	Mechanical Soft/Ground	Puree	Full Liquid	Clear Liquid
Dairy	Any that are well tolerated	All milk and milk drinks Yogurt Custard Ice cream Sherbet Grated/melted cheese	All milk and milk drinks Cultured milk beverages Ice cream Sherbet	None
Protein (Meat and Meat Substitutes)	Soft meats and fish should be canned or cut up small with all bones removed Beef should be very tender, chopped fine or ground Cooked dry beans, mashed Peanut butter Tofu	Cook and cut meat into small cubes before blending. Blend with milk, gravy, or sauces until smooth Lightly cooked eggs Cooked dry beans, mashed Peanut butter if very soft "Baby food" meat	(Dairy products also provide protein) Peanut butter melted in milk Soy Milk	None
Fruits and Vegetables	All juices Canned or stewed fruit or vegetables Fresh vegetables, cooked Fresh fruit, peeled, seeded, cut-up	All juices Tomato sauce Canned products blended in juice from can Fresh fruit, chopped & blended Fresh vegetables, well cooked before blending "Baby" fruit, vegetables	All juices	Clear juices (apple, cranberry, white grape juice)
Grains and Cereals	Any that are well tolerated	All hot cereals Soften bread in sauce, gravy, milk; blend pasta with cream soups Rice pudding	None	None
Other	Any that are well tolerated	Soup, blended Sauces, seasonings	All beverages (alcohol may not be permitted)	Carbonated beverages Jello Ices Ice
Comments		Add gravies or milk for extra protein; margarine or light cream for extra calories Pureed food should be seasoned to personal preferences		Diet is not nutritionally adequate. Commercial clear, elemental formulas may help provide needed protein, vitamins, and minerals if diet will be long-term

All These Diets May Be Low In Fiber, Resulting In Constipation: See Text.

the oral phase (food in the mouth); (2) the pharyngeal phase (the reflex that channels food into the esophagus and not into the lungs), and (3) the esophageal phase (food is carried down the esophagus to enter the stomach).[1] In a complete swallow, each phase may take 5 to 10 seconds to complete. During the first two stages the larynx or windpipe is shut off; this prevents breathing and talking. Once the food passes the larynx into the esophagus, the airway to the lungs opens once again and breathing resumes. Persons who talk and laugh with food in their mouths are in danger of "aspirating" or inhaling the food into the lungs or regurgitating it up through the nose because the larynx is forced open when it would naturally close itself off. Certain positions, such as lying down or tilting back the head also make swallowing difficult, due to the position of these two channels.

Swallowing problems occur in many different circumstances. Paralysis may affect one or both sides of the throat. Neurologic disorders or head trauma may affect the muscles that work in swallowing. Cancer may create an obstruction. Radiation treatments and drugs may make the throat too dry and too sore to swallow easily. Drooling can be a sign of a swallowing dysfunction. Sometimes the problem continues or worsens for weeks or months before it is treated. Persons who finally come to the doctor because of a swallowing problem may have lost much weight and need aggressive nutrition therapy early in their treatment.

Treatments depend on individual abilities. They include correcting the disorder; compensating for it by using other related functioning abilities, or finding an alternate method of feeding. The three may be combined; an individual may meet daily with a therapist to regain functions lost in a stroke, but receive a tube feeding until these lessons help him regain sufficient skills to obtain adequate nutrients. He may need the tube feeding to develop strength to go on with therapy. In therapy he will regain as much ability as possible.

Correcting

Sometimes paralysis is temporary, for example with a stroke. The person will be able to swallow again, but he must *learn* how to do so. This usually involves regular work with a speech pathologist and occupational or physical therapist. These professionals help teach the client how to swallow, gradually advancing the textures of food involved.[2] Thick, soft foods are easier to swallow than fluids.[3] So the diet frequently begins with puréed foods, then progresses to liquids and, much later to solids. This is usually a long process and the person, as above, will obtain needed nutrition in some other way, usually by tube feeding. Sometimes corrective surgery can also help an individual regain feeding and swallowing skills.

Compensating

It is not always possible to completely correct a dysphagia and sometimes long-term compensation is the best alternative. This takes time, consistent physical therapy and, sometimes, surgery. Food is advanced as far as possible, in an attempt to return the person completely to oral feeding. The individual may be able to compensate for some lost abilities by using other muscles, or by limiting all food to a particular texture.

Finding Alternatives

When physical therapy (PT) has helped a client regain as much swallowing control as possible and it is still not sufficient, long-term alternatives are considered. A feeding tube and a stoma of some kind may be necessary. The stoma, a permanent surgical opening, is formed in some part of the digestive tract, usually the esophagus or the jejunum. Commercial formulas are often the chosen nutrition because they are complete and there is less risk of malnutrition. Many insurance providers will cover the cost of this formula for the client who is totally unable to eat.

TEXTURE-CONTROLLED DIETS

When a person has a limited feeding ability but is able to eat certain foods and textures, diets must be planned carefully. The four food groups is one way to plan a varied but adequate diet. Clients need the same nutrients as usual and texture may be altered in all four groups. This is illustrated in Table 35-1.

Texture-modified diets are usually divided into several major categories: mechanical soft or ground; puree; full liquid, and clear liquids. The specific restriction depends on the person's abilities, which may change. Below is a brief description of each of these diets.

Mechanical soft is recommended for persons who need a soft diet for mechanical reasons. An individual may be edentulous (without teeth) or have had dental surgery or some other difficulty in chewing. The diet includes any food that can be easily masticated. High-fiber foods, such as bran cereals or vegetables, are allowed if they are soft. Fish and tender meats, such as ground beef and poultry, are permitted. Seasonings are not restricted. This mechanical soft diet may also be called a "ground meat" diet since tough meats must be ground and often soft meats must be cut up into small pieces.

Pureed food is recommended when persons are unable to chew anything. This may be the result of paralysis, throat or mouth cancer, or an otherwise tender, inflamed mouth and esophagus. Pureed food should be as appealing as possible in smell and in taste. Persons will enjoy favorite foods and seasonings. Almost any food can be pureed in a food processor or blender. Adding appropriate liquids (*e.g.,* seasoned bouillon to meat dishes, sauces, milk, or juice to well-cooked vegetables) softens otherwise dry foods and adds the calories the person may need.

Full-liquid diets are often recommended as one of the stages after surgery, as the diet is advanced from clear liquids to normal. A full-liquid diet allows all liquids or foods that are in liquid form at body temperature. Liquids can be fed by cup, straw, or tube. Most full-liquid diets are temporary; a liquid diet that will be long-term often includes commercial supplements to help meet the Recommended Dietary Allowances.

Clear-liquid diets are the least demanding of the four on the intestines. Clear liquids are easily absorbed. They are usually the first foods recommended after surgery or after a period of fasting. A clear-liquid diet (described in Table 35-1) is almost always nutritionally inadequate. Clear, sweetened beverages, jellos, ices, and meat broths all contain very few vitamins and minerals. Commercial supplements that are clear (*e.g.,* Vivonex®, Citrotein®) are available to provide extra nutrients, but this diet is usually not followed for long because it is so inadequate and monotonous. The person with a mechanical feeding problem usually does not need a clear-liquid diet except after surgery and in other unusual, short-term circumstances. And, as discussed in Chapter 38, clear liquid formulas are very elemental and unpalatable; they may, in addition, cause problems with hyperosmolar diarrhea.

TEXTURE-RELATED PROBLEMS

When textures are modified, as they are in these diets, texture-related problems sometimes develop. These may include tooth decay and gum disease; constipation, weight loss or malnutrition.

Dental Problems

A soft diet may not use the teeth or stimulate blood flow in the gums. Frequent oral feeding can encourage bacteria and promote cavities. Dry mouth often increases the risk of caries; this will be discussed in more detail in Chapter 41. This problem may be prevented by brushing teeth frequently, flossing when appropriate, and encouraging the use of plain water and ice chips to keep the mouth moist.

Constipation

Constipation may be a result of the low fiber or fluid content of the diet or some physiological problem, such as partial damage to the muscles along the digestive tract. Inactivity can also contribute to constipation. Constipation may be extremely uncomfortable, especially for someone whose disease may have left him immobile and/or wheelchair-bound.

Diet treatment for constipation has been discussed in Chapter 24. If diet is the problem, soft, high-fiber cereals and juices, with plenty of fluids, may help alleviate the discomfort. Physicians sometimes recommend laxatives, although usually with caution; the gut may become "dependent" on them. Some liquid supplements "with fiber" are also available in the hospital and through pharmacies for the individual on a full-liquid diet. Activity should be encouraged as much as possible.

Weight Loss and Malnutrition

When eating stops being a pleasure, persons may eat less and eat a limited selection of foods. Many of the diets that adjust texture quickly become monotonous and persons may lose interest in eating. The disability itself or some medication that is part of therapy may promote anorexia. Eating may become associated with pain or with the humiliation of being fed. Whatever the reason, individuals with mechanical feeding problems often lose weight and may, after a long period of time on a very restricted diet, develop a vitamin or mineral deficiency. They may become less resistant to infection and more lethargic about eating.

This should be prevented if at all possible. Food should be made especially appealing, and alternate feeding methods should be considered (and discussed with the client) if oral feeding is just not working well enough.

Planning is a very important part of compensating for a feeding disorder. Therapy, menus, variety, and ways to help the person become as independent as possible all need to be planned. Progress toward an acceptable, lifelong feeding pattern is often slow and discouraging, but it does happen. With hard work, the client may well regain at least some lost feeding skills or become equally adept with new skills.

STUDY QUESTIONS

1. Define:
   - Mechanical feeding problem
   - Dysphagia
   - Esophagostomy
   - Stoma
   - Full liquid diet
   - Nasogastric tube
2. What are some causes of mechanical feeding problems?
3. Why may mechanical feeding problems lead to nutrition problems?
4. List at least four categories of health profes-

sionals who may be helpful in the treatment of a mechanical feeding problem.
5. List at least five of the seven skills required for self-feeding.
6. Why do some people choke when they try to swallow food?
7. Try lying flat on a floor, bed, or other flat surface. Instruct a friend to try and feed you custard or a milkshake. You cannot raise your head. Describe your experience.
8. How is dysphagia treated?
9. Janie is 15 years old and has just become blind. She was admitted to the hospital with a high fever, underwent surgery, and is now in her first day of recovery. She may or may not regain her sight. The doctor has prescribed a clear liquid diet for two days.
   - What beverages and foods are permitted?
   - How would you begin to help her mother think about ways to make mealtimes easier after Janie goes home?
   - What are some of the other concerns Janie and her mother are probably thinking about right now?

REFERENCES

1. Dobie RA: Rehabilitation of swallowing disorders. Am Fam Physician 17(5): 84–95, 1978
2. Griffin KM: Swallowing training for dysphagic patients. Arch Phys Med Rehabil 55:465ff, October 1974
3. Silverman EH, Elfant IL: Dysphagia: An evaluation and treatment program for the adult. Am J Occup Ther 33(6): 382–392, 1979

RESOURCES

Two companies that sell eating-related utensils for mechanical problems are:

Fred Sammons, Inc.
Professional Self-Help Aids Catalog
Box 32
Brookfield, IL 60513

American Foundation for the Blind
15 W. 16th Street
New York, NY 10011

CHAPTER 36

Nutrition and Drugs

OBJECTIVES

1. To introduce briefly the historic role of nutrition in pharmacology

2. To discuss "herbal" or "natural" medicine, its place in history, and the risks involved in its current application among some cultures and subgroups

3. To introduce the interaction of nutrients and drugs and, in general, why and how they interact

4. To discuss the effects of drugs on nutritional status, with specific examples
   a. As they relate to absorption, metabolism, and excretion
   b. Common side-effects that influence nutrition:
      Appetite changes
      Sensory changes
      Secretory changes

5. To discuss food factors that influence drug status, providing specific examples of
   a. Absorption, metabolism, and excretion
   b. Timing
   c. The pH of the digestive tract
   d. Combinations and competition

6. To discuss the interaction of drugs with drugs, especially drugs commonly accepted as food:
   a. Alcohol
   b. Caffeine

   c. Vitamin-mineral or protein supplements
   d. Natural sources of drugs in foods, such as tyramine in foods that may trigger monoamine oxidase inhibitor (MAOI) reactions

7. To discuss the special considerations of drug use in the elderly population and the effect of aging on drug sensitivity.

8. To emphasize specific ways to prevent undesirable interactions

9. To provide references for further study

HISTORY

From very ancient times man has used unusual nonfood substances in an effort to cure diseases. These substances have included ash, root, herbs, dust, and many other odd products of the earth. Treatment depended on what the specific culture believed about the illness. Sometimes the treatment worked, but sometimes the patient worsened and died, often no doubt from the disease but certainly sometimes from a toxic dose of the "medicine." This early study of what substances worked in illness and what did not was the beginning of pharmacology.

Hippocrates, the "father of medicine," a Greek who lived about 400 BC, believed illness was based on imbalances in the body and prescribed fresh air, good food, and an opportunity to let the body heal itself. A century later another Greek, Theophrastus, compiled a history of plants and their medicinal properties. Both nutrition and medicinal substances have long been partners in the treatment of disease. The Bible refers in several places to trees whose "fruit will be for food and their leaves for healing."[1] "Herbals," books listing potential healing properties of different herbs, have been used by physicians and lay people for centuries, until modern medicine has made it possible to test the claims of the herbal and refine into purer forms the substances that truly work most effectively.

HERBAL MEDICINE TODAY

Some persons who reject modern medicine still use "natural therapy," including the old herbals (one common text frequently used is *Culpeper's Complete Herbal,* first published in 1826) for treating disease and illness. Unfortunately there is a far greater risk with these treatments than modern medicine. "Herbals" list what worked for a few people at some forgotten time. They do not provide success rates and have never been updated to include current knowledge of the body cells and functions. Further, the herbs themselves are not drugs in pure forms. They contain a mixture of many unknown and poorly understood substances. The content of plants varies according to the season and the species. Substances may be toxic at certain times of the year or if the plant is handled in a particular way. Many modern drugs (*e.g.,* penicillin) have been extracted from plants and purified. Their synthetic forms are chemically pure, unlike their natural counterparts, which may be a mixture of several substances. It is illegal to make a written claim for a natural product that its "natural" source is biologically superior to the form made in the laboratory.[2] In the laboratory, there is no need to be concerned with foreign, unwelcome substances. The exact effects of the isolated substances are known and understood. Any person who chooses herbal treatment rather than the more exact modern medicine should be aware that he is working with variable substances that may range from harmless to toxic. The problem being "treated" may become worse when simple, available medical treatment is ignored. And if a medical problem improves on any "natural" treatment it may (up to one third of the time) be

the result of the "placebo effect" discussed in Chapter 40, faith in the treatment, and not actually benefit in the substance.*

Interactions

Drugs, whether from herbs (*e.g.,* digitalis in foxgloves, laxative substances in some herb teas), prescribed medications, or foods (caffeine, alcohol, and other natural druglike substances) can interact with nutrients in positive or negative ways. Sometimes the drugs come from the diet; that is, they are contained within the nutrients in food. Sometimes they are not beneficial drugs but rather social or addictive (as in alcohol, cocaine, and other "controlled" or illegal substances). Sometimes they are over-the-counter substances used for minor complaints and concerns (multivitamin substances, laxatives, decongestants). Or they have been prescribed for treatment of diseases. Nutrition has many benefits but it cannot always guarantee health. Sometimes drugs are essential. And yet these same essential substances may interact with food to cause both nutrient- and medication-related problems.

There are four general areas of interactions between nutrition and drugs:

1. The diet may affect the way the drug is used
2. The drug may upset the body's normal ingestion, or use of nutrients
3. The body may not use the drug properly because it is already malnourished
4. Drugs and foods may "cancel out" each other, due to mutually negating interaction in the digestive tract.[3]

These interactions vary widely. Sometimes they can be used to help both medication and nutrition. At other times they cause damage or interference.

Drug-diet interactions are extremely com-

---

* Most of the information presented here on pharmacology and current risks of herbal medicine is based on a lecture by Wayne Bidlack, "Overview of Basic Pharmacy," delivered at the American Dietetic Association's conference on Pharmacology Applications for Dietitians, Boston, Sept. 7, 1984

plex. This chapter is intended only as an introduction to the subject. There are hundreds of different drugs and many different nutrients and food substances. Each nutrient may interact in a specific way with each drug. Various combinations may interact is different ways. The interaction depends on the specific drug, the food or nutrient, and the unique characteristics of the individual person. The more medications a person uses, the more interactions are possible. This makes the study of drug-diet interactions particularly difficult, and makes it especially vital for the dietitian and the pharmacist to work together with the rest of the health care team to provide adequate support to the client who has been placed on a combination of prescription medications.

THE EFFECT OF DRUGS ON NUTRITION

The action of a drug in the body may affect nutrition. A drug may affect appetite, absorption, metabolism, or excretion of nutrients. It may affect one, several, or all of these. Below are a few common examples:

Appetite

Appetite changes, including nausea and vomiting, are commonly listed as possible side-effects of many drugs. Drugs known to increase appetite include steroids (*e.g.,* Prednisone) used to minimize hypersensitive reactions, antihistamines (often used for asthma or allergy), psychotropic drugs (used for depression or other mental or emotional disturbances), some birth control pills, and oral hypoglycemic agents (used to help control blood sugar in type II diabetes mellitus).[3,4]

Drugs that suppress the appetite include amphetamines, alcohol, cough medication, caffeine, antacids, cardiac glycosides (*e.g.,* digitalis) and drugs used for cancer chemotherapy.[3,5] Chapter 29 discussed the problems of drugs and prolonged anorexia.

Absorption

The most common interactions occur where drugs and nutrients first meet: in the gut. It is here, especially in the stomach and small intestine, that drugs impair absorption.

One example is mineral oil. Sometimes used as a laxative, mineral oil is not absorbed into the body. However it coats the lining of the small intestines. This prevents nutrients from being absorbed. Chronic use of mineral oil may lead to vitamin deficiencies, especially fat-soluble vitamins A or D, which may dissolve in the oil and never reach the cells. Mineral oil has occasionally been used as a substitute for vegetable oil in cooking. This is not a wise practice because of the potential for this deficiency.[3,4]

The action of many other drugs in the gut can inhibit absorption. Other laxatives may stimulate peristalsis. If food moves through the system too quickly, nutrients may not have time for proper absorption. Calcium and potassium absorption may suffer. Neomycin (an antibiotic) may actually damage the mucous surface of the small intestine. This damage may impair absorption of fat, protein, lactose, several electrolytes, calcium, iron, and vitamin B_{12}. Cholestyramine (used to lower lipid levels) acts by "binding" or combining with bile acids. When fewer bile acids are available, absorption of fat, iron, and vitamins A, D, K and B_{12} is affected. Steroids or glucocorticoids impair the way in which potassium and calcium are carried across the wall of the digestive tract.

Sometimes the pH or acidity of the gut affects absorption. Drugs can change the pH of the intestine. Potassium chloride (KCl), used as a salt substitute, lowers the pH of the ileum, making B_{12} absorption more difficult. Antacids, on the other hand, increase the pH of the gut, affecting the absorption of several nutrients, especially folacin.[3]

Metabolism

Drugs may also affect the nutrient balance within the cells. Anticonvulsants (for example dilantin) used in controlling seizures cause the body to use vitamin D and folate more quickly. This can lead to folate deficiency, megaloblastic anemia (described in Chapter 27), and may affect calcium absorption as well, since calcium metabolism depends heavily on vitamin D.

Oral contraceptives also seem to change the

way in which the body distributes several nutrients. Women on the Pill often have low blood levels of folate, riboflavin, B_6, B_{12} and vitamin C. However, such women rarely develop the symptoms of an acute deficiency of these vitamins, so it is not clear whether the body levels of the vitamins are really being wasted. This may be a special concern for women whose normal diet might be low in these nutrients, particularly teens and/or low-income women. Since vitamin supplements are also a type of drug with possible interactions of their own, women concerned about their nutrition while on the Pill are probably safest choosing food sources high in these vitamins.

Another drug that seems to impair the metabolism of B_6 is isoniazid (INH), which is used to treat tuberculosis. Vitamin B_6 is often prescribed when clients with tuberculosis must be on INH.

Excretion

Drugs that prevent a nutrient from being properly absorbed will cause it to be excreted. Laxatives are chief offenders in the malabsorption and excessive excretion of nutrients. Sometimes these losses lead to major metabolic imbalances.

Oral contraceptives may lead to a loss of tryptophan, often treated and corrected by extra B_6.[6]

Some diuretics that are used to help rid the body of extra fluid (often used in heart diseases and hypertension) "waste" potassium. Persons on these medications are sometimes told to eat a banana or drink orange juice daily to prevent the heart irregularities and other complications of low-serum potassium levels. This is *not* necessary with all diuretics. Some of them "spare" or conserve potassium. Potassium imbalance can be serious, so clients who are on a diuretic should check with their physician before using any high-potassium product, including salt substitutes (which are usually potassium chloride).

Chronic use of aspirin can irritate the stomach and intestinal wall, wear a hole in it, and cause bleeding. When blood is lost, iron is also lost and excreted, and anemia may result.

Side-Effects

Drugs affect nutrition in other ways as well. Appetite changes, discussed above and in Chapter 29, are a common side-effect. Sensory changes are another common side-effect. Clients on chemotherapy sometimes complain that food "feels" different, like "cotton" or "steel wool." Drugs that use up zinc can lead to taste changes. Secretory changes may also occur. The glands that secrete saliva and the digestive enzymes may work less effectively. If there are not enough enzymes to digest food, the food is not well-absorbed. Table 36-1 outlines the major drug side-effects that may influence nutrition.

FOOD FACTORS THAT INFLUENCE DRUG STATUS

Food-drug interactions work both ways. Drugs may affect nutrition but diet and nutritional status can also affect the way the body uses drugs. Many other factors also play a part in how the body uses a drug. These factors include age, blood flow, nutritional status and the individual characteristics of the GI tract, including enzyme status and diseases.

Like the effects of drugs on nutrition, nutritional status can also affect the absorption, metabolism, and excretion of substances, including drugs. The same factors may be involved; that is:

a. pH of the gut

b. Combinations that bind substances and prevent absorption

c. Competition for the same absorption site

In addition, malnutrition can also affect drugs, causing them to function abnormally or inadequately.

Absorption/Excretion

The simple presence or absence of a recent meal in the gut can affect drug absorption and excretion. There are many different ways food can influence medication. Drugs taken on an empty stomach will encounter nothing but the digestive fluids and walls of the GI tract. Sometimes

Table 36-1

Common Drug-Related Side-Effects

Side-Effect	Comments
Anorexia	See Chapter 29
Constipation	See Chapter 24
Diarrhea	Increase liquids to prevent dehydration
	Avoid foods that obviously aggravate diarrhea
	Very cold or very hot food may stimulate the colon; avoid extreme temperatures
	Frequent, small meals help replace lost nutrients
	Pectin (in apples) and gums (in oatmeal) may help form stool
	Include high-potassium foods, since potassium is often lost in diarrhea
Dry, sore mouth	Keep teeth and mouth moist, clean; may be at risk for tooth decay
	Use sugarless gum, low-sugar beverages
	Lemon, lime, and citrus drinks (if tolerated) may stimulate saliva
	Use sauces, liquids to keep all foods moist
	Avoid spicy, dry, sharp, or rough-textured foods that may irritate
	Have beverages with all meals
	Cold, soft dairy products or fruit are often soothing
Heartburn	See Chapter 13
Hyperphagia, weight gain	Limit intake to foods low in nutrient density
	Increase activity and regular exercise, if possible
	Boil, broil, or bake foods without added fat
Nausea	See Chapter 13
Taste changes	See Chapter 29

(Adapted from Smith CH, Bidlack WR: Dietary concerns associated with the use of medications. J Am Diet Assoc 84 (8): 901–904, 1984)

this helps absorption and sometimes drugs are more effective when they travel along the GI tract with food.

Food helps protect the gut against drugs that may irritate its delicate lining. When food is present in the stomach or small intestine, drugs are absorbed more slowly. This is one reason alcohol may be less intoxicating if it is consumed together with a meal.[4] Sometimes food *delays* absorption but does not cause less *total* absorption. For example cimetidine, used in the treatment of ulcers, is given with food because the food causes only some of the drug to be absorbed. The rest is absorbed later, when the gut is empty. This simple mechanism helps control the blood level of this drug. However not all drugs "wait around" for the gut to clear. If penicillin, for example, is taken with food, some of the drug is lost because of impaired absorption;

penicillin is most effective on an empty stomach.

Specific nutrients also affect absorption. A high-carbohydrate meal slows down absorption of many drugs. A high-fat meal, on the other hand, increases absorption of griseofulvin, a drug used to treat fungus infections. Fiber can bind with drugs and prevent absorption; calcium can do the same. When tetracycline (an antibiotic) is taken while milk or dairy products are still present in the gut, the calcium binds the drug so that neither calcium nor tetracycline is absorbed. Persons who are on tetracycline should never take it with a milk product and should let 2 to 3 hours elapse between taking the drug and drinking milk or eating a high-calcium food.[3,7]

Acidic juices and sodas taken with medication may cause some drugs to be dissolved too quickly. A drug that is absorbed best in the distal jejunum may not be effective if it is dissolved and broken down too soon, for example, in the stomach. On the other hand, some acids help enhance absorption: citrus juices (high in vitamin C) should be taken with iron supplements because they enhance the absorption of the supplemental mineral (discussed in Chapter 27).

Metabolism

Once in the blood, nutrients may still interfere with drug action. Warfarin (or coumadin) is an anticoagulant; it may be used to help prevent blood clotting. Vitamin K promotes clotting. Therefore, Warfarin may not be effective if the diet is high in vitamin K foods.

Natural licorice contains a drug called *glycirrhizic acid*. This drug causes the body to hold sodium and excrete potassium. People on diuretics and other medications for hypertension may complicate their own treatment if they eat as much as 100 grams (3 ½ oz) per day of natural licorice.[8]

Indoles, substances present in vegetables such as sprouts and cabbage, can increase drug absorption.

Goitrogens, discussed in Chapter 27, should not be eaten in large amounts by persons on thyroid medication.

Alcohol, a depressant, is technically a drug. It can lower the body's metabolism; this in turn may mean a drug is not "cleared" from the system quickly and may result in excessively high blood levels (since the medication will take longer to move out of the blood and into the cells). This is most dangerous when the medication is another type of depressant, for example, sedatives or tranquilizers, or an oral hypoglycemic agent. Too much of the drug in the blood at a time can cause serious problems.

Malnutrition may also affect the metabolism of drugs. For example, the blood normally contains proteins that act to carry substances such as drugs into the cells. Protein (especially albumin) levels often drop in malnourished persons. If there is too little protein to carry medication effectively from blood to cell, the levels in the blood may rise too high, causing a toxic reaction.

On the other hand, a high level of protein causes liver enzymes to work more rapidly than usual and some drugs are metabolized quickly, while the presence of protein may actually interfere with the absorption of other drugs.[9]

DRUG/DRUG INTERACTIONS

Drugs also interact with each other. The interactions are highly variable and sometimes unpredictable. They depend on what drugs and how many drugs are present, and the actions of each. A registered pharmacist is the professional member of the health care team who is best qualified to answer any questions about these interactions. *The Lippincott Nurses' Drug Manual* and the annual *Physicians' Desk Reference (PDR)* are two publications that also discuss specific drug actions (and possible side-effects) in detail.

But the line between drugs and food is sometimes a fuzzy one. Alcohol and caffeine are both drugs that are also considered in nutrition. Supplements of vitamins, minerals, protein, or fatty acids technically may contain nutrients but may be used as drugs. Supplements that contain more than 100% of the Recommended Dietary Allowances may act as drugs in the body. And many foods contain natural substances that act as drugs, including the glycirrhizic acid in natural licorice (discussed above), natural salicylates (discussed in Chapter 40), and tyramine, dopamine, and phenylethylamine.

Tyramine, dopamine, and *phenylethylamine* are protein substances present in many aged and fermented foods. These substances have a natural effect on blood vessels, causing them to constrict. As a result, blood pressure may rise slightly, and this reaction is not usually significant. But when a person is on drugs called Monoamine oxidase (MAO) inhibitors, usually to treat depression, phobic anxieties[4] and sometimes hypertension,[10] a dangerous reaction may result. The drug interacts with the food substance, causing blood pressure to rise quickly and dangerously. Symptoms of these reactions include headaches, palpitations, nausea, vomiting, and even occasional strokes. The reaction depends on the dose both of medication and tyramine substance.

FOODS CONTAINING TYRAMINE SUBSTANCES

Must Be Avoided
Red wine (especially Chianti)
Pickled herring
Other pickled or smoked fish
Dry summer sausage
Fava or broad bean pods
All aged cheeses
Liver, especially beef or chicken
Italian green beans
Yeast vitamin supplements (Brewer's yeast)

Large Quantities May Cause Problems
Other alcoholic beverages
Ripe avocado
Ripe banana
Sour cream
Yogurt
Fermented soy products (soy sauce, miso)

Many foods contain these substances but certain foods may have levels high enough to cause serious side-effects. Persons on MAO inhibitors should avoid these foods. Listed above are foods known to be highest in these substances. The more aged (or spoiled) a food, the more of these substances it may contain. Aged cheese has more tyramine closer to the rind than closer to the center of the same block.[11] Some foods may have small amounts of these substances but have been safely enjoyed by many persons taking these drugs. These foods include chocolate, figs, meat tenderizers, raisins, yeast breads, coffee, tea, and other caffeine-containing beverages.[11] Cheeses that are not aged, such as cottage cheese and ricotta, contain little or none of the substances.

Vitamin, mineral, and protein supplements may also interact with medications just as drugs do. Megadoses of vitamin A can lead to severe headaches in persons who are on tetracycline.[9] Folate supplements may interfere with methotrexate treatment in chemotherapy. Certain mineral supplements may interfere with antibi-

otics. Protein supplements of PABA (para-aminobenzoic acid) may cause drug-related problems for some persons.[9] On the other hand, some drugs such as pyridoxine (vitamin B_6) may be helpful in some drug treatments but should be given only with the approval of a physician.

AGING AND DRUGS

As the body grows older it changes. The manner in which it absorbs, metabolizes, and excretes both nutrients and drugs may also change. The elderly often have several other risk factors as well:

1. They often have limited resources and thus may not be able to afford an adequate diet. Borderline, "subclinical" malnutrition may result.

2. They often have mechanical eating problems. They may be handicapped, unable to shop often, or prepare a variety of foods. They may depend on canned, convenience, or highly processed foods. Dentures or digestive problems may limit the textures of foods they choose.

3. They may be on several prescription and over-the-counter medications. At least 50% of all drugs are taken by the elderly and the elderly in nursing homes may take as many as ten different drugs.[12] The elderly who live independently frequently purchase over-the-counter drugs, such as analgesics, laxatives, and vitamin supplements, in addition to their prescribed medications. Some medications should be taken on an empty stomach; others, with foods. Some should not be taken at the same time. Planning an adequate menu around these proscriptions may be more bother than some persons want and many are not aware that food and medication may interact, affecting both their nutrition and the ability of the drugs to do their job.

These factors place the elderly at special nutritional risk. In addition, the way their bodies react to a drug may be quite different than the reaction they might have had 30 years earlier.

GUIDELINES FOR THE INDEPENDENT ELDERLY PERSON ON PRESCRIBED MEDICATION

---

1. Report all side-effects to the doctor, especially after beginning a new medication. If you are not sure whether or not it is a side-effect but it is a recent change, tell the doctor.

2. Know which drugs to take on an empty stomach and which to take with meals.

3. Ask the doctor and the pharmacist about possible drug-nutrient interactions and how to prevent them.

4. Choose a diet containing foods high in all major vitamins and minerals. Ask for help, if necessary, from a dietitian or visiting nurse.

5. Never take medicine that has been prescribed for someone else.

6. If you stop taking a prescribed medication for any reason, notify the doctor. It is cheaper to keep in touch with the doctor and stay healthy than to develop problems from "treating" yourself.

7. Tell the doctor about all the over-the-counter medications you take, even occasionally. They may affect the way your prescription drugs work.

8. If you drink, say so. Long-term effects of alcohol can change the way the body uses drugs, and even a small drink may have a large effect on the body in reaction to some medications.

Alcohol abuse (current or past) or other diseases may have damaged the liver and the liver enzymes that metabolize drugs and nutrients. Or the medications may be taken incorrectly, due to a misunderstanding, confusion, or other factors. The elderly may alter their own doses or use other persons' medications rather than go to the doctor. Smoking may also affect their metabolism of certain nutrients, notably vitamins B_6, B_{12} and C.[5]

There are many ways to prevent undesirable interactions and drug-related malnutrition in the elderly. Some suggestions are listed above.

Many elderly do not live independently or with family members, but live in long-term care facilities, such as nursing homes. Many are hospitalized frequently. Sometimes diet prescriptions are changed. Drugs are changed. The elderly may be on parenteral or enteral tube feedings. Disease or poor eating habits may have resulted in subclinical malnutrition. These are all special situations that can affect drug-nutrient interactions. New medications bring new problems. Illness changes the nutrient status of

the patient. Malnutrition becomes more likely. Tube feedings usually keep some food in the gut at all times, making it hard to coordinate with medication that may work best on an empty stomach. Medications that come in liquid forms ('elixirs') are sometimes "flushed" through a feeding tube. If the elixir has a pH of less than 4, it may gel in the tube, blocking it, and causing even more problems.[12] Each of these problems must be worked out to help the elderly client obtain the best, most effective nutrition and drug treatment for optimal health in these later years.

STUDY QUESTIONS

---

1. Define
- "Natural therapy,"
- "Placebo effect"

2. Iris E. is a 70-year-old unmarried, retired schoolteacher who is afraid of doctors. Lately she has had many unusual symptoms of illness and has begun to read the "herbals" she finds in her health food store. She has also begun to collect natural products from the woods behind her house to treat her symptoms. She believes this is better for her than anything a doctor might give. How would you respond?

3. What are the four general areas of drug-nutrient interactions?

4. List several drugs or drug types that
   - Commonly cause anorexia
   - Change absorption as a result of altered *p*H
   - May irritate the gut and cause bleeding

5. Describe some drug-nutrient problems that may develop from the use of the following:
   - Mineral oil
   - Oral contraceptives
   - Diuretics
   - Alcohol

6. Which food(s)
   - May dissolve medication before drugs reach the area on the small intestine where their action is needed?
   - Should not be taken with tetracycline? Why?
   - May complicate medications used in blood clotting?
   - Are dangerous for people on MAO inhibitors? Why?

7. What are at least three reasons drug-nutrient interactions are of special concern for the elderly?

8. Why might tube feeding make medication therapy difficult?

REFERENCES

1. Old Testament: Ezekiel 47:12. New Testament: Revelation 22:2
2. Mead Johnson Laboratories: Nutritional Perspectives No. 3: Liquid Diets, p 9. Evansville, IN, Mead Johnson, 1974
3. Roe DA: Nutrient and drug reactions. Nutr Rev 42(4): 141–154, 1984
4. Roe DA: Interactions between drugs and nutrients. Med Clin North Am 63(5): 985–1007, September 1979
5. Winick M: Drug-nutrition interaction in the elderly. Institute of Human Nutrition Newsletter. New York, Columbia University, 1982
6. Goodhart RE, Shils ME: Modern Nutrition in Health and Disease, 6th ed, p 224. Philadelphia, Lea & Febiger, 1980
7. Smith CH, Bidlack WR: Food and drug interactions. Food Technology, pp 99–103, October 1982
8. Hartshorn EA: Food and drug interactions. J Am Diet Assoc 70:15–19, January 1977
9. Smith CH, Bidlack WR: Dietary concerns associated with the use of medications. J Am Diet Assoc 84(8): 901–904, 1984
10. Food and Drug Administration: Food and Drug Interaction. Pueblo, CO, Consumer Information Center, Department 698F
11. Powers DE, Moore AO: Food Medication Interactions, 4th ed., 1983. Available from F-MI Publishing, P.O. Box 26464, Tempe, AZ, 85282, 1983
12. Roe DA: Therapeutic effects of drug-nutrient interactions in the elderly. J Am Diet Assoc 85(2): 174–181, 1985

CHAPTER 37

Eating Disorders: Anorexia Nervosa, Bulimia, and Failure-to-Thrive

OBJECTIVES

1. To define
  a. Anorexia nervosa
  b. Bulimia
  c. Bulimarexia
  d. Failure-to-thrive

2. To discuss briefly the historical development of anorexia nervosa

3. To describe the common characteristics of a person with an eating disorder and to discuss the severity of the problem

4. To distinguish between thin, amenorrheic athletes and athletic anorexics

5. To list and discuss the dangers and complications that can develop and threaten the life of anyone with an eating disorder

6. To define and discuss the family characteristics and dynamics that intensify eating disorders

7. To outline and discuss basic treatment choices and prognosis

8. To provide specific guidelines to help the friends of a person with an eating disorder

9. To discuss the common symptoms, causes, and nutrition treatment of nonorganic failure-to-thrive in young children

Since the late 1970's, the eating disorders of anorexia nervosa and bulimia have become more and more endemic among otherwise

healthy young women and teenagers. At least one popular singer, Karen Carpenter, died from complications of *anorexia nervosa*. Others who feel they have recovered (or who continue to struggle) have written about it.[1-3] The increased (or increasingly public) numbers of anorectic women have made them more visible: half-skeletons seen jogging down streets, through parks, or shivering, covered in bulky sweaters but with the most unlikely bones showing through. In fact they may be seen doing almost anything — except eating. Some women who do eat in public and whose weight is normal may also suffer from the partner of anorexia nervosa: *bulimia,* or from a combination of the two conditions called *bulimarexia*. These are the women who disappear after a meal in order to induce vomiting, to rid themselves of extra calories.

Another type of "eating disorder" that also has a social and psychological base is that of nonorganic failure-to-thrive in children, often very young children. This condition, too, will be discussed in this chapter, although it is otherwise unrelated to anorexia nervosa or bulimia.

ANOREXIA NERVOSA

Anorexia nervosa is very different from the simple anorexia discussed in Chapter 29, although the term anorexia is commonly used to refer to the eating disorder rather than a loss of appetite. The woman with anorexia nervosa (and almost 90% of those with this condition *are* women) is also called "anorexic," but her attitude is different. She has a perfectly normal appetite but ignores and suppresses it. The person with simple anorexia has lost interest in food; a woman with an eating disorder is often fascinated by it. She may spend a great deal of time cooking, studying nutrition, cutting out pictures of food, and dreaming about it, but the amount she actually allows herself to eat is minute. In spite of this, she sees herself as fat, not thin. This is vividly illustrated by Figure 37-1.

History is vague, even silent, concerning this syndrome. The first medical description of it appeared in 1689 when an English physician referred to "a nervous consumption."[4] Only in 1873 was it identified by both a French physician and a British physician as a distinct medical entity and named "anorexia nervosa."[5-6]

Psychiatry has defined anorexia nervosa (AN) and bulimarexia by what is called the "DSM–III Criteria." This is a type of checklist psychiatrists can use to determine whether or not a woman actually has the disorder. Listed on page 338 are these criteria for anorexia nervosa (AN). Figure 37-2 also outlines some of the factors that influence the disorder, as well as some of the symptoms.

The woman who develops an eating disorder may be any age, but she is usually in her teens or early twenties. Sometimes the event that triggers the sudden starvation is menarche, sometimes it is a loss, or a family separation such as divorce or leaving home for school. There are certain common characteristics in the type of woman who develops the disorder. She is usually eager to please people and is an "over-achiever." She pushes herself to do her best in everything. She may be considered a "leader" and a "model child."

Beneath this surface success is an unhappy, insecure, and fearful little girl. Her self acceptance depends on her ability to be perfect and she fails. Perfection includes her body image: she must be as thin as the most attractive model. She may begin to work toward this goal with a sensible diet and exercise. But at some point, something happens. Thin is not thin enough. Regular exercise is not enough. And the food she is eating is definitely too much.

The anorexic's family influences the development of the disorder. Studies of these families find they usually have several characteristics in common. They are often overly protective. Communication in the home may be poor. The

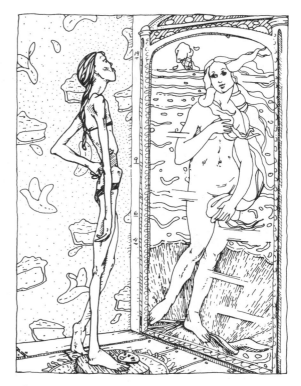

Figure 37-1
The phenomenon of anorexia nervosa. (Illustration for *The Boston Globe* by S.J. Shue. Used with permission)

family exercises a tight control on behavior. And it usually has highly unrealistic expectations for the daughter, expectations she cannot meet, but feels she must.[7]

The point where diet becomes eating disorder is not clear or scientifically well-defined. Many anorexics, however, can pinpoint a specific comment or event that triggered them to begin their dieting.[8] Diet became obsession at some point on a continuum where the body and mind begin to act abnormally, in a way that can quickly become destructive.

The woman feels a lack of control in her life and fights to gain it. She is desperately afraid she will lose all control and gain weight. She would rather die than gain weight—and she may. She becomes more and more obsessive about food and exercise, unable to relax or eat more than, for example, one Cheerio or one sliver of cheese

DIAGNOSTIC CRITERIA FOR ANOREXIA NERVOSA

1. Age of onset under 25 years

2. Anorexia with weight loss of at least 25% of original body weight

3. A distorted attitude toward food, eating, or weight that overrides even the instinctive responses to hunger and threats
   The above three may be associated with
   a. Denial of illness
   b. Apparent enjoyment in losing weight
   c. Desired body image of extreme thinness
   d. Unusual avoiding of or handling of food

4. No known medical illness that would account for the extreme loss of weight

5. No overt psychiatric illness

6. At least two of the following:
   a. Amenorrhea
   b. Bradycardia (persistent resting pulse less than 60 bpm)
   c. Hyperactivity despite severe weight loss
   d. Bulimia
   e. Self-induced vomiting

---

at a meal or snack. She may deny her developing sexuality, happy with the fact that menstruation stops. She is often so obsessed with food that all other activities — clubs, parties, meetings, dates — suffer or are abandoned. The less she eats the more control she feels. And, frequently, the thinner she becomes, the heavier she may see herself.

This distorted body image is well documented. The woman genuinely does not see herself as others see her. She may deny established weight and calorie standards and believe she is "different." She works hard to maintain control, to remain anorectic, despite intense misery and often suicidal feelings. Hilde Bruch, a psychiatrist who has worked with anorectics for many years, describes the experience this way:

"The real difference lies in the extraordinary pride and pleasure they take in being able to do something so hard. Suddenly it is easy and the conviction comes that it can go on forever; and this quickly turns into the feeling of "I enjoy being hungry." Now it is no longer ordinary dieting — the secondary biological effects of hunger begin to take place and bodily sensations get transformed. As one girl described it, 'When it becomes a plea-

sure to pursue, then something happens. One feels intoxicated . . .' Developing the anorexic state is not a process that takes place suddenly and automatically; it demands active and alert attention from its victim, every hour. It is not just a habit they cannot break; to maintain it requires suffering and continuous hard work. They struggle hard to change, deny, misperceive the evidence of their senses . . . The longer the illness lasts and the more weight they lose, the more anorexics become convinced that they are special and different; each one has a private word to describe the state of superiority she strives for. Then they feel they are no longer able to communicate with ordinary people who won't understand." [9]

In treatment, the anorexic is often called "manipulative." This means she is fighting to maintain complete, absolute control, short of open refusal, at all costs. She may want control over her body or over a whole environment. Treatment (discussed below) is long, arduous, and complex. It essentially means helping the woman to use her control in bringing *herself* back to health and honestly, sensitively working through the underlying personality problems without allowing her to manipulate her counselors.

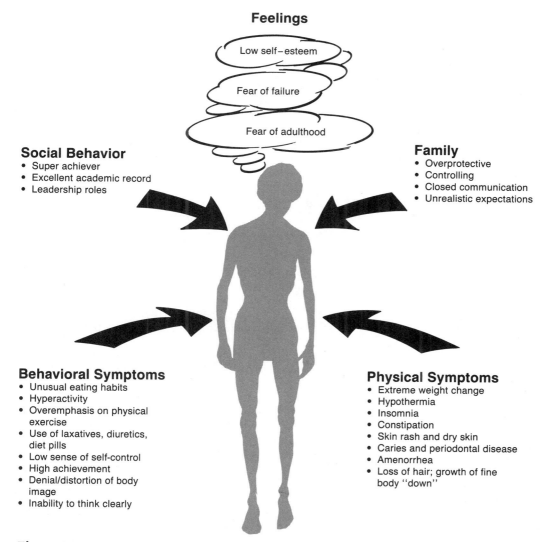

Feelings

Low self–esteem

Fear of failure

Fear of adulthood

Social Behavior
- Super achiever
- Excellent academic record
- Leadership roles

Family
- Overprotective
- Controlling
- Closed communication
- Unrealistic expectations

Behavioral Symptoms
- Unusual eating habits
- Hyperactivity
- Overemphasis on physical exercise
- Use of laxatives, diuretics, diet pills
- Low sense of self-control
- High achievement
- Denial/distortion of body image
- Inability to think clearly

Physical Symptoms
- Extreme weight change
- Hypothermia
- Insomnia
- Constipation
- Skin rash and dry skin
- Caries and periodontal disease
- Amenorrhea
- Loss of hair; growth of fine body ''down''

Figure 37-2
Factors and symptoms in the development of eating disorders. (Adapted from Block PJ: Working with anorexic and bulimic adolescents. Food and Nutrition News 56(5), 33–34, Nov–Dec 1984)

BULIMIA AND BULIMAREXIA

Bulimia is "the condition whereby an individual repeatedly loses control of the impulse to binge and rapidly consumes a large amount of food in a short period of time. Vomiting is then self-induced in an attempt to lose weight." [10] Laxative abuse is also a common practice in bulimia. As a symptom, bulimia may or may not be a part of anorexia. Both groups of women struggle for control of their weight and their food intake. While anorexics are normally emaciated, bulimics may be at their normal weight or slightly overweight. A bulimic may never have that distorted body image that is common in anorexics, but the same factors may be behind her practices.

Anorexics may often practice bulimia when they "lose control." "Binge" is followed by "purge." This is repeated until a destructive cycle, called bulimarexia, is well established.

Bulimia as a practice may be much more common than simple AN or bulimarexia. It is easy to begin and may easily become a compulsion and/or a reflex. Bulimia may easily lead into bulimarexia for some women. When bulimia is involved, a woman will often eat more than she claims (unlike the anorexic who may eat one and a half Cheerios and claim she had a bowlful). Binges can become expensive, and deception, lying, hiding foods, and shoplifting are common. Because of the complexities of the disorder, bulimarexia is the most difficult of the three to treat, with a very slow recovery accompanied by many setbacks.

WHAT ABOUT THE SUPER ATHLETE?

Are many women athletes actually borderline bulimics or anorexics? Some persons may think so because of the stress that many athletics, especially running and dancing, place on leanness. Many athletes, too, stop menstruating, also a sign of anorexia nervosa.

It is possible that some athletes struggle with an eating disorder. The factors outlined in Figure 37-2 may actually be their motivators for training and competition. The intensity of the food conflict may vary greatly. But a thin, amenorrheic runner or dancer does not necessarily have anorexia nervosa or practice bulimia. She may be naturally thin or seek to be so in order to become a better athlete. Bulimia may become a temptation at times for some athletes but it should never be assumed that the athlete does practice bulimia. Most athletes are in perfectly normal health and have excellent appetites.

Researchers who have looked at this issue in dancers find both similarities and differences between anorectics and dancers.[11] The groups may easily overlap, though, and dancers should be warned and educated about the subtle temptations and serious risks of eating disorders.

Amenorrhea is a predictable development of extreme weight loss, not just of anorexia nervosa. It was an almost universal development among the women in starvation areas or concentration camps during World War II. The body requires a certain level of fat in order that menstruation may begin. In athletes, muscle may replace fat. Gaining a few pounds may make all the difference, and menstruation may begin again. So amenorrhea is by no means a sure sign of an eating disorder. It may not even occur in bulimia and, in anorexics, may relate more to psychological factors than to fat since it may stop even before critical fat is lost.[10]

DANGERS AND COMPLICATIONS OF EATING DISORDERS

As visible (or secretive) as she is, the bulimic or anorexic woman is more than a curiosity: she is a person caught up in behaviors that could destroy her. She desperately wants control but, in reality, her fears control her. She may be happy about her thinness but overwhelmed with guilt when she eats anything at all. She tries to break loose of a family that has always controlled everything and fed her its expectations, often without hearing or giving value to her own thoughts and feelings. Yet she seeks tight control. Oddly enough, her family may come to depend on her abnormal behavior to remain intact as a unit.

This could continue for months, years, or a lifetime. The longer it continues, the poorer the chances for full — or functional — recovery. A young teen with a concerned family is more likely to resolve the problem issues and to recover than is an older counterpart whose family revolves around "her problem."

The major medical dangers of these disorders are physical and psychological. Women with any of the disorders need in-depth, trustworthy counseling. The eating behavior is only the outward sign of the inner disorder; changing the eating behavior is not enough. Weight gain is no sign of cure and has even been followed by suicide when the real, deeper problems were not resolved. Competent psychological counseling is essential. Many major medical centers have an "eating disorders" team or clinic; several national, lay support groups could help individuals find the nearest counselors in their area.

As critical as counseling is, the physical complications of the disorders are often serious. Karen Carpenter died of a heart attack at age 32—a heart attack brought on by complications of anorexia nervosa. Often the complications that develop and may prove fatal are some type of chemical imbalance, often an electrolyte disturbance. In long-term starvation, an electrolyte imbalance can develop quickly. Other complications may include collapsed lungs, degenerating heart fibers, kidney insufficiency, infection, and acute gastric dilatation (expansion) after refeeding.[12]

With the chronic vomiting of bulimia, very specific problems can develop. The digestive tract is not designed to empty "up." Stomach acid can burn holes in the walls of the esophagus, and "eat away" tooth enamel, especially on the back of the front teeth, which are in frequent contact with vomit. Long-term bulimics usually develop serious dental problems and may be so secretive about their behavior that the first person who may "find them out" could be their dentist.[13]

Vomiting may also upset the body's fluid and electrolyte balance and lead to serious disturbances that can develop quickly and, in extreme situations, lead to death.

PROGNOSIS

Currently there is only about a 33% chance of complete recovery for a woman with an eating disorder.[13] Another one third of these women will be chronically ill, unable to work or function productively in society, and the remaining third will walk a lifelong tightrope, constantly struggling in some measure with the disorder. Studies that look at the outcome of women with eating disorders find that many of them are eventually well educated and employed as professionals.

A key feature of the disorder is a denial of sexuality, and according to some researchers, only about 50% of the women are eventually able to sustain a long-term relationship.[12]

Mortality varies, with statistics ranging from 3% to 15% and even up to 25%.

The relationship between the psychological and physical manifestation of the disorder is a very tight one, and some of the psychological disorders are "normal" psychological responses to starvation. Hallucinations, voices, obsession with food, sleep disorders, and some fears may disappear or improve when the body is refed.

PARENTS AND FAMILIES

As mentioned earlier, family members are usually deeply involved in the development of the eating disorder and almost always have strong feelings about it. Their influence in the development of the disorder has been considerable. As Hilde Bruch describes it:

"Often the children were well cared for in every detail, physically, emotionally, and culturally, but everything was done according to the parents' decision without regard for the child's need . . . [As a result the anorexic suffers from] a lack of autonomy, having difficulties with decision-making and self-assertion . . . these short-comings become dramatically apparent with adolescence but subtle expressions were present throughout their childhood but were overlooked or praised."[8]

Because families cannot see this, they often deny that there is any problem, except that of the anorexic. This is often a difficulty, because treatment is most successful when it involves working together with the entire family and with disordered family relationships:

"The development of anorexia nervosa is so closely related to abnormal patterns of family interaction that successful treatment must always involve resolution of the underlying family problems, which may not be identifiable as open conflicts; on the contrary, quite often excessive closeness and overintense involvement lie at the roots.[9]

Because the parent-child relationship is so close, parents of anorexics or bulimarexics respond to the growing illness with anger, frustration, and resentment. Their "perfect child" is causing them pain and problems. They may blame the child. They may feel great guilt themselves. They may or may not deny their own responsibility. The mechanisms developed to cope with family problems now begin to crumble and parents may fight hard to restore that image of a happy, intact family. The image may be more important to them than coping with this real illness in their daughter. They may benefit greatly from counseling for their own troubles, but usually deny them. They may react with depression.

Some parents do work through the therapy with their daughter, admitting that all has not been well and, by doing so, consequently enrich their personal and family relationships. Many lay support groups for anorexics include support for parents, encouraging them "in spite of all odds, to forgive themselves and their family members for the disruptions associated with eating disorders, [taking] care of themselves gently, lovingly and honestly." [14]

TREATMENT

Treatment depends on the severity of the problem. Success is most likely for the young adolescent who has had anorexia nervosa a short time and who is not also bulimic. The bulimarexic, for whom this lifestyle is well-established and whose family has established some mechanism (often unhealthy) to cope with her, will find healing and recovery the hardest. Years of treatment are often needed.

One enormous danger in treatment is to believe that a woman is recovered when she has gained a certain amount of weight. An eating disorder is a psychological disorder; it cannot be measured on bathroom scales. Weight must change, simply to draw the woman away from physical danger, but the most successful treatment is therapy that helps the woman learn and want to change her behavior and attitudes.

Below is a brief description of some of the common treatment methods and resources.

Trained Counseling, Usually Psychotherapy. In counseling, the woman meets on a regular basis with a counselor whom she can trust. These sessions usually continue for months or years. Often a nutritionist is involved in education and ongoing nutrition counseling[15]. Many publications are available with more detailed counseling information than can be included in this chapter.*

Hospitalization. Usually a woman is only hospitalized when her weight has become critically low and her life may be in danger if she loses any more weight. Treatment begins or continues during hospitalization. She may be force-fed or some type of behavior modification may be used so that she might gain weight.

Force-Feeding. For an anorexic or bulimarexic, force-feeding may seem like rape, although it may at times be the only way to save her life. At best it is a short-term, emergency measure that may help the client survive to enter other types of therapy with long-term effects.

Behavior Modification. In behavior modification, all privileges are usually taken from the client (phone, bathroom, visitors, TV, privacy). Weight gain is rewarded with the return of certain privileges. What and how the client eats to gain the weight may not matter as long as she does gain the weight. This may encourage binge eating and spell disaster for the bulimarexic when she is discharged. She learns how to comply with authorities and receive rewards, but she may learn nothing about a healthy control of her impulses and may leave the hospital more depressed, suicidal and helpless than before. Behavior modification may work for a while, but it should never be the only treatment method.

Drugs. Sometimes drugs are used as part of therapy. Antidepressants have helped some.[1,12] Appetite stimulants are usually not used because appetite is not the problem. The role of drugs in treatment of eating disorders is a minor and controversial one. If a mineral or vitamin deficiency exists those supplements may be part of the drug treatment.

Nutrition Counseling. A nutritionist can help an anorexic to better understand food and how it works in the body. She can help teach principles that might, intellectually, help the client learn control in maintaining her weight at

---

* e.g.: Anorexia Nervosa and Bulimia: A Handbook for Counselors and Therapists by P. Neuman and P. Halvorsen. Published by Van Nostrand Reinhold, New York, N.Y. 10020.

a safe level. Exchange diets may be very helpful. In addition, a nutritionist may be able to help an anorexic see food as a source of health and energy. But, as mentioned above, nutrition counseling is not enough. The client may already know nutrition well. Above all, she needs a healed relationship with, and a deeper understanding of, herself and her feelings. This seems to be best accomplished by some type of trained, honest, consistent, sensitive psychotherapy.

Self-Help Groups. Some persons with eating disorders find help in self-help groups, such as Overeaters' Anonymous® or a local, lay support group formed by and for recovering anorexics, bulimics, bulimarexics and, sometimes, their families. These groups may be the most helpful when the disorder is mild, life is not threatened, or the client is also in some other type of therapy. Persons may be able to locate local groups by contacting national groups.

An eating disorder is a serious problem for many. One third of this population may remain seriously handicapped or die from their pain, self-hatred, and destructive behaviors. The other two thirds need consistent support to struggle toward recovery.

Friends of women with an eating disorder can help. Specific guidelines are outlined below. But ultimately the person with the disorder must help herself. Early treatment and consistent therapy hold the most hope for complete recovery.

SENSIBLE GUIDELINES FOR THE FRIENDS OF ANOREXICS

Be Honest

Be honest with your feelings. Are you trying to make her feel guilty because she makes you feel angry?

You are not (wholly or partly) to blame. Her disorder is the result of many years of patterns, events, and responses in her and in her family.

You do not possess the miracle cure.

Let her be honest about her true feelings, thoughts, and desires. They hurt her more than they can hurt you. But the more she is able to be totally honest about them, the closer she is to recovery.

Help her, within your limits. When you can't (or don't want to) be available, tell her.

Be Empathetic

Respect her as an individual. She is not helpless. She will not break.

Remain separate and strong—for both of you.

Listen and care. She may want nothing more from you than a caring ear and a warm hug. A caring touch can do wonders.

If you are afraid she will reject your concern, ask her what she wants. Be willing to risk rejection. Keep caring.

Be Consistent

She lives in a mentally confusing and inconsistent world. Her emotions swing and her desires are ignored in self-deprivation. She needs friends and family who are honest, empathetic, sensitive, *predictable*, and *stable*. If you give too much time one day or week or month and burn out the next, this is inconsistent. She will misunderstand. If you seem to understand one day but tease another, you may lose her and her trust.

(continued)

Be Sensitive

Don't try to make her eat. If she has good medical and psychiatric care, let
the professionals help her deal with the issue of weight. Trust the doctors
to do their job well.

Never tease her about her weight or eating. Jokes and laughter are important, but not teasing. She will take your teasing seriously.

Try to understand that she feels her low weight is a treasure. Suggestions
that she should gain back some fat may be dismissed as an archaic and
deep misunderstanding of her greatest concern.

Her final goal weight will probably be lower than you think is best for her. It
is her weight; let her work it out with her counselors. There is nothing
unhealthy about a weight that is even 10% below adult standards if it can
be maintained with healthy, bulimia-free eating habits.

(Adapted in part from "What Can I Do to Help" by Judith Weisman, Anorexia Nervosa Aid
Society, Lincoln, MA.)

FAILURE-TO-THRIVE

Nonorganic Failure-to-thrive (FTT) which occurs in infants and young children, *not* adolescents, is not commonly considered an "eating
disorder" but it shares with the other eating disorders a basis in some psychological upset. FTT
may also be stress-related: a very young child's
reaction to stress in his environment or the result of poor interaction with parents as a result
of parental stress or other social problems.

Technically, FTT is a symptom describing a
child whose weight is below the third percentile
or 80% of the median for age.[16] A child may fail
to thrive because of some undiagnosed disease
(in which case, the cause is *organic*) or because
of some other, *inorganic* factor. When a child
grows poorly, and no disease can be found,
"nonorganic FTT" is usually diagnosed.

This type of FTT is usually caused by a problem in the child's environment, some emotional
disorder in the relationships of the family.
Sometimes these problems are present from
birth. Sometimes an upset such as divorce,
death, or some other trauma causes sudden disorder. The child is affected physically and emotionally; growth slows. Because FTT may involve an entire family, treatment also must
involve the family.

When children stop growing, low weight for
age is usually the first sign of a problem. If they
continue underweight, malnutrition may affect
bone growth and the children soon become too
short for their age. This is called "short stature."
It may be a sign of chronic undernutrition. A
child who is also underweight for his length is at
high risk for serious malnutrition and needs immediate attention. If the problem is detected
early, recovery may be rapid and complete. Figure 37-3 charts the growth of an FTT child during and after diagnosis.

FTT is not isolated to poor or single-parent
families. It does not mean that parents pur-
posely have been abusing or neglecting their
children. It may mean they have been concentrating on other stresses and concerns and have
not given their children the emotional support
needed to grow and thrive; it does not mean they
are "bad" parents. In fact, parents need as much
encouragement and support in this disorder as
their children, since the parents often feel tremendous guilt.[16]

FTT does not result only in a small child,
although children may remain smaller than
peers even after treatment. What *is* affected
most seriously, in long term, is the learning
function. In some studies, half of the FTT children grew up to have below normal cognitive
function. Their biggest problem was developing
verbal skills: speaking and finding words to express themselves. They had trouble adjusting to

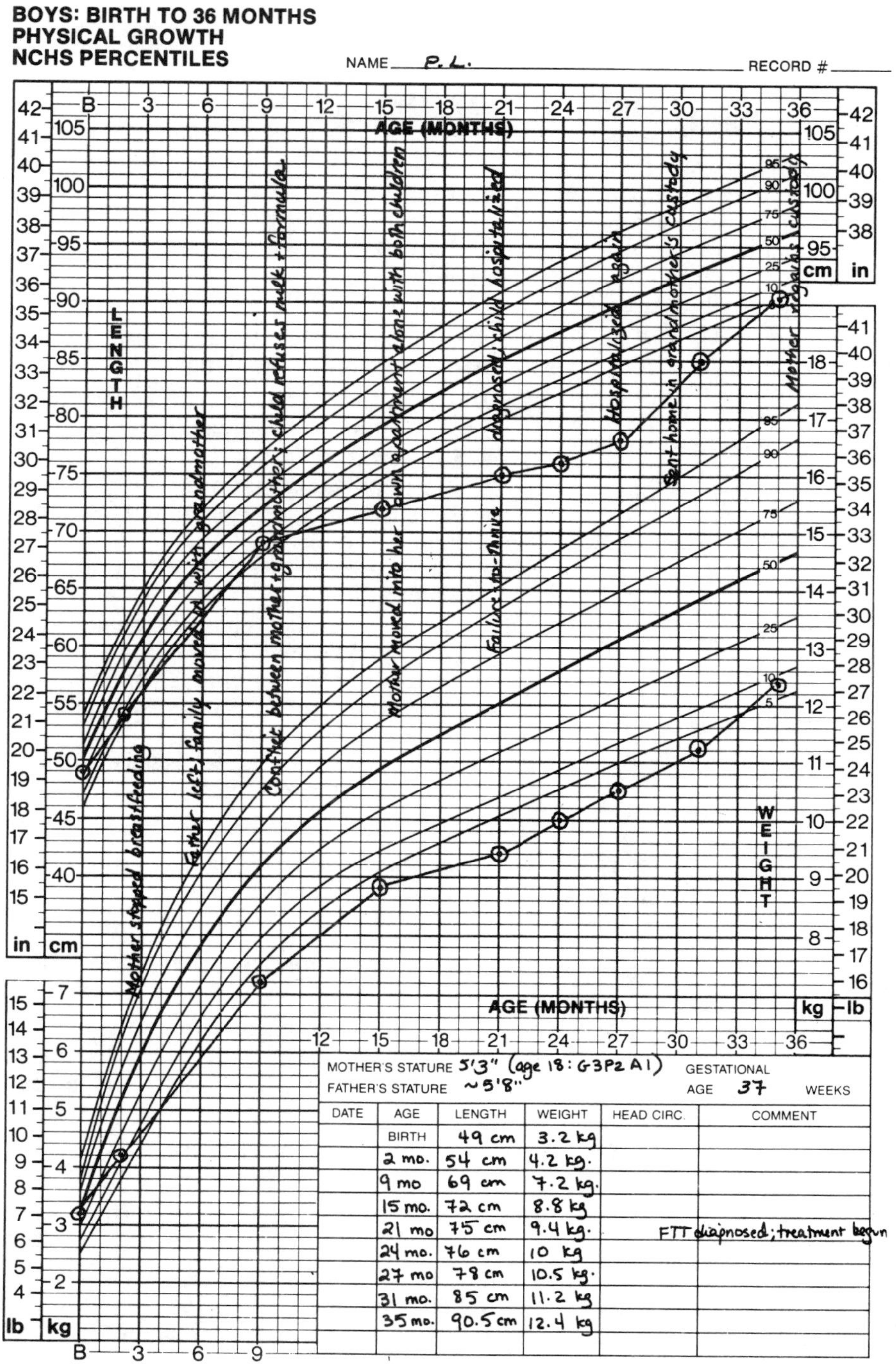

NAME **P. L.**   RECORD # _____

AGE (MONTHS) — B, 3, 6, 9, 12, 15, 18, 21, 24, 27, 30, 33, 36

LENGTH (cm): 105, 100, 95, 90, 85, 80, 75, 70, 65, 60, 55, 50, 45, 40
LENGTH (in): 42, 41, 40, 39, 38, 37, 36, 35, 34, 33, 32, 31, 30, 29, 28, 27, 26, 25, 24, 23, 22, 21, 20, 19, 18, 17, 16, 15

Percentile labels: 95, 90, 75, 50, 25, 10, 5

Handwritten annotations on chart:
- Mother stopped breastfeeding
- Father left; family moved in with grandmother
- Conflict between mother & grandmother; child refused milk + formula
- Mother moved into her own apartment alone with both children
- Failure-to-thrive
- diagnosed; child hospitalized
- Hospitalized again
- Sent home in grandmother's custody
- Mother
- FTT diagnosed; treatment begun

AGE (MONTHS) — 12, 15, 18, 21, 24, 27, 30, 33, 36

WEIGHT (kg): 16, 15, 14, 13, 12, 11, 10, 9, 8, 7, 6, 5, 4, 3, 2
WEIGHT (lb): 41, 40, 39, 38, 37, 36, 35, 34, 33, 32, 31, 30, 29, 28, 27, 26, 25, 24, 23, 22, 21, 20, 19, 18, 17, 16

MOTHER'S STATURE 5'3" (age 18: G3 P2 A1)
FATHER'S STATURE ~5'8"
GESTATIONAL AGE **37** WEEKS

DATE	AGE	LENGTH	WEIGHT	HEAD CIRC.	COMMENT
	BIRTH	49 cm	3.2 kg		
	2 mo.	54 cm	4.2 kg.		
	9 mo	69 cm	7.2 kg.		
	15 mo.	72 cm	8.8 kg		
	21 mo	75 cm	9.4 kg.		FTT diagnosed; treatment begun
	24 mo.	76 cm	10 kg		
	27 mo	78 cm	10.5 kg.		
	31 mo.	85 cm	11.2 kg		
	35 mo.	90.5 cm	12.4 kg		

Figure 37-3
Sample: Failure-To-Thrive. (Adapted from Hamill PVV, Drizd TA, Johnson CL, Reed RB et al: Physical growth: National Center for Health Statistics percentiles. Am J Clin Nutr 32:607–629, 1979.

elementary school, with many behavior problems.[16] It is important to remember, though, that the other half of the group did well. FTT children can be treated successfully when parents and the entire medical team are thoroughly involved from the time the problem is diagnosed.

Food and emotions are often closely related, especially in childhood. The FTT child may have lost interest in food. He may be listless, anorexic, and show signs of other nutrient deficiencies. The child needs to be refed, to begin to grow again, and to grow quickly enough to catch up to growth for age. The FTT child is usually kept in the hospital while this initial refeeding occurs. Parents are involved in feeding and treatment. Children may need up to 50% more calories than usual, plus more protein in order to catch up.[17] Parents who have had trouble feeding the child enough for normal growth will need very specific support to feed the child enough for catch-up growth. Guidelines must be practical, not discussing merely how to give *enough foods* but how to give *emotional support* as well. What is taught in the hospital must be tried at home and the results then tested back in the hospital or clinic. Parents need close follow-up after they take the child home and many hospitals have "FTT teams" who can help treat and coordinate this kind of support; nutritionists on the team meet with parents at follow-up visits to discuss weight and height gain and feeding times.

Growth is usually measured at every visit. It is very important that the measurements be correct. Page 83 illustrates the basic guidelines for obtaining accurate, consistently reliable measurements. If arm circumference and triceps skinfold thickness are measured, the same trained person should always measure the same children.

Nonorganic FTT is a serious stress-related disorder that affects the growth and mental development of a child. Nutritional therapy is part of treatment and is aggressive but tailored to the individual child's needs. The sooner the problem is caught and the more the parent is involved in hospital treatment and refeeding, the more likely it is that the child will go home to grow well, physically and emotionally.

STUDY QUESTIONS

1. Define:
   - Anorexia
   - Anorexia nervosa
   - Bulimia
   - Bulimarexia
   - Failure-to-Thrive

2. How many clients with eating disorders are male? How many are female?

3. Which of the following criteria may indicate a woman has anorexia nervosa:
   - She vomits after a large meal
   - She stops menstruating
   - She suddenly loses weight, but her appetite is normal
   - She exercises more than her athletic boyfriend
   - She is seeing a psychiatrist regularly
   - Her "goal weight" is 85 pounds
   - She insists that nothing is wrong
   - Her eating problems begin when she is 36
   - She appears thin but takes seriously any teasing that she is "fat"

4. Describe the typical feelings of an anorexic.

5. What are the potential dangers of anorexia nervosa? Of bulimia?

6. How might a dentist help a bulimic?

7. What are an anorexic's chances for complete recovery?

8. List and describe at least three types of therapy used for clients with eating disorders. What are the benefits of each? The limitations?

9. How can a nutritionist help a client with an eating disorder?

10. Do you know anyone with an eating disorder? How do you know the disorder exists? How can her friends help her?

11. What may cause FTT? How important is nutrition in treatment? Explain your answers.

12. Kim N. is a 3-year-old whose parents arrived in this country as refugees 2 months ago. They bring Kim to the hospital because she has severe diarrhea and vomiting.

She is treated but is obviously malnourished as well. In their home country, her parents were poor farmers; they have six older children and are now on welfare until they can learn enough English to find jobs.
- What are some problems that may be the causes for Kim's GI distress?
- For her malnutrition?
- How could you help Kim's parents?

REFERENCES

Autobiographies of Anorexics:

1. O'Neill CB: Starving for Attention. New York, Continuum Books, 1982
2. Barrile J: Confessions of a Closet Eater. Wheaton, IL, Tyndale House, 1983
3. MacLeod, S: The Art of Starvation: A Story of Anorexia and Survival. New York, Schocken Books, 1982

Original Anorexia Nervosa References:

4. Morton R: Phthisiologica, or a Treatise of Consumptions. Printed for Sam Smith and Benjamin Walford at the Prince's Arms in St. Paul's Churchyard, London, 1689
5. Laseque C: On Hysterical Anorexia. Medical Times Hospital Gazette 2:265, 1873
6. Gull WW: Anorexia Hysteria (Apepsia Hysteria.) Br Med J 2:527, 1873

Other References:

7. Block PJ: Working with anorexic and bulimic adolescents. Food and Nutrition News 56(5):33–34, November–December 1984
8. Bruch H: Anorexia nervosa. Nutrition Today, pp 14–18, September–October 1978
9. Bruch H: The Golden Cage: The Enigma of Anorexia Nervosa, p 112 New York, Vintage Books, 1978
10. Golden N. Sacker IM: An overview of the etiology, diagnosis and management of anorexia nervosa. Clin Pediatr 23(4):209–214, April 1984
11. Cohen MA: Eating disorders and the world of dance. Consuming Passions 3(1):3–5, January–February 1985
12. Mansfield J: Lecture Notes. Conference on Food: Use and Abuse. Boston, Children's Hospital Medical Center, September 21, 1983
13. Wynn DR, Martin MJ (Letter to the Editor): A physical sign of bulimia. Proc. Mayo Clinic 59:722, October 1984
14. Anorexia nervosa and related disorders: A personal and professional focus. Conference notes: In newsletter: Anorexia Nervosa Aid Society of Massachusetts 60:5, June–July 1984
15. Huse DM, Lucas AR: Dietary treatment of anorexia nervosa. J Am Diet Assoc 83(6):687–690, December 1983
16. Berwick DM: Nonorganic Failure-to-Thrive. Pediatrics in Review 1(9):265–270, March 1980
17. Peterson RE, Washington J, Rathbun JM: Team management of failure-to-thrive. J Am Diet Assoc 84(7):810–815, 1984

RESOURCES

For more information on the physical effects of starvation on fertility and prenatal growth and development, the following are suggested:

Keys A et al: The Biology of Human Starvation. Minneapolis, University of Minnesota Press, 1950

Smith CA: The effect of wartime starvation in Holland upon pregnancy and its product. Am J Obstet Gynecol 53(1947b):599–608

Stein Z et al: Famine and Human Development. The Dutch Hunger Winter, 1944–45. New York, Oxford University Press, 1975

Swyer GIM: Nutrition and human fertility. Br J Nutr 3(1949):100–107

Winick M (ed): Hunger Disease: Studies by Jewish Physicians in the Warsaw Ghetto. New York, John Wiley and Sons, 1979

Two national lay support groups are:

National Association of Anorexia Nervosa and Associated Disorders (ANAD)
P.O. Box 271
Highland Park, IL 60035

American Anorexia/Bulimia Association
Department P
133 Cedar Lane
Teaneck, NJ 07666

CHAPTER 38

Enteral and Parenteral Nutrition

OBJECTIVES

1. To define common terms used in enteral and parenteral nutrition, such as
   a. Enteral
   b. Parenteral
   c. Hyperalimentation
   d. TPN
   e. IVH
2. To describe briefly the use of tube feeding in history
3. To discuss and illustrate the following essentials of enteral and parenteral nutrition:
   a. Entry sites and feeding methods
   b. Types of formulas
   c. Frequency of feeds
   d. Common physical complications
   e. Common problems with patient acceptance
   f. Practical guidelines for initiating tube feeding
   g. Practical calculations to determine energy and protein needs
   h. Basic methods to evaluate enteral and parenteral nutrition in a patient
4. To discuss the alternative of home enteral nutrition, its advantages, and its risks

Whenever a hospitalized patient cannot or will not eat enough to meet basic nutrient needs, the medical team considers providing nutrition in some other way. They may decide to feed the patient through a tube or by a surgical opening into some part of the gut or into the veins. Feeding through the digestive tract (by mouth or tube, solid or liquid) is called *enteral nutrition.* Providing necessary nutrients directly into the blood is called *parenteral nutrition.* Enteral and parenteral nutrition are sometimes called *hyperalimentation,* although this term is technically incorrect because the medical team is not feeding the patient too much, as "hyper" implies. Another common term is *total parenteral nutrition* (TPN). A person is receiving TPN when all the nutrients he receives are taken through an intravenous needle or "line." TPN is sometimes called "intravenous hyperalimentation" or IVH. Both tube and intravenous feedings are chosen when, for some reason, the patient cannot receive the nutrients he needs in the normal way.

TPN of some type is used when enteral feeding is not possible due to some obstruction, disease, or the physician's desire that the client receive nothing by mouth (NPO) for more than five days.[1] Sometimes the gut cannot or should not be used. Most surgeons want it empty before surgery. Sometimes diseases such as active Crohn's ileitis have left the gut raw, with tissue easily damaged (friable) by irritation. Sometimes areas have been damaged and need time —and rest—to heal. Or the client may have developed severe diarrhea from malabsorption in the gut. Often these situations mean that a client must go days or weeks or more without eating. This kind of fasting could lead to serious malnutrition, slower wound healing, and poorer resistance to infection, making it necessary to prolong the hospital stay.[2]

Although enteral and parenteral nutrition have become safer and more widely used since the 1960s, the concept is not completely new. Centuries ago, tube feeding was given by rectum and contained mixtures such as eggs, milk, fresh ground pancreas, barley broth, and wine or brandy.[3] This was common in ancient Greece, Egypt and, into the twentieth century, in the Western World. Tubes from the nose into the stomach were probably introduced in the late sixteenth century and were made of lead or silver and animal bladders, rubber, or eel skin. Sometimes they seemed to work remarkably well, enabling a patient to survive and begin to feed himself once again.

However, intravenous feedings are more recent, developing in this century with modern medicine, syringes, and a more exact understanding of human nutrition and the types of liquids that can be administered safely directly into the blood.

SITE AND FEEDING METHODS

Figure 38-1 summarizes the different categories of enteral and parenteral feeding. The methods depend on the problem, on the limits of the client, and on his *willingness* and *ability* to receive and digest nutrients. There are three basic feeding methods, each with different feeding *sites,* or places where the food enters the body.

Tube Feeding

Tube feeding utilizes the gut, the digestive tract. Formulas that are fed through tubes contain nutrients in a liquid form. The nutrients may be in the same form as they exist in ordinary liquids or they may be broken down in some way to be more easily digested; types of enteral formulas will be discussed in further detail below.

Enteral or tube feeding is used when the digestive tract works well, but the client cannot or will not eat. This might happen:

a. When chewing or swallowing is impossible as a result of coma, a head, jaw, or face injury, mouth or throat cancer, numbness from disease or radiation therapy

b. When there is refusal to eat, as in anorexia nervosa

c. When the gut is damaged and will only tolerate certain basic forms of the nutrients

d. When the gut works well but nutrient needs are so high the client cannot possibly eat

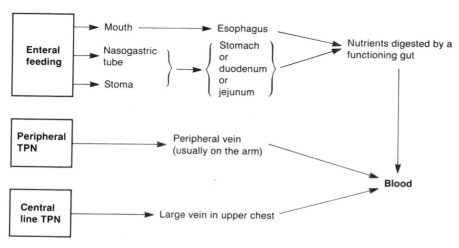

Figure 38-1
Basic routes of enteral and parenteral nutrition.

enough. This might happen in malnutrition, in burns, in high fever, in cancer, after surgery, or in some diseases.

The site of entry is the point at which the tube enters the body. Most tubes are first guided into the nose, down the throat, then into the stomach or beyond. But sometimes they enter the body through other, surgically created openings called *stomas*. This usually occurs when disease or surgery has made it impossible for food to travel the entire route, uninterrupted. A stoma may be created through the neck into the esophagus; this is called an "esophagostomy." Or it may be an opening directly into the stomach, a "gastrostomy." Or it may channel the tube through the abdomen directly into the jejunum; this is called a "jejunostomy."

Not all tubes that go through the nose are designed to stop in the stomach. The point in the digestive tract where they stop is the point where the enteral formula will enter the system. If part of the gut is missing or malfunctioning, the tube can bypass it to the area where digestion will be normal. Three routes from the nose are common:

1. The nasogastric tube (into the stomach)
2. The nasoduodenal tube (into the duodenum)
3. The nasojejunal tube (into the jejunum)

Tubes for tube feeding are made by several commercial companies. Ideally, nasogastric tubes should be as pliable and as thin as possible (slightly wider than a strand of spaghetti but not as wide as a strand of macaroni). Thin tubes are easier to swallow. A thick tube may cause irritation in the esophagus and even necrosis (cells dying from lack of proper blood supply) from constant irritation and pressure. A tube should never be any thicker than is absolutely necessary to allow the formula to flow easily.

Many *nasogastric* tubes (also called NG tubes) have a small weight made of mercury on the end of the tube. This weight helps draw the tube through the digestive tract to the desired site. Other tubes may be treated with substances to make them slippery when wet, and easier to swallow. Some include a stainless steel wire that can be threaded into the tube before it is swallowed to help guide it. Without some type of weight, tubes may simply curl up on themselves in some part of the gut and never reach their destination. Consequently, it is very important to "confirm" that the end of the tube is where it belongs in either the stomach, duodenum, or jejunum. This is usually done by x-ray film. A tube that is accidentally aspirated into the lungs can quickly lead to fever, confusion, septic shock and, at worst, death; at best it will cost the patient a setback of more days in the hospital. So proper placement is critical and is usually done by a trained team including the physician, and experienced nursing staff. The dietitian is rarely directly involved but may help recommend the type and size of tube that the patient may find least irritating.

When a feeding tube is being used, it is important to help the client keep nose, mouth, and teeth as clean as possible. Unless comatose, the client still needs sips of water to keep the mouth moist and to lubricate the area around the tube. In fact the tube-fed patient should receive as much as 2 quarts daily of free water. This promotes normal bowel and kidney function and helps prevent fluid and electrolyte imbalances that may develop.[4]

Tubes should be replaced every few days. They are not designed to stay in the gut for a long period of time and problems can develop if they do so.

Peripheral TPN

Peripheral TPN is TPN that enters the blood at some "peripheral" site, usually a blood vessel on the arm or hand. It leaves the individual free to eat whenever eating is possible. The needle enters the vein and is taped to the area for as long as it is needed. The TPN solution then "drips" into the blood at some steady rate. Peripheral TPN is often used to keep the client who will be going without food, short-term, from developing these problems by providing some needed energy and nutrients.

TPN alone is usually not sufficient. It rarely provides all the calories needed. So peripheral TPN is not usually used long-term. When it is used for an extended period, especially if eating is impossible, a fat solution is added. This helps ensure extra energy and prevents essential fatty acid deficiencies. TPN may be used together with enteral feeding. But when a client needs intravenous feeding on a very long-term basis, the choice is usually central line TPN.

Central Line TPN

A *central line* is an injected catheter-type tube that goes directly into a surgically opened vein under the collarbone. The central line is more permanent than the peripheral TPN line, and more solution at a time can be fed through it because the vein is larger. However, whenever a needle remains in the body, under the skin, there is always a risk of infection entering the blood and causing septicemia. If an infection develops, the "line" has to come out and the client's nutrition is stopped. Infection that enters the central line is extremely serious; every possible precaution must be taken to prevent it.

Figure 38-2 illustrates peripheral and central TPN.

The three feeding methods are not always mutually exclusive. Enteral and parenteral nutrition are often combined, usually when nutrient needs exceed what can reasonably be taken via the digestive tract. It may also be beneficial for the client on TPN to receive some nutrients through the gut on a regular basis, even if it is only by a tube. This continued feeding stimulates hormones and the digestive organs to continue functioning at optimum level and makes refeeding easier.[5]

FORMULAS

The formulas that enter the gut through an enteral route (mouth or a tube) are very different from the formulas used in parenteral nutrition. Formulas that enter the blood must help maintain the careful chemical, electrolyte, and osmolar balance of the blood. They are called TPN solutions and are available from the hospital pharmacy or from a formula company. Formulas that enter the gut, on the other hand, contain nutrients in the forms common in the gut. They may still need some digestion.

Enteral formulas vary widely. The right formula for a client depends on the gut function for digestive ability that exists. Enteral formulas usually fit into one of five basic categories,[6] depending on how completely they have been broken down into their basic parts. The more poorly the gut works, the more "elemental" the formula must be.

1. General formulas. These contain puréed foods, sometimes including meat, often diluted to flow through a tube. The nutrients are all "intact;" they have not previously been broken down by any process. A general formula is used when the digestive tract works well, but food must be fed in puréed liquid form for some mechanical reason. Individuals who can swallow may receive general formulas, but need not be tube-fed.

2. Milk-based formulas. These are vitamin- and mineral-fortified formulas that supply protein and calcium from a milk base. Carbohydrate and sometimes fat sources are often added to the formula. Most common infant formulas and "instant breakfast drinks" are examples of milk-based formulas.

3. Lactose-free formulas. Many persons who have a damaged digestive tract have lost the ability to digest lactose; they have become (or may be genetically) lactose intolerant. These persons need a lactose-free formula. The formula provides carbohydrate in some other form as well as protein, fat, and all the necessary vitamins and minerals.

4. Chemically defined formulas. These are fluids with a protein, carbohydrate, and fat source that is already digested into its molecular parts. The digestive tract must work at least partially and be capable of breaking down these formulas into their most basic, elemental components. These formulas may also be called "isotonic" and their ingredients will sound more like a chemistry list than a grocery list. Like the other three, these chemically defined formulas may be taken orally if a tube feeding is not necessary.

5. Elemental formulas. The elemental or completely defined formula is composed of carbohydrate, protein, and fat sources in their most basic, completely predigested forms.

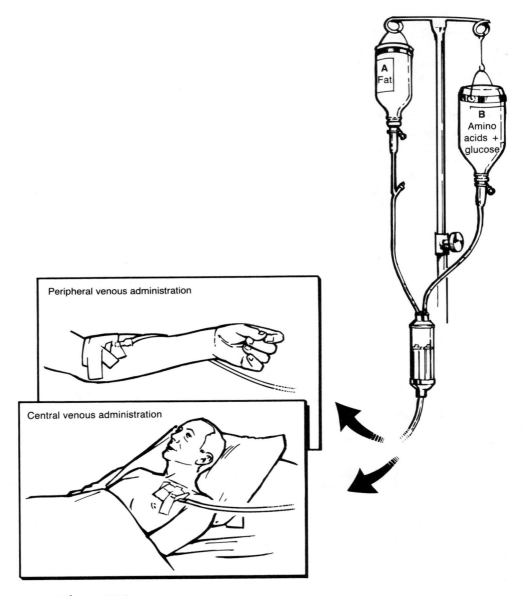

Labels within figure: A Fat; B Amino acids + glucose; Peripheral venous administration; Central venous administration

Figure 38-2
In peripheral and central TPN, fluids flow by gravity or pump directly into the blood. (Redrawn after Balanced Parenteral Nutrition, pp 44–45. Abbott Laboratories Hospital Products Division, 1982)

Even though they are fed into the gut, the digestive tract can simply absorb them; it need not digest them first. These formulas are usually nonallergenic. They may be given by mouth (although their taste is very objectionable), or by a feeding tube. They are expensive and may cause hyperosmolar diarrhea and discomfort when they are introduced too suddenly.

There are many different brand name products available for each of these five types of enteral formulas. Many are special in some other way, providing carbohydrate, protein, or fat in a particular form for certain disease states. Precisely which ones are used in the individual institution depends on the pharmacy and the department of dietetics, and these, in turn, may be influenced by the choices of the physicians.

Very few institutions prepare their own formulas for enteral tube feeding. Most prefer to use commercial brands. Not only is this more convenient but it is also more likely that (1) every preparation is identical, (2) bacterial contamination is prevented, and (3) vitamin and mineral deficiency is less likely to occur, since most formulas provide at least 100% of the Recommended Dietary Allowance and often more per liter.

FREQUENCY OF FEEDS

A tube feeding team must also consider the frequency and timing of feeding. There are three basic methods: bolus, intermittent, and continuous administration.

1. *Bolus* feeds are feeds that provide a large amount of food at one time, followed by an interval of several hours before feeding begins again. "Three meals a day" is a type of bolus feeding schedule since a large "bolus" of food is consumed in a short time.

   Bolus feeding combines regular meals and some tube feeding. The digestive tract must function very well to handle a bolus of food. In general, bolus feeding is not recommended for tube feeding because it usually leads to great discomfort and diarrhea. Intravenous feedings are never given by bolus.

2. Intermittent feeds occur more frequently than bolus feeds, with a smaller volume given at each feed. A person on an intermittent tube feeding schedule may, for example, receive a prescribed amount of formula that is released into the digestive tract every hour for 15 or 20 minutes.

3. Continuous feeds are usually given by some machine or chemical device. In TPN this may be an intravenous "drip," a process in which the fluid is dripped slowly, constantly, from a bottle(s) hanging on an IV pole, to descend by gravity into the bloodstream. Continuous feeds in enteral nutrition are regulated by a "pump." The pump is attached to the tube and releases a certain constant quantity of formula into the tube.

Combinations of these three methods exist. For example, some persons may receive continuous feeding through the night as they sleep, but they may also be able to disconnect themselves from the machine every morning to go to work. Some people who will never have enough functioning gut due, for example, to Crohn's ileitis, can survive this way and never need to eat. This is usually done at home and is called "home enteral feeding," discussed in greater detail below. Others may receive a continuous IV drip but may also be encouraged to eat at meal or snack time.

PROBLEMS

There are two general types of problems that can interfere with adequate nutrition in enteral and parenteral feeding: (1) physical complications and (2) problems that result from poor acceptance of the feeding method. Table 38-1 lists some of these common problems.

Physical Problems

Infection is the most immediately serious problem. Placing and caring for a tube or an IV line should always be done with sterile techniques to prevent all contamination. If a client on TPN develops fever or any infection, the line is removed and checked for contamination and measures are taken to prevent sepsis (contamination in the blood). When this happens, the

Table 38-1

___

Some Common Complications of Enteral and Parenteral Nutrition

Problem	Comment
I. Mechanical Problems	
Infection	Can lead to sepsis in TPN; TPN usually stopped
	Can lead to diarrhea in tube feeding; tube may be removed or replaced and formula may be changed
Aspiration	Caused by tube in wrong place or gastroesophageal reflux up into trachea from overfull stomach or stasis
Stasis	Formula unable to flow because normal peristalsis has slowed or stopped; excess "residual" formula left in stomach; residual should be checked before each feeding
GI erosion	From constant wearing and pressure on walls of digestive tract caused by a feeding tube that is too wide
Blocked tube	From solid obstruction in tube; often caused by medications that are crushed and then given through the tube; tube must be replaced. Medication given by tube feeding should always be in liquid form
Diarrhea	May be caused by infection, medication, impacted stool, and/or hyperosmolar formula
Nausea	Tube feeding given too fast
Cramps	Tube feeding formula too cold
Undernutrition	Formula overdiluted; given too slowly; not given for some reason
II. Problems with Client Acceptance	
Pulling out tube	Especially if hostile or disoriented; client must understand and consent to tube; family may be able to help monitor if client is disoriented
Pulling up part of tube	Can lead to lost nutrients, aspiration, tissue damage; placement must be checked before each feeding
Refusal to eat	If client able to eat, removal of tube may be contingent on calorie intake by mouth
Depression	Cause needs to be discovered and discussed
Inadequate water	Water necessary to keep tube lubricated and comfortable (as possible) in digestive tract and to keep mouth and teeth clean; encourage water
Inadequate sleep	May be a problem if tube feedings given at night; work with client and team to minimize nighttime disturbance; sleep is important for recovery

client does not receive essential nutrients at a time when these nutrients are especially important. Bacteria can enter the system through an IV line (which would cause sepsis) or by growing on the inside of a feeding tube that has not been changed often enough or that has been handled improperly. Not all infection is caused by the feeding tube or line but these sites must be checked.

Aspiration may occur when the tube or tube feeding flows into the lungs. This can happen if a tube is placed incorrectly and can lead quickly to such serious complications as pneumonia. Aspiration may also occur if the stomach does not empty quickly enough; "gastroesophageal reflux" can force the excess liquid up, out of the stomach and into the trachea, especially in a person who has poor control of swallowing.

Stasis occurs when peristalsis slows down. *Stasis* means lack of movement. Food in the digestive tract stops moving or slows down. When this happens, the stomach cannot empty quickly enough and may leave a large "residual" of formula in the stomach between feedings. This "residual" should always be checked before the next formula feeding is given.

GI erosion has already been mentioned. A tube that is too large to be comfortable in the throat and esophagus can seriously irritate the tissue walls.

Blockage may occur when particles (which should not be there) stop the flow of liquid through the tube. This sometimes happens when medication is crushed and given through the tube. In general, the tube is NOT to be used for medication; the physician must decide what other route is most appropriate. Some medications, even if they are in liquid form, congeal into a gel in the tube and cause blocks as effective as though they were solids.

Diarrhea is a common problem for clients on tube feeding and is often blamed on the tube feed itself. Diarrhea may occur as the result of a tube feeding with a high osmolarity; the medical team can usually adjust the feeding to a more dilute or less osmolar solution. But diarrhea is not always caused by the formula. It may also result from an infection, from medication, or from liquid forcing itself around stool that is impacted in the bowel.

Nausea may result from feeding a client too much too quickly. Or it may be a side effect of a new medication.

Cramps sometimes occur when the tube feeding is too cold.

Inadequate nutrition is the resulting problem that can easily develop with any of these complications. Whenever tube feeding or TPN must be stopped or slowed for any reason, the client misses essential nutrients. Clients' needs during enteral and parenteral nutrition are carefully calculated by the dietitian, but many events can interfere with these feedings. To ensure sufficient energy and nutrients to meet basic needs, the client must receive all of the recommended formulas at the recommended strength (dilution) and rate. When any of the above complications prevent this from happening, they put nutrition at risk.

Acceptance

Other problems that may cause a person to receive less than the optimum nutrition from enteral or parenteral feeds stem from the problems of client acceptance. Many persons object to swallowing a tube, no matter how thin and flexible it may be. Many object to being attached to a needle and an IV "pole" with its hanging bottles of liquids.

To help a client accept this method of feeding, he should understand, as completely as possible, why such feeding is necessary and how long it may be used. The family should also understand these reasons, before the tube or needle is inserted. If the client is disoriented, the family may be able to help the medical team keep the feeding tube or needle in place. A client who is hostile to the feeding method may

Pull out the tube or needle, making replacement necessary, interrupting nutrition, and creating the potential for tissue damage and infection

Pull up only part of the feeding tube. This is less detectable, and is why placement should be checked with every feeding

Refuse to eat, even if he is able to do so. It may help to encourage the client by pointing out that the better he adapts to their nourishment, the sooner the tube or line can be removed

Become depressed for any number of reasons, depending on the need for this particular feeding method

Refuse to take necessary water

Refuse to brush teeth and keep mouth clean

In addition most patients (whether they accept the feeding tube or not) may have trouble sleeping if the feeding schedule interferes with normal sleeping habits

The medical team must work closely with the

client and family to avoid as many of these problems as possible.

CALCULATING NEEDS FOR ENTERAL AND PARENTERAL NUTRITION

As mentioned earlier, most tube feedings and TPN formulas are commercially prepared, available from the dietary department, or the pharmacy of an institution. There are many options available, depending on the needs of the client. Before tube or IV feeding begins, the dietitian helps to determine what the client needs and therefore what amounts of what formulas are most appropriate. This determination includes calculations of the client's energy and protein needs, and development of concrete ways to meet these needs within any existing fluid restriction.

Energy is usually calculated by the Harris–Benedict equation with factors added to allow

A. ENERGY

Total energy requirement = REE × Activity Factor × Stress Factor

1. REE (Resting Energy Expenditure) =

Men:	66.42 + 13.75 (W) + 5 (H) − 6.78 (A)	W = weight (kg)
		H = height (cm)
Women:	655.1 + 9.65 (W) + 1.85 (H) − 4.68 (A)	A = age (years)

×

2. Activity Factor

Out of bed — 1.3
Confined to bed — 1.2

×

3. Stress Factor

Mild starvation:	0.85 – 1.0
Postoperative:	1.0 – 1.5
Cancer:	1.1 – 1.45
Fractured bone:	1.15 – 1.3
Severe trauma/infection:	1.3 – 1.55
Severe burns:	2.0

B. PROTEIN

1. RDA = − 0.8 g protein per kilogram per day (g/kg/d)

2. 6.25 g of protein = 1 g of nitrogen

3. Energy: Nitrogen ratio for normal or undernourished individual: 300 : 1.
   For hypermetabolic individual: 120 : 1 – 180 : 1

Figure 38-3
Calculating energy and protein needs for enteral and parenteral nutrition. (From MacBurney M, Wilmore DW: Rational decision-making in nutritional care. Surg Clin North Am 61(3):571–581, June 1981. Elwyn DH, Kinney JM, Askanazi J: Energy expenditure in surgical patients. Surg Clin North Am 61(3):545–555, June 1981. Enteral Nutrition Handbook for the Pharmacist, Ross Laboratories, 1982)

for *activity* (usually very little) and *injury* or *illness.*

Daily protein needs are normally 0.8 grams of protein per kilogram of body weight. Injury or illness may increase this need for protein in a different proportion than energy needs. The ratio of needed calories to nitrogen changes with illness. The normal, healthy person needs about 300 kcals for every 1 gram of nitrogen (1 g N = 6.25 g protein). Figure 38-3 outlines these basic energy and protein ratios commonly used in calculating needs for enteral and parenteral feeding.

EVALUATION

Calculation and treatment are not enough. The only way to measure success is to evaluate progress. This is especially important when an artificial method of feeding is being used: if an evaluation is ignored, problems may develop. The easiest way the team can tell if a client is getting enough energy is to check weight. This should be done every day.[7] Often this is compared with a daily record of exactly how much formula or TPN solution was administered. Daily weight will also indicate if the client is retaining excess water.

There are several ways to evaluate the adequacy of the protein. These, too, involve all the members of the medical team in some way and may include any of the following:

1. Anthropometrics, especially triceps skinfold thickness and midarm muscle circumference (TSF and MAMC). These were briefly described in Chapter 12 and are rarely done routinely. When they are done, they must be done by a trained nutrition support team and preferably all measures should be done by the same person. They help measure how much reserve fat and muscle is available.

2. Laboratory tests. Blood tests measuring total albumin, creatinine, total lymphocytes, and serum transferrin all indirectly measure protein status (although albumin levels may naturally drop after several days in bed due to changes in fluid balance with the changed posture and activity).[8]

3. Urine collection to measure 24-hour creati-

nine, which can then be compared to height to assess total body protein status. (This is called a creatinine height index.)

4. Nitrogen balance studies, measuring nitrogen lost with dietary nitrogen consumed.

Of these four, the laboratory tests are the easiest, fastest, and most common evaluation measures. Each institution may use slightly different standards for normal values and may also use one or more of the other methods. Whatever the standard, regular evaluation of some kind is essential. This evaluation requires accurate daily records of weight and at least one accurate measure of height, as well as detailed records of how much formula or IV solution — at what strength — the client actually received each day. This kind of attention to the client on enteral or parenteral feedings goes a long way toward helping prevent hospital malnutrition from developing, and may save both the client and institution a great deal of trouble, time, and money.

TUBE FEEDING AT HOME

Some persons have diseases or problems that are under control except that the individual cannot eat. This might mean death or a lifetime in the hospital if home tube feeding were not an option.

"Home enteral nutrition" is now financially and practically possible for many people. If tube feeding is the ONLY feeding option, many health insurance companies will now cover the cost of formula for treatment of many different diseases.[9] Some of these include Crohn's ileitis, fistulas, pancreatitis, short gut syndrome, colon or head and neck cancer, and neurologic diseases that impair the ability to swallow. The client who is well enough may work during the day and begin tube feeding when he gets home. Some clients find continuous tube feeding during the night most convenient. All home enteral feeding programs include the continued support of professional medical care, so there is always someone a client can call for help or advice.

Many national companies now offer home enteral feeding support of varying quality. In some communities, local pharmacies may have developed similar services[9] that usually include any of the following: trained nurses to teach the client self care and to regularly visit and monitor the feeding; the resources of a pharmacist; reliable delivery systems; maintenance of the formula feeding pumps (if pumps are used); regular laboratory evaluations of the client; a consultant dietitian, and a clear policy on third party reimbursement procedures. These companies provide supportive services but should never replace the client's primary physician or medical care.

Planning home enteral feeding begins in the hospital before the client goes home. It requires careful teaching and supervision for at least three to five days before discharge and should involve the whole family. The family needs to know who to call when questions or problems develop. If a feeding pump (a small machine that mechanically releases a controlled amount of formula for intermittent or continuous drip feeds) is used, its operation should be familiar to everyone involved in feeding before the client goes home.

Infections and GI problems can develop quickly in a less sterile, less closely supervised home environment. Families need to be aware of this and to call the physician as soon as any problems (such as a fever) begin to develop.

Home tube feeding allows for much freedom in the life of someone who is well enough to go home but not well enough to eat. Many of these clients can live an otherwise normal life. Home tube feeding is a welcome option, saving discomfort and unnecessary hospital costs for many with serious, chronic bowel problems.

STUDY QUESTIONS

1. Define the following terms:
  * Total parenteral nutrition
  * Hyperalimentation
  * Enteral nutrition
  * Fistula
  * Hyperosmolar diarrhea
  * IVH

2. List at least three circumstances when a hospitalized individual may need
  * Enteral nutrition
  * Parenteral nutrition

3. A feeding tube may empty into one of what four areas along the digestive tract?

4. What are the five basic categories of enteral formulas? Explain each group. Which, if any, can be taken by mouth? By NG tube?

5. List at least five problems common in enteral and parenteral nutrition. What is the ultimate problem that may result from any of these complications? Why is it a serious problem?

6. True or false: Explain your answer.
  * Tubes used for NG feedings should be as thick as possible to allow as much formula per feeding as possible.
  * Medications should not be crushed and given by tube.
  * Many tubes are weighted with lead to help keep them in the digestive tract.
  * Diarrhea is usually caused by a high-formula osmolarity.
  * In general, the more elemental a formula, the higher its osmolarity.

7. Rosemary G. is a 32-year-old mother of three who is in the hospital following minor surgery. She is confined to bed but otherwise well. She is 160 cm tall and weighs 54 kg.
  * How many calories does she need?
  * How much protein does she need?

REFERENCES

1. Mailler JO: Calculated parenteral feedings: A programmed instruction. J Am Diet Assoc 84(11): 1312–1323, November 1984
2. Bistrian BR, Blackburn CL, Vitale J: Prevalence of malnutrition in general medical patients. JAMA 235: 1567–1570, 1976
3. Randall HT: Enteral nutrition: Tube feeding in acute and chronic illness. J Parenter Enter Nutr 8(2): 113–136, March–April 1984
4. MacBurney M, Wilmore DW: Rational decision-making in nutritional care. Surg Clin North Am 61(3): 571–581, June 1981
5. Enteral Nutrition Handbook for the Pharmacist (1982). Columbus, Ohio, Ross Laboratories
6. Steffee WP, Krey SH: Enteral hyperalimentation

for patients with head and neck cancer. Otolaryngol Clin North Am 13:437–448, 1980

7. Blackburn GL, et al: Nutrition and metabolic assessment of the hospitalized patient. J Parenter Enter Nutr 1(1): 11–22, 1977

8. Courtney ME, et al: Rapidly declining serum albumin values in newly hospitalized patients: Prevalence, severity and contributory factors. J Parenter Enter Nutr 6(2): 143–145, March–April 1982

9. Adams MM, Wirsching RG: Guidelines for planning home enteral feedings. J Am Diet Assoc 84(1): 68–71, 1984

CHAPTER 39

Surgery, Stress, and Trauma

OBJECTIVES

1. To define common terms such as trauma, sepsis, stress, and shock
2. To illustrate and discuss the altered metabolism and special energy and protein needs of
   a. Mild starvation
   b. Elective surgery
   c. Infection
   d. Major injury
   e. Severe sepsis
   f. Burns
3. To discuss the goal and rationale of intervention to prevent complications
4. To list and describe briefly measures of preventive intervention
   a. Immediate and ongoing medical attention
   b. Restore and maintain fluid/electrolyte balance
   c. Provide energy, protein, and other nutrients to conserve body tissue
   d. Provide insulin, if necessary
5. To discuss 4(c) above, outlining ways these needs are met
6. To outline diets commonly recommended prior to surgery

Several conditions place the body in a state that changes basic nutrient needs in a major way.

Most of these conditions involve hospitalization. These conditions add some type of *stress* or *trauma* to the body; they include starvation, surgery, infection, sepsis, major injury, burns, and shock.

A trauma is a physical injury or wound. It may be intentional, as is surgery, or accidental, as are burns, fractures, and any other type of accident. All trauma causes physical *stress* to the body; the organism must work harder than usual to compensate for the damage. The degree of stress depends on the degree of trauma and how well a person is prepared to meet the increased needs. A person who was well-nourished and healthy before the trauma may be able to recover quickly, with minimal damage. A person who has already been weakened by other stressors, such as disease, infection, or starvation, may take longer to recover and need much more medical and nutritional support.

NUTRIENT NEEDS IN TRAUMA AND STRESS

All the physical stressors listed above may change the body's need for energy and protein. This is clearly illustrated in Figure 39-1. The body must continue to meet its basal metabolic needs in order to maintain basic functions, but it may also need to work at a hypermetabolic rate to meet the demands placed on it by the stressor. These high metabolic needs may continue for days or weeks. Below is a brief description of the unique needs in each of the common stress and trauma states.

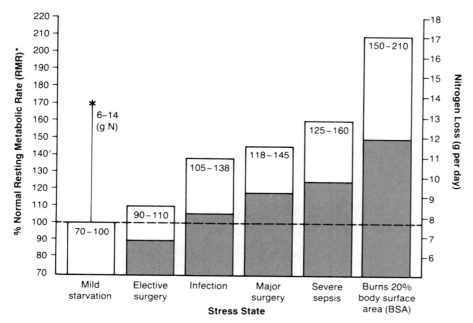

Figure 39-1

Increased energy and protein needs in trauma, stress, and surgery. (Adapted from Blackburn GL: Adaptation to starvation. Intake: Perspectives in Clinical Nutrition 5, Norwich, NY, Eaton Laboratories, May 1973. MacBurney M, Wilmore DW: Rational decision-making in nutritional care. Surg Clin North Am 61(3):571–581, June 1981. Gastineau CF (exec ed): Nutrition care of the critically ill patient; selection of appropriate feeding modalities. Dialogues in Nutrition 3(2), Health Learning Systems, 1979. Elwyn DH, Kinney JM, Askanazi J: Energy expenditures in surgical patients. Surg Clin North Am 61(3):545–555, June 1981; Medical Directions: Contemporary Parenteral Nutrition: Protein Sparing. North Chicago, IL, Abbott Laboratories, 1981)

---

* This data is based on *resting,* not *basal,* metabolic rate. The RMR may be about 5% to 10% higher than BMR, since it is based on slightly more activity.

Starvation

As Figure 39-1 indicates, mild starvation (not complicated by any other stress) actually *lowers* the body's demands for energy. BMR drops, probably in an effort to compensate for the lack of necessary food. This is a natural mechanism that has probably helped man survive throughout his existence when food was scarce.

When fasting begins, the body depends on the glycogen stored in the liver. This is only a

200 to 300 gram supply: 800 to 1200 Kcals,[1] not even a full day's supply of energy. It may take longer to exhaust this supply, however, since fat and muscle stores may be used as well, even before glycogen is totally exhausted. When glycogen is gone, the body switches over to a total dependency on fat and muscle tissue for energy, producing high levels of ketones and using up large supplies of protein.

This high nitrogen, low energy loss is what

makes starvation different from other types of stress. Even though metabolism is low, between 6 grams and 14 grams of nitrogen may be excreted daily,[1] as much as a person might lose in severe infection. This high loss can be slowed, however, by feedings of carbohydrate and/or protein even if these foods are not meeting energy needs. This is the philosophy behind "protein-sparing modified fasts:" the severely overweight person fasts under close medical supervision, but is supplied daily with a certain amount of protein to prevent serious loss of muscle mass.

Sometimes mild starvation occurs in the hospital or prior to admission, while a patient is also undergoing some other stress. This is much more serious; weight loss and protein loss may be much more severe than in simple starvation. The body is being starved at a time when nutrient and protein needs are especially high. Often hospitals permit a patient to go several days without adequate nutrition, and some wait ten days before they begin special nutritional support. Someone who enters the hospital already malnourished or whose needs are so high they probably will not be met by normal meals should receive aggressive nutritional support much sooner; that ten-day period may already be used up.[2] Otherwise, the person may be so weakened by starvation that he may develop complications, take much longer to recover, and have to stay in the hospital longer than usual.

Surgery

Surgical patients are examples of persons with increased needs who may inadvertently be starved. (As Figure 39-1 illustrates, resting metabolism may increase 15%). Often a surgical patient must be "NPO" 8 hours to 24 hours before surgery. In the process of anesthesia for surgery, the peristalsis of the gut slows down. All muscle movement, including the swallowing mechanisms, are anesthetized. It is not safe for a patient to try to eat a normal meal immediately after surgery because the digestive tract needs time to begin functioning normally again. Ordinarily this means that the diet provided is inadequate to meet the patient's elevated needs. Depending on the surgery, recovery may be slow

and some studies have indicated that up to 50% of all surgical patients have some degree of protein-calorie malnutrition.[3,4] Malnutrition may result from increased needs, difficulty getting, digesting, or absorbing nutrients, starvation, or the complications that can result from surgery. The most common—and potentially most dangerous—complication is infection.

Infection and Sepsis

Sepsis is infection that has spread throughout the body; it is always caused by bacteria. Infection can affect a small area, such as the area directly opened by the surgery, or it can become severe. If the bacteria that causes the infection spreads to other areas or enters the blood (septicemia), it may become very difficult to control, cause great damage, and lead to many more days in the hospital before the patient will have recovered fully. Fever is usually a sign that infection is present somewhere. Minor infection may raise the resting metabolism 15%–40%, but severe sepsis may cause basic needs to rise 40%–70% and almost double nitrogen losses. Since the body's immune system is composed of proteins that will work well only as long as they do not need to be used for energy, nutrition is a vital partner to medical (usually antibiotic) treatment used in fighting sepsis.

Sepsis is a serious complication and almost always lengthens the patient's hospital stay. A longer stay means more costs and more risks. Sepsis may lead to shock, discussed below. It may lead to pulmonary edema, or excess water in the lungs. When the lungs hold excess fluid, a person may continue to depend on a respirator to breathe. Fluids are a stress when kidney function may be poor. Sepsis may also cause liver or other organ dysfunction. Forty percent of all intensive care unit (ICU) deaths may be caused by sepsis.[5] The body may be more susceptible to sepsis after an injury, making precautions especially important. The environment and food must be kept as completely germ-free as possible.

Major Injury

Most trauma is caused by major injury or accidents and may increase energy needs 20%–

45%. Trauma is a leading cause of death for ages 1 year to 38 years in the USA and comprises one third of all hospitalizations.[6] There are three stages to trauma:

1. The acute stage is the first 24 hours, when the body may go into shock and stress needs are high. Usually trauma patients are not able to eat during this period because other life support systems are more important to assure immediate survival.

2. The intermediate or adaptive phase, when the body adapts to the new state, nutrition support is introduced, and the long process begins of preventing complications and promoting healing. The body continues to be hypermetabolic during this period, with high energy and protein needs.

3. The chronic stage, when the patient may go home or to rehabilitation to recover and regain skills and/or strength that was lost. In this phase metabolism has returned to normal but recovery is not complete.[6,7]

There are many potential complications of injury. Natural immunities drop at first so infection is more likely. The lungs may fail. An intestinal block (which is called an *ileus*) or *fistulas* (abnormal openings between areas) may develop. And shock may prevent organs from functioning, causing great damage.

Burns

The greatest traumas and injuries of all are the major burns. A burn physically tears apart tissue, cell by cell, burning through the three major skin layers that protect the body.

Burns are classified according to *degree* and *extent* (or percentage). A first-degree burn affects only the surface skin layer, the epidermis. Second-degree burns pierce through to damage the corium, the second layer. Third-degree burns destroy all skin layers and require grafting.[8] The extent of the burn is a measure of the percentage of the total body surface area that is affected.

Burns cause tremendous losses. The greatest loss is fluids, and fluid replacement is usually the first, most immediate treatment. Fluid losses can quickly lead to electrolyte imbalances,

shock, and death. Treatment, therefore, usually begins with fluids, often the fluid called *Ringer's Lactate Solution* (or "lactated ringer's solution"), a mixture of sterile water and electrolytes but without any nutrients providing energy. As soon as the immediate crisis is over, nutrition support is started.

As Figure 39-1 illustrates, the trauma of burns may more than double energy needs. It is not unusual for a severely burned patient to need 5000 calories per day. The needs depend on the extent of the burn and may be estimated by *Curreri's equation:*

$$\text{Kcals needed} = (25 \times \text{weight[kg]}) + (40 \times \% \text{ total body surface [TBS] burned})$$

This equation was developed by Curreri and is commonly used when working with burn patients.[7,8,9] Protein needs may double or even quadruple.[8] Eating is usually difficult or impossible so TPN, tube feedings, or both are started. Sometimes energy and protein needs are so high that all three methods may be used simultaneously (see Figure 39-2). Of the other nutrients required, zinc is the most important because it helps encourage wound healing. Nutrition is so critical in burn treatments because the needs are so high. "Survival depends on the effectiveness of the nutritional program."[7] Refeeding is usually aggressive and is discussed in more detail under "Intervention," below.

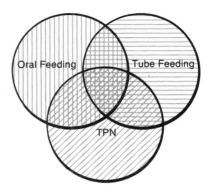

Figure 39-2
Feeding method combinations. Different methods of feeding may be used in combinations to meet very high nutrient needs.

Recovery takes a long time; over 10% weight loss may prolong the recovery period and increase the risks for complications. Large sections of raw, open, grafted tissue make infection a serious risk. The burn may cause damage to the organs and lead to internal bleeding (hemorrhage). Bones may break. The three stages of recovery from general trauma are also applicable in burn treatment.

1. Treatment for the immediate, life-threatening injury
2. Continued hypermetabolism as therapy begins and skin is grafted (BMR continues very high)
3. Long recovery and repletion of lost nutrients, beginning when BMR finally returns to normal.

Shock

Like infection, *shock* is a natural, physical and life-threatening response to severe trauma. Its position in the process and treatment of trauma is illustrated in Figure 39-3. Shock is most commonly caused by prolonged bleeding, although it may develop quickly even after trauma where bleeding is not obvious. The body that goes into shock *suddenly slows down.* Nutrients, oxygen, and fluids stop flowing through the cells at their normal rate. The digestive tract slows. Blood pressure drops rapidly; other muscle action slows and changes. The body becomes warm with fever and chills; it is dry, and the heart beats irregularly and rapidly. Heat is being lost quickly.

The oxygen deficit and hypothermia that result from shock may quickly lead to death unless they are treated immediately. Anyone who has a major accident, burn or other trauma may quickly go into shock. The person must be kept warm and must receive immediate medical care.

Shock affects the way in which the body uses nutrients. Electrolyte imbalances develop quickly. Protein and fat are rapidly broken down as the body turns on itself for energy, unable to obtain oxygen to break down other sources.

Since the 1940s, parenteral glucose has been one of the critical aspects of treatment for shock.[10] Glucose can be used as food by all the cells, so muscle and fat stores are protected and conserved. Other essentials in the parenteral nutrition used for shock include insulin and replacement of lost electrolytes, amino acids, vitamins, and minerals.

PREVENTIVE INTERVENTION

Figure 39-3 illustrates one model of trauma, its major causes, complications, and the interventions used in treatment.

Trauma cannot always be prevented. Once it occurs, however, treatment is important to aid in healing and recovery, and to prevent further complications from developing.

Shock and sepsis are the most common, preventable complications. Intervention is designed to prevent these conditions and to stop them from leading to organ failure and death when they do develop.

As mentioned, there are four key parts to intervention: (1) immediate medical attention; (2) restoration of electrolyte and fluid balance; (3) administration of insulin, if necessary, and (4) providing necessary energy, protein, vitamins, and minerals to protect body tissue and allow for healing.

Immediate Medical Attention

Nutrition may help *prevent* disease and infection, but once these disorders occur, food is not enough. Immediate and consistent medical care is essential to help restore the body to health. Such care may involve medicines, surgery, correcting fluid/electrolyte imbalances, and supplying insulin or other essential substances.

Restoration of Electrolyte and Fluid Balance

Any stress or trauma that causes blood or water loss may upset the body's careful fluid and electrolyte balance. Imbalances can rapidly lead to coma and death (see Chapter 28). Balance is usually restored by blood transfusions and intravenous and oral fluids and electrolyte solutions.

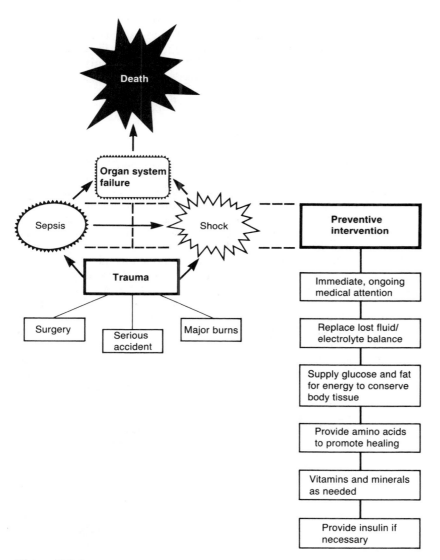

Figure 39-3
Model of trauma and preventive interventions.

Administration of Insulin, if Necessary

The traumatized system needs glucose for energy. Glucose has to be carried into the cells by insulin. Sometimes hyperglycemia in stress and trauma is a sign that natural insulin production (or sensitivity) may be low or inadequate and more insulin is necessary.

Provision for Needed Nutrients

When nutrients are not available, the body uses its own supplies for energy. Needs may be so high that body tissue is wasted rapidly. Fat and protein are lost. The body may use up high levels of protein, leading to low levels of serum albumin, red blood cells, and a lowered immunity to infection.

Calories are needed to prevent the body from using necessary protein for energy and to prevent weight loss. The trauma patient needs a baseline of about 25 Kcals per kg per day[6-8] plus a certain added "stress factor" (which was discussed in Chapter 38 and which can be determined by the dietitian) to meet the additional energy needs of the particular stress. Both energy and protein may be provided by (1) regular meals and snacks, (2) tube feedings, (3) TPN (discussed in Chapter 38) or a combination of the three, illustrated in Figure 39-2. Because needs are highest in burns, nutrition in burn therapy is especially aggressive and will involve as many feeding routes as can be used. Often tube feedings are essential because TPN — even with added lipid emulsions — is usually not sufficient and oral feeding is sometimes difficult or impossible.

When eating is possible for a burn patient, food must be available at all times. Patients may have refrigerators and be able to request almost any foods they want. Often all fluids must contain calories. As much energy and protein as possible (short of causing hyperosmotic diarrhea) may be concentrated into every food and fluid. Everyone who cares for the patient — nursing, dietary staff, and family — as well as the patient himself is involved in the feeding process. Daily records, especially I and O (intake and output) records and weight records, *must* be kept to evaluate progress.

It is possible to overfeed trauma patients. Overfeeding can cause still more trauma and complications. Carbohydrate breaks down into carbon dioxide that is released by the lungs. Excess carbohydrate may produce excess CO_2 and make breathing and recovery even more difficult for someone who is already having problems with lung function or fluid balance. A high glucose load may also lead to liver dysfunction[11] and a hyperosmolar diet may lead to diarrhea and severe discomfort if it is above the patient's tolerance. This is why tube feedings are usually begun slowly and advanced from dilutions to full strength over several days. Sometimes carbohydrate content is limited to keep CO_2 production at a certain level and diet is altered to maintain as low an osmolarity as necessary. Overfeeding that leads to any of these complica-

tions may cause as much trouble as malnutrition, so continued medical supervision, monitoring, and evaluation are very important. Enteral formulas are more effective when they are started slowly.[12]

Protein is needed to fill many roles in tissue conservation, healing, and the immune response. Protein balance is most difficult for the patient who is only able to have TPN therapy. The glucose in TPN solutions helps to protect body nitrogen. Fat emulsions may also work together to help maximize the conservation of nitrogen.[13] A patient on TPN may also receive "amino acid infusions," special amino acid formulas added to the glucose-electrolyte TPN solution. These infusions help prevent some protein loss. However, they do not usually provide enough nitrogen to prevent a net nitrogen loss from the body.[2] A basic TPN solution of D_5W (water that contains 5% dextrose) may only provide 200 calories per liter, so supplemental nutrients from protein and fat are essential to prevent complete starvation. Amino acid infusions, together with glucose water and fat emulsions, help to spare as much protein as possible. An individual in trauma may need 1 to 3 grams of protein or 400 to 500 mg nitrogen per kilogram per day.[6]

Vitamin and mineral needs in trauma do not increase as greatly as energy and protein needs. In fact, there is no clear evidence that a person needs any more vitamins and minerals than usual, although most physicians prescribe extra "to be safe."[13] Extra vitamins and minerals have little benefit in nutrition therapy unless a particular deficiency has developed. Even the extra body need for zinc in burn therapy is not clear, although it seems very likely it is necessary because the damage of burns on tissue is so severe.

PRESURGERY

Surgery is a minor trauma. It involves the shock of anesthesia, the trauma suffered by the organ itself, opened tissue with the risk of infection, and the high demands of recovery from the surgery as well as from whatever problem made surgery necessary in the first place. Added to all this, the surgical patient is usually unable to obtain any food for up to 24 hours before surgery and often 24 hours afterwards as well, because the gut must be empty before surgery and may be sluggish afterwards. As a result, the body is in stress and must rely on its own stores to initiate recovery. Sometimes eating is difficult, even after surgery, and there is real risk of malnutrition—unless the patient started off with sufficient protein and energy stores to get through this crisis period.

Many studies have shown that the surgical patient who starts off with adequate muscle, protein, and energy stores is better able to survive surgery, with rapid wound healing and improved resistance to infection and other complications than could someone who starts out with depleted stores.*[4,14-16] There are many different ways for the medical team to measure this risk before surgery.[15,17-18] The most effective methods consider muscle strength, weight for height, percent of ideal body weight (IBW), triceps skinfold thickness (TSF), midarm muscle circumference (MAMC) —both of the latter are indirect measures of fat and muscle stores, creatinine height index (CHI), serum albumin, and other serum protein measures. Probably the most critical risk factor is a preoperative weight loss of 10% or more.[11] Patients who are at nutritional risk should be nourished *before* they go through the trauma of surgery. This will help provide them with the stores they will need to recover quickly, with as few complications as possible. Often this aspect of preventive nutrition therapy is ignored or not considered to be cost-effective. When it *is* employed, the patient may be able to continue postoperative buildup at home. More often, however, he will receive some type of hyperalimentation over a period of several days while he is still in the hospital.[11,14] Preoperative feeding can help build up the "emergency" energy stores of liver glycogen that may be low in the malnourished patient. However, most aggressive nutrition therapy begins postoperatively, rather than before surgery.

---

* Adequate glycogen stores help protect the liver against anesthesia and provide energy for the postoperative period.[9]

STUDY QUESTIONS

1. Define
   - Stress
   - Trauma
   - Protein-sparing modified fast
   - Ileus
   - Fistula
   - Ringer's Lactate Solution

2. In simple starvation, how do energy needs change? Why? How do protein needs change? Why?

3. How much storage glycogen does the liver usually hold? Is it in the form of fat, protein, or carbohydrate? How much energy does this represent?

4. What nutrition risks may develop when stress is combined with starvation?

5. Why is nutrition important in
   - Surgery
   - Sepsis
   - Shock

6. Describe specific ways nutrient needs may be met for a burn patient by
   - Oral feeding
   - Tube feeding
   - TPN

7. Why is food withheld immediately before and after surgery? List at least three reasons.

8. Mr. G. is a 62-year-old 60 kg man who is scheduled for surgery next week for stomach cancer.
   - What might you need to know in order to assess his nutritional status?
   - What nutritional problems might he develop after surgery?

REFERENCES

1. Blackburn GL: Adaptation to starvation. Eaton Laboratories' Intake: Perspectives in Clinical Nutrition, Vol. 5, May 1973
2. Gastineau CF (ed): Nutrition in stress and starvation. Health Learning Systems' Dialogues in Nutrition 1(3), September 1976
3. Hill GL, et al: Malnutrition in surgical patients: An unrecognized problem pp 689–692 Lancet, March 26, 1977

4. Bistrian BR, et al: Protein status of general surgical patients. JAMA 230(6): 858–860, 1974

5. McLean APH, Meakins, JL: Nutritional support in sepsis. Surg Clin North Am 61(3): 681–689, June 1981

6. Kudsk KA, Stone J, Sheldon GF: Nutrition in Trauma. Surg Clin North Am 61(3): 671–679, June 1981

7. Gastineau CF (ed): Nutrition in Trauma and burns. Health Learning Systems' Dialogues in Nutrition 2(1): March 1977

8. Ross Laboratories: Dietary Modifications in Disease: Major Body Burns/ Columbus, Ohio, Ross Laboratories, 1977

9. Thiele VF: Clinical Nutrition, pp 144–146. St. Louis, CV Mosby, 1976

10. Schumer W: The nutritional basis of the therapy of shock. Eaton Laboratories Intake: Perspectives in Clinical Nutrition, Vol. 4, September 1975

11. MacBurney M, Wilmore DW: Rational decision-making in nutritional care. Surg Clin North Am 61(3): 571–581, June 1981

12. Trunkey D, Grzyb S, Sheldon GF: Nutrition in trauma. Eaton Laboratories' Intake: Perspectives in Clinical Nutrition, Vol. 6, September 1975

13. Shils ME, Randall HT: Diet and Nutrition in the care of the surgical patient. In Goodhart RE, Shils ME (eds): Modern Nutrition in Health and Disease, 6th ed, pp 1082–1124. Philadelphia, Lea & Febiger, 1980

14. Parenteral Nutrition before Surgery? (editorial): Br Med J 6204: 1529, December 15, 1979

15. Klidjian AM, et al: Relation of anthropometric and dynamometric variables to serious postoperative complications. Br Med J 281: 899–901, October 4, 1980

16. Gastineau CF (ed): Malnutrition in the hospital. Health Learning Systems' Dialogues in Nutrition 2(2), June 1977

17. Blackburn GL, et al: Nutritional and metabolic assessment of the hospitalized patient. J Parenter Enter Nutr 1(1): 11–22, 1977

18. Buzby GP: Prognostic nutritional index in gastrointestinal surgery. Am J Surg 139: 160–167, January 1980

CHAPTER 40

Allergies and Food Sensitivities

OBJECTIVES

1. To discuss common definitions of food-related allergies and hypersensitivities

2. To discuss the frequency and occurrence of common food-related sensitivities

3. To list and discuss briefly substances, symptoms, and diet treatment of common

   a. Food Sensitivities
     1. Milk
     2. Eggs
     3. Nuts
     4. Soy
     5. Wheat
     6. Citrus
     7. Tomato
     8. Strawberry
     9. Other, including shellfish and other fruits and vegetables

   b. Food and Additive-Related sensitivities
     1. Additives
       — Tartrazine and salicylates
       — Sulfite agents
       — Monosodium glutamate
       — Sodium benzoate
       — BHA, BHT
       — Nitrates and nitrites
       — Dyes
     2. Contaminants and Toxins
       — Insect parts
       — Mushrooms
       — Shellfish
       — Molds/aflatoxins

     3. Drugs
       — Histamines
       — Methyl xanthines
       — Alcohol
       — Tyramine

4. To discuss the role of diet in behavior, including a critique of the "Feingold" diet sometimes used for hyperactivity

5. To define and explain common objective methods used to test for food sensitivities

6. To emphasize nutrient adequacy as a key part of all treatment of food allergies and hypersensitivities

Two extremes are common in discussing food allergies. At one extreme is the person who blames every medical and food problem on an allergy. "Offending" foods are blamed for depression, anger at a spouse, poor judgment that causes a car accident, and the normal behavior of a tired four-year old a half hour before dinner.

At the other extreme is the individual who persistently ignores the symptoms and nearly dies of suffocation brought on by a genuine hypersensitive or allergic reaction to a specific food. Some persons may not believe allergies truly exist.

The subject is further confused by the way emotions may play a role in allergic reactions. For example, one housewife was tested and found to be allergic to celery; celery brought on a skin rash. The rash was worse, though, early in the month when she was most anxious about household bills. When the financial stress was resolved, so was her allergy.[1a]

Many others "have a food allergy" simply because they believe they have one. They exhibit symptoms if they knowingly eat a particular food. However, when they are objectively tested for this, by swallowing the food in a form they cannot recognize — a capsule or through a stomach tube — they show no symptoms.[2a] This is why physicians may identify three possible causes of a food allergy: biochemical, immunological or psychological.[2a]

DEFINITIONS

Many terms are commonly used, including *allergy,* food intolerance, *food sensitivity,* and hypersensitivity. There is still much debate over these terms, since this particular area of food reactions is still not completely understood, and there are many unanswered questions. This chapter will discuss this issue in terms of: *allergy* and *food sensitivity.*

An allergy occurs when the body's immune system overreacts to something. Normally, the immune system functions by manufacturing *antibodies* to fight off a foreign agent in the body (usually bacteria or a virus). The foreign agent is called an *antigen.*

An allergy develops when the body is conditioned or taught to recognize some normal, otherwise nonthreatening substance as an antigen, and to produce antibodies against it. This may happen later in life. More often, however, the stage may be set in the first few months after birth when the immune system and the mucus barrier in the small intestine are too immature to know which absorbed substances (especially protein) are normal and which are foreign.[3] This is one reason infants may tolerate breast milk better than formula and is partially why they should not be fed any solids until they are at least 4 months old.

Once an allergic response is developed, subsequent exposures to this substance will cause the body to overreact, to produce more antibodies, and to show stronger symptoms of allergy. Allergic reactions may affect the skin, the lungs, or the intestines, as shown elsewhere on this page. An antigen that seems to be the culprit in

COMMON SYMPTOMS OF ALLERGIES AND HYPERSENSITIVITIES

Skin

Urticaria (hives)
Skin rash (except palms and soles)
Angiodema (swelling of lips, ears, eyes, face, larynx. Can cause suffocation)
Eczema

Lungs

Dyspnea (shortness of breath)
Asthma

Intestines

Nausea
Abdominal pain (sometimes so severe it leads to surgery)
Vomiting
Colic (especially in infants)
Fatty stools, diarrhea

---

an allergy is called an *allergen.* Pollen and goldenrod are common allergens. Unlike them, however, food allergies may not cause all the allergic symptoms listed here. In fact, it has never been clearly proven that asthma and eczema are caused by foods, although these conditions may be exaggerated after the ingestion of some foods.[4] A person who avoids some known allergen (*e.g.,* egg) may obtain some relief, but eczema or asthma will usually not be cured.

Frequently, there is a relationship between allergies to plants and allergies to foods, so that a person's immune system may overreact to several different substances with no apparent relationship. For example, someone "allergic" to grass pollen may also react to wheat; ragweed to melon; birch to apple; carrot to potato.[2b] The body seems to relate these substances to each other in some yet unknown way.

Many food sensitivities do not seem to be related to the immune system, however. Some are the result of an inborn error in metabolism (see Chapter 34), an enzyme deficiency (such as lactase, discussed in Chapter 24), or a disease, such as Crohn's ileitis, that has somehow damaged the intestinal area where the substance is normally absorbed. Some sensitivities relate to drugs. For example, people on monoamine oxidase (MAO) inhibitors (for psychiatric problems or treatment of hypertension) should not eat foods high in tyramines. Drug-nutrient interactions are discussed in more detail in Chapter 36.

The many foods sensitivities that do not fit into these categories and are not caused by allergic reactions are simply called food sensitivities. The outward signs of a food sensitivity are usually similar to those of an allergy. Treatment is also the same: the individual (or his parents) is taught the sources of the offending food(s) and told to avoid them.

Another term often encountered in discussions of allergies, hypersensitivities, and drug treatments is the term *placebo.* A placebo is an inactive substance that will neither cure nor aggravate the medical situation in which it is used. Placebos are common in research: One group is given a test drug and the other group is given a placebo that looks like the test drug. No one knows what he is taking, so results are more likely to be objective. Many people believe they feel better after taking the placebo; this is called the "placebo effect." Persons feel certain results (sometimes) because they *believe* the medicine will cause the results. Placebos (*e.g.,* capsules filled with sugar) are sometimes used to test food allergies; they are given alternately with capsules filled with the suspected food. Sugar is a common placebo.

Listed below are many of the common substances that may be allergenic or cause hypersensitivities in some people.

OFFENDING SUBSTANCES IN MANY COMMON FOOD ALLERGIES AND RELATED SENSITIVITIES

Foods

Milk	Wheat	Chocolate
Eggs	Citrus	Herb teas that contain common
Soy	Tomato	plant allergens
Nuts	Strawberry	Fish and shellfish

Additives

Tartrazines	MSG	Nitrites, nitrates
Salicylates	Sodium benzoate	FD & C Red #5
Metabisulfites	BHA, BHT	

Contaminants and Toxins

Insect parts
Mushrooms
Improperly selected or prepared wild plants, flowers
Shellfish
Molds

Drugs

Histamines
Methyl xanthines
Alcohol
Tyramine

FOODS

Food allergies are most commonly caused by milk, eggs, soy, and nuts. Many sensitivities and allergies may be caused by proteins and all four of these foods are high in protein.

Milk

Milk "allergy" is most common in infants. One to two percent of all infants are estimated to be allergic to cow's milk during their first two years.[4] The allergy is almost always triggered by some part of the protein in cow's milk, not breast milk. However, some breast-fed infants are so sensitive that they develop colic or diarrhea because of the cow's milk their *mother* is drinking.[5] Women who are breast-feeding infants with this food sensitivity are usually told to drink less milk and sometimes the missing calcium is supplied in a supplement. Since the infant is allergic to protein, not to a sugar (such as lactose), all forms of dairy products may cause problems; foods to avoid are listed below. Cooked and sour milk may cause fewer problems than unprocessed milk. The diarrhea, malabsorption, and intestinal damage that results from an uncontrolled milk allergy may lead to a "secondary" lactase deficiency. The infant develops a temporary lactose intolerance because the lactase enzymes in the intestines have been destroyed. But the enzyme will grow back once the diet is controlled, and the intestines heal.

"HIDDEN" SOURCES OF MILK

Butter	Ice Cream
Calcium caseinate	Junket
Casein	Lactose
Caseinate	Malted milk
Cheese	Milk added to
Chocolate	casseroles, cakes,
Cottage cheese	pancakes
Cream soups	Puddings
Curds	Sauces
Custard	Sodium caseinate
Dry milk solids in	Whey
baked goods,	Yogurt
margarine	
Gravy (some)	

Cow's milk is never recommended in the first 6 months of life (see Chapter 15), but often an infant becomes allergic to milk-based formulas. These infants are usually switched to soy-based formulas. If allergy is a severe problem or if the infants are also allergic to soy, the next alternative is usually a meat-based formula or one specially treated to remove all the possible allergens (*e.g.,* Nutramigen®).

A milk allergy is usually temporary. Sixty percent to ninety percent of children can tolerate cow's milk with few problems by age 2 (unless they are also lactase deficient).[2c,6] But while the allergy is present, it is very important that the substitute formula contain necessary calcium. It is vital that infants—with or without allergies—acquire the calcium and other nutrients they need for growth during their first few years. Many milk-free recipes are available from dietitians or special cookbooks, and formula companies may also provide recipes and guidelines to help identify hidden sources of milk and to substitute an alternative product.[7]

Soy

Another common allergen is soy. The child allergic to both cow's milk and soy requires close attention from both pediatrician and dietitian to make sure he is receiving the necessary nutrients. Individuals allergic to soy may also need to avoid lecithin made from soy and soy oils.[2d] Lecithin is a common emulsifier added to many processed foods. As with milk, a soy allergy may also be temporary.

Eggs

The white of the egg, not the yolk, may cause allergic reactions in some persons. It is difficult to avoid eggs because they are added to so many foods. They are often used as emulsifiers in water–oil mixtures, and in baked goods, and are frequently used in baking powders.

Powdered egg substitutes are available in many grocery stores. One teaspoon of baking powder in a recipe can be replaced with one and an eighth teaspoons of cream of tartar plus a half teaspoon of baking soda. Add an additional teaspoon of baking powder or its substitute for each egg omitted from a recipe.[7] It is often impossible to find an acceptable substitute for foods that depend on eggs for their texture (such as custards, quiche, and some breads).

Nuts

Nuts, especially peanuts, are another common food allergen. The nut allergy may be caused by a sensitivity to some protein in the nut or it may be due to a toxin that has grown from mold. Aflatoxins on peanuts sometimes cause severe reactions, and may even be fatal in highly sensitive individuals. Persons allergic to nuts should also avoid nut butters and perhaps oils made from the nut.

Many other foods cause some persons difficulties. The common allergenic foods include wheat, citrus fruits, tomato, shellfish, and strawberries. A genetic intolerance to the gluten in wheat is called celiac disease, nontropical sprue, or gluten-sensitive enteropathy, and was discussed in Chapter 24. It is not a wheat allergy but a gluten sensitivity; all gluten products (and gluten is present in wheat, oats, rye, and barley) must be avoided. A wheat allergy may be simpler to treat than a gluten sensitivity, as it is easier to identify sources of wheat than all the sources of gluten. Shown on this page are some acceptable substitutes for one cup of wheat flour.

To avoid these foods and substances, the sensitive person must know *where* to find them. This means knowing "hidden" sources, reading labels, using special products, and/or modifying recipes. Food and plant allergies may overlap, and a person allergic to certain plants but not to foods may need to avoid certain herb teas that might contain the offending plant. For example, anyone sensitive to ragweed, asters, chrysanthemums, and related plants should avoid herb teas that contain chamomile, goldenrod, marigold, or yarrow.[8]

Food allergies may run in families. Doctors are divided about what to tell a pregnant woman whose family members have problems with certain foods. Some suggest a high exposure to the food very early in pregnancy, believing that this may help the developing infant accept the substance and prevent allergies.[2e] Most physicians, however, suggest that a woman avoid these

SUBSTITUTES FOR WHEAT FLOUR*

½ cup Barley flour
¾ cup Buckwheat flour
1 cup Corn flour
¾ cup Coarse cornmeal
1 scant cup Cornmeal
½ cup Cornstarch
1-⅓ cup Ground rolled oats
⅞ cup Rice flour
1 cup Rye flour
¾ Soy flour
½ cup Potato flour + ½ cup Rye flour
⅝ cup Rice flour + ⅓ cup Rye flour

---

*Product will probably need to bake at a lower temperature and for 10–20 minutes more than if it were made with wheat flour. This is because gluten, the substance in wheat flour that stretches and holds baked goods together, is missing or minimal in these other types of flours.
(From Wyeth Laboratories:Nursing Cookery: Milk-Free Recipes for Patients Allergic to Cow's Milk, p 4. Philadelphia, Wyeth Laboratories, July 1982)

---

foods during her pregnancy, believing that early exposure may make an allergic reaction more likely.

ADDITIVES

Some persons are especially sensitive to certain additives or substances found in foods, and the most common of these are listed on page 371. This chapter will focus only on *tartrazines* and *salicylates, sulfites* and *monosodium glutamate (MSG)*.

Tartrazine is the same as yellow food dye (FD & C Yellow #5). It is related chemically to salicylates, so a diet that omits salicylates should usually omit tartrazine as well. Because of the risk of hypersensitivity, the dye currently is illegal in Sweden; it is, however, allowed in the US and most other countries.

Salicylates are natural substances found in many foods. They are also commonly added to many drugs, beverages, and flavorings. The active ingredient in aspirin is acetyl salicylic acid

(ASA). As a drug, salicylates can be controlled by law, but they are also a natural compound in many foods (see the listing below). Sensitive persons may react to small amounts with severe asthmatic symptoms. Sometimes this inability to breathe (resulting from angioedema or swelling of the lips, eyes, and sometimes the larynx) is life-threatening. Some sensitive individuals also develop a rash. Asthmatics are more likely than nonasthmatics to be sensitive to these substances. A person who is very sensitive to the salicylate in aspirin will almost certainly be sensitive to other, natural salicylates and tartrazine. Tartrazine is usually listed on product labels as FD & C Yellow #5; salicylates are not listed because they occur naturally. When in doubt, it is wise to avoid the food until more detailed information can be obtained from the manufacturer.

Sulfites are preservatives that have been used in food preparations for many years. It was only recently recognized that some asthmatics — and even nonasthmatics — may react in a hypersensitive way to these substances.[9] These agents include the terms sodium *metabisulfite* ($Na_2S_2O_5$), *sodium bisulfite,* sodium sulfite, potassium bisulfite, potassium metabisulfite, or *sulfur dioxide.*[10] Soon after contact with these substances, a sensitive person may experience itchy palms, hives (called urticaria), abdominal pain, severe diarrhea, facial and laryngeal edema, flushing of the skin and, in severe cases, loss of consciousness and shock.[11]

In spite of this, sulfiting agents have been on the Food and Drug Administration's "generally recognized as safe" *(GRAS) list* since 1959. They are powerful antioxidants (a type of preservative) that help keep foods from browning and spoiling. They are often used in a spray form to keep fruits and vegetables looking fresh in restaurants and salad bars, and are also used in many other processed foods and beverages (see the guide found on page 375). Since sulfites used on produce are frequently in aerosol form, persons may be sensitive not only to the treated foods but also to the very air around them.[2f,11]

Sulfites are most widely used in restaurants. Sensitive persons would be wise to ask if sulfites have been added to foods, to choose foods least likely to contain any preservatives, and perhaps to choose restaurants as carefully — or rarely — as possible. Some restaurants may have written information identifying those of their foods that do contain sulfites. Sulfites may also commonly be used on produce in cafeteria salad bars, which may cause problems for sensitive college students who depend on them for meals. Since many beers and wines are also treated with sul-

SALICYLATES IN FOODS AND SPICES

Foods That Naturally Contain Salicylates*†

Almonds	Licorice
Apples	Nectarines
Apricots	Oranges
Bananas	Peaches
Blackberries	Peas, green
Boysenberries	Peppers
Cherries	Pickles
Cucumbers	Potatoes
Currants	Plums
Dewberries	Prunes
Gooseberries	Raisins
Grapes	Raspberries
Grapefruit	Strawberries
Lemons	Tomatoes

Spices That Naturally Contain Salicylates

Allspice	Oregano
Almond flavoring	Paprika
Cloves	Rosemary
Oil of wintergreen	Thyme

* Many medications and processed food may also contain salicylates, tartrazine (FD & C Yellow #5) or both. A person suspected of hypersensitivity to these substances should check with a physician and dietitian for more detailed guidelines.

† These include many foods high in vitamin C. If all these foods are omitted, alternative sources of C may be needed.

(From Food Sensitivity: Report of Proceedings of Tenth annual Marabou Symposium. Nutr Rev 42(3):110–111, and Guidelines for Eliminating Tartrazine and Reducing Salicylate Intake. Printed by Frances Stern Nutrition Center, New England Medical Center, Boston, MA)

WHERE ARE THE SULFITES?

Sulfites are added during the processing of many foods, as preservatives (antioxidants) to help improve their appearance and texture. They may be sprayed in aerosol form onto fresh fruits and vegetables used in salad bars, cafeterias, and restaurants. A "sulfite sensitivity" reaction may occur in some very sensitive people simply from breathing this aerosol, not just from eating the sulfite-containing foods.

Below is a partial list prepared by the National Restaurant Association in cooperation with the American College of Allergists. These are foods very likely to contain sulfites. Because the preservative may legally be added to any food, the sulfite-sensitive consumer must read labels, ask questions, and sometimes avoid foods that may possibly contain the substances. Sulfites may also be added to these foods before they are shipped to the restaurant or store, so a manager may not know if some foods already contain the preservative. Whole or well-cooked fruits and vegetables are less likely to have sulfites than their raw, cut, or unprocessed forms.

Sulfites are often added to

Avocado dip and guacamole
Baked goods*
Beer
Cider
Coconut "milk" (imported)
Cod (dried)
Coleslaw
Fruit (cut up, fresh, dried, or maraschino)
Fruit juices, purees, fillings*
Gelatin*
Potatoes (cut up, fresh, frozen, dried, or canned)
Raisins
Salad dressing (dry mix,)* relishes

Salads, especially at salad bars
Sauces and gravies, canned or dried*
Sauerkraut
Shellfish (fresh, frozen, canned, or dried), clams, crab, lobster, scallops, shrimp
Soups, canned or dried*
Vegetables (cut up fresh, frozen, canned, or dried)
Fresh mushrooms
Wine vinegar*
Wine, wine coolers*

---

*Read labels and look for any of the following terms: sulfur dioxide, potassium bisulfite or potassium metabisulfite, sodium bisulfite, sodium metabisulfite, or sodium sulfite.
Food that probably do NOT contain sulfites include all fruits and vegetables that are free of additives or that can be peeled at home, fresh meats and fish, breads and cereals, oils, eggs, dry beans, and nuts.
(From Sulfite Sensitivity and Eating Out: A leaflet available from the National Restaurant Association and the Food Allergy Committee of the American College of Allergists)

---

fiting agents, a consumer should look for sulfite-free brands, or write to the manufacturers and ask if sulfites are ever added to their products. Any reactions should be reported to a physician. It is ironic that many drugs (including some used to treat asthma itself) may also contain sulfites.

Monosodium Glutamate or *MSG* sensitivity is commonly called *Chinese restaurant syndrome.* This seasoning is found in oriental foods more often than in other, more particularly western foods. MSG is a form of sodium and, like salt, enhances the flavor of the food it seasons. Persons sensitive to MSG experience a severe headache, chest pain, facial flush (sudden heat and reddened skin), and pressure. The sensitivity is not well understood but it may be dangerous. People susceptible to "Chinese restaurant syndrome" should always order Chinese food prepared *without* MSG; most restaurants are aware of the problem and should comply with this request.

Oriental food is most likely to cause a reaction because so much MSG is added in its preparation, but the substance may also be added to many other, nonOriental foods. MSG is part of many kitchen seasonings (especially those that "enhance flavors") and may also be found in many processed foods. It is considered safe for general use by the FDA, and many sensitive consumers may be able to tolerate small quantities.

CONTAMINANTS AND TOXINS

Some reactions to foods are not allergies or sensitivities. They are, to some degree, food poisoning from contaminants and toxins that get or grow in the food. There are several ways foods can be contaminated.

1. The toxin may be a natural part of the food. In these instances, the food should never be a part of the diet. Four examples of these natural toxins include

   a. Fava beans, which may lead to a hemolytic anemia (*i.e.,* red blood cells are destroyed) in some persons who are deficient in the enzyme glucose-6-phosphate dehydrogenase (G6PD) and who eat a large quantity of fava beans.

   b. Flour made from the cycad nut, which may cause fatal amyotrophic lateral sclerosis (ALS). This has occurred most commonly in Guam, where the nut was used for flour when other food supplies were short.

   c. The lathyrus sativus seed, a chicken or cattle feed used by man in some parts of the world when wheat is in short supply. The toxin in the seeds affects the nervous

system and leads to loss of muscle control, tingling, convulsions, and even death.[1b] Attempts to extract the toxin from the seed so that it can be used safely by humans have not been completely successful.

   d. Mushrooms picked by an amateur may not be what they seem. Many poisonous mushrooms look just like other safe, edible types. Only an expert with many years of field experience can tell the difference. The same is also true of other herbs and plants: one part of a plant may be edible while another section of the same plant may be toxic.

2. The environment may add or concentrate a poison in a food. This has happened in fish and shellfish. One of the best known and tragic examples of this is "Minamata Disease," mercury poisoning that affected the mental development of many unborn children in Japan's Minamata Bay area, whose mothers ate fish from the bay during their pregnancy. Adults were affected as well, often suffering from collapsed vertebrae caused by the poisoning. The fish had become concentrated sources of the mercury that was in the water from industrial waste.[1c]

   Other environmental poisons include saxitoxins from a parasite in the shrimp, dinoflagellates from some shellfish that may cause a paralytic poisoning, and the aflotoxin mold that may grow on peanuts.[6]

3. Food may also contain contaminants resulting from poor cleaning, pesticide residues, or from insects that entered into the food during processing, packaging, or shipping.

DRUGS

Some people react with an apparent allergy or food sensitivity to substances that are actually drugs. These may include the methyl xanthines (*e.g.,* caffeine or theobromine in coffee, tea, cocoa, cola, or chocolate products), alcohol, and vasoactive amines such as tryptamine, tyramine (see Chapter 36), dopamine, phenylethylamine (chocolate), norepinephrine, serotonin, and histamine (which is in tuna, mackerel, and swiss cheese where bacteria has chemically acted on natural substances).[28] The major symptom for many of these types of sensitivities is headache, sometimes a result of increased blood pressure. The reaction may occur immediately or it may take several hours and appear slowly. Many of these natural substances in foods cannot be controlled, and content varies widely. But anyone who is on medication should ask his physician about any side-effects he might experience. He should also know if there are any foods to be avoided, since drugs and food can antagonize each other (Chapter 36). Anyone (on medication or not) who has some type of sensitivity reaction should discuss it with his physician and keep a careful record of both diet and symptoms. This will be discussed in greater detail below.

DIET AND BEHAVIOR

One of the most popular and controversial areas of food allergy and hypersensitivities is that of behavior, especially hyperactivity in children. Many persons blame food allergies for a wide range of vague symptoms (such as depression, fatigue, chronic coughing, poor concentration, dry mouth, and muscle cramps). Some blame vitamin deficiencies for the development of allergies.[12] Unfortunately, neither of these theories has any reputable, scientific basis to support it.

In 1973 Dr. Benjamin Feingold, an allergist, proposed what became one of the most controversial diets in the field of allergy and sensitivity. His *Feingold diet* suggests that hyperactivity in children may be caused by a sensitivity to natural salicylates and all artificial colors, flavors, and preservatives. Most of his "evidence" is anecdotal rather than carefully tested; that is, it is composed of personal testimonies from parents who believed they noticed a change in their child when he began the diet. Anecdotal evidence is not accepted as scientific because it comes from an environment (the home, the parents who want and expect a change, and so forth) where the trial is not tightly enough controlled to tell if there is indeed a change and what really has caused whatever change does appear. The diet itself may simply have a "placebo effect." The few controlled studies that have been done do not support Feingold's theory.[13,14]

Feingold believed his diet worked for 50% of hyperactive children. But in 1982 the National Institutes of Health held a Consensus Development Conference to examine the limited evidence for the effectiveness of this diet. The Conference concluded that

1. The diet may help a small percentage of children, but not as much as 50% of them.
2. It may be most helpful in young children.
3. Susceptible children may have a druglike sensitivity to high doses of food coloring. This sensitivity may affect their learning abilities (this was most evident with FD & C Red #5).
4. Allergies and sensitivities to foods and additives are probably completely unrelated to the effect diet may seem to have on [hyperactive] behavior.[14]

TESTING FOR ALLERGIES AND FOOD SENSITIVITIES

Whenever a person suspects or seems to have an allergy or food sensitivity, treatment involves one or more of the following:

1. A detailed food record for days or weeks. The client records time and content of all meals and snacks, and time and details of any symptoms.
2. *Elimination diets.* The suspected foods or substances are totally eliminated from the diet. A physician and often a nutritionist may need to help teach the client what foods and "hidden sources" to avoid. The food and symptom record may continue.

   When the person continues to have symptoms, he may be put on a severely restricted diet. This diet usually consists of only three or four foods that are known to be nonallergenic. The diet is inadequate in most nutrients and should never be followed for a long period of time.
3. "Double-blind challenges" with suspected foods. In a "challenge," the food that might cause a reaction is given in quantity. A double-blind test is one in which neither the person taking the food nor the person giving it knows *what* is given *when*. The food and sim-

ilar-appearing placebos are hidden inside gelatin capsules that are swallowed whole. Sometimes a "single-blind" challenge is given, in which the client does not know what is being given, but the physician does know. The method prevents any reactions that may be based on what the person believes about the substance.

4. Skin testing. Some allergists test for allergies by lightly scraping the skin with the substance. This is common for pollen, dust, and other nonfood allergies but is not a reliable method for food allergies.[2h] The skin reacts to substances in quite a different manner than the warm, soft, moist, enzyme-laden wall of the small intestine. By means of skin test a person may seem to be allergic to foods he actually may continue to enjoy. This is called a "false positive" testing error.

Sometimes, for example with sulfites or MSG, it is quite clear what substance is causing the reaction. Some persons are often so sensitive to a food that it would be dangerous to test them with a skin or oral challenge.[15] For these persons, the safest treatment is a diet that eliminates the offending food. They know what they should not eat and it is now their responsibility to avoid these foods. Often this severe reaction occurs in response to only one or two foods or a particular method of preparation and the offender is not critical for adequate nutrition.

Children may find it most difficult to stick to a diet for their allergies or sensitivities, esecially the common milk, wheat, or egg allergies. Children may not understand the importance of diet nor have the maturity to follow a specific diet. But the need to do so should be explained to them in the simplest possible terms. Gradually all children, including those who have special needs, must take responsibility for their own food choices. Fortunately, many children will outgrow their food allergies.

ELIMINATION DIETS AND GOOD NUTRITION

Persons allergic or hypersensitive to certain foods may be at risk of developing a nutrient deficiency, especially if they simply eliminate the food entirely and do not work to replace the missing nutrients. For example, children with milk allergies must have other sources of calcium. Anyone sensitive to salicylates and tartrazines may be unconsciously avoiding all the best sources of vitamin C. These persons need to know what nutrients they may be missing and to find other good food sources for them or to ask their physician about using a vitamin or mineral supplement. A balanced diet may have no effect on the allergy but it is important for continued good health.

STUDY QUESTIONS

1. How does a food allergy differ from other types of food sensitivities?

2. Which of the following symptoms may be signs of a food allergy/hypersensitivity?
   Hives
   Depression
   Chronic cough
   Asthma
   Swollen face and larynx
   Skin rash
   Poor concentration
   Abdominal pain
   Muscle cramps
   Vitamin deficiency
   Dry mouth
   Diarrhea

3. What three factors may cause a food "allergy?"

4. What is the "placebo effect?"

5. How may eczema and asthma relate to food sensitivities?

6. List six foods and three additives to which some people may have allergies or sensitivities.

7. For each of the additives listed above, explain what types of foods contain them and ways a sensitive person might avoid them.

8. Discuss cow's milk allergies:
   - How common are they in infants?
   - Why might a breast-fed infant show symptoms?
   - What is the usual treatment for an infant who is taking formula?

- Is an infant with a cow's milk allergy also lactose intolerant? Why or why not?
- Will the infant ever outgrow this allergy?
- What key nutrient in cow's milk must be replaced to make sure the infant will grow normally?

9. Someone allergic to eggs should avoid what foods?

10. What types of foods might be a problem for a person sensitive to the pollen of wild flowers?

11. What is tartrazine? Where is it found?

12. People sensitive to salicylates might need to find other sources of what vitamin?

13. List at least four names (which might be found on food labels) for the sulfiting agents.

14. What is "Chinese restaurant syndrome?"

15. List and discuss at least three foods that may contain natural toxins or poisons.

16. How might a food be contaminated?

17. Mrs. P's son, Tommy, is 3½ and has recently become difficult to handle. He started nursery school several months ago, just as the Ps were finalizing their divorce. He eats well but refuses to take naps, sleeps about 7 hours every night, and is constantly "into everything" in loud and destructive ways. Mrs. P believes he is hyperactive and wants to try the Feingold diet. What would you tell her?

18. Describe at least two objective tests used when food allergy or hypersensitivity is suspected.

19. How important are the essential vitamins and minerals in treating food allergies?

REFERENCES

1. Goodhart RE, Shils ME: Modern Nutrition in Health and Disease, 6th ed, a, p 1077; b, pp 463–493; c, pp 485–486; Philadelphia, Lea & Febiger, 1980

2. Food Sensitivity. Proc Tenth Annual Marabou Symposium. Nutr Rev 42(3): a, pp 70–139; b, p 90; c, p 129; d, pp 102–103; d, p 71; e. p 112 f, p 111; g, p 95; h, p 95

3. Walker WA: Absorption of protein and protein fragments in the developing intestine: Role in immunologic/allergic reactions. Pediatrics (Suppl)75: 167–171, January 1985

4. Foucard T: Development of food allergies with special reference to cow's milk allergy. Pediatrics (Suppl)75: 177–181, January 1985

5. Colicky Babies and Breast Milk. Tufts University Diet and Nutrition Letter 1(9): 1, November 1983

6. Bock SA: Food sensitivity. Nutrition News 47(3):9–11, October 1984

7. Wyeth Laboratories: Nursoy Cookery: Milk-Free Recipes for Patients Allergic to Cow's Milk. Philadelphia, Wyeth Laboratories, July 1982

8. Brody J: Jane Brody's Nutrition Book, p 246. New York, WW Norton & Co, 1982

9. Fraser WM, Huang AS: Letter to the Editor. Are sulfite additives really safe? N Engl J Med 311:542, August 9, 1984

10. Sulfite Sensitivity and Eating Out. A leaflet available from the National Restaurant Association and the Food Allergy Committee of the American College of Allergists

11. Hecht A, Willis J: Sulfites: Preservatives that can go wrong. Food and Drug Administration Consumer (HHS Publ No. (FDA) 83–2178), September 1983

12. Davis A: Let's Eat Right to Keep Fit, pp 123, 210. New York, New American Library/Harcourt Brace Jovanovich, 1970

13. Mayer J, Goldberg J: Does the Feingold Diet Help Hyperactivity? The Boston Globe, p 56N October 3, 1984

14. Defined Diets in Childhood Hyperactivity. National Institutes of Health Consensus Development Conference. Office for Medical Applications of Research, Bethesda, Md., Washington, DC, January 13–15, 1982

15. Knight CB: Canary in a Coal Mine. Placentia, CA, Aristan Press, 1984

CHAPTER 41

Nutrition and Dental Health

Dental health is dependent on four normal ingredients of the mouth: the teeth, the gums (or periodontal tissue), the production of saliva, and the particular bacteria that thrive in the mouth. The health of the first three depends very much on adequate nutrition and protects against harm by the fourth, the germ or bacteria.

Good nutrition is important even *in utero* for proper gum and tooth formation. Before birth, cells that will become teeth and gum tissues are multiplying. Under the gum, the teeth are already forming, months or even years before the teeth erupt. The glands that produce saliva are being formed. All these cells multiply and grow, using important nutrients from the placental blood to develop properly. If the mother is malnourished, the fetus suffers as well.[1] This may play a role in many lifelong areas of dental health, including the normal formation of the jaw and teeth. Teeth that are not as strong, straight, or big as they should be because of poor prenatal nutrition may affect appearance as well as health.

Figure 41-1 shows a cross-section of healthy and diseased tooth and gum tissue. The tooth is not simply a piece of bone set into the jaw, but has several layers:

Center *pulp,* filled with blood vessels and nerve fibers. These blood vessels help keep the teeth healthy, while the nerves allow sensation in the tooth and "set off" the pain caused by toothache

Dentin, a softer substance surrounding the pulp

Cementum, a thin protective covering over the "root," between the dentin and the gums

Enamel, the hard white surface (harder even than the cementum) that protects the inner portions of the tooth from damage.

Like a glacier, only a small part of the whole tooth is visible above the surface. The rest, the "root," is surrounded and protected by the gums. Gum tissue also has several layers:

Alveolar bone that helps to form the jaw

Periodontal membranes, between the cementum and the bone

Gingiva or surface tissue made of thin epithelial cells

The normal, healthy mouth is also continuously producing saliva. This fluid is made by several glands around the face. Saliva plays several very important roles in dental health: it rinses out substances, helps keep the *p*H (or acidity) of the mouth minimal, keeps tissues

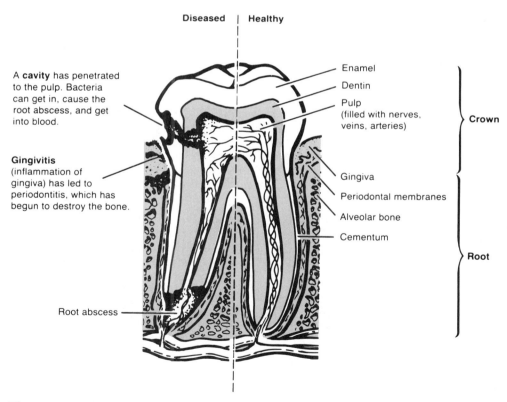

Figure 41-1
The healthy versus the diseased tooth. (Adapted from DePaola DP, Alfano MC: Diet and oral health. Nutrition Today, pp 6ff, May–June 1977)

moist, flushes the teeth and gums with nutrients, including minerals, and plays a role in protecting against infection.[2,3] Enzymes in saliva work with the teeth to help break down food into smaller particles before they enter the esophagus and stomach. Without saliva, dental disease can set in very quickly.

Bacteria is naturally present in the mouth. Without food, the bacteria can do little damage; the role of bacteria in cavities and gum disease will be discussed in detail below. The most common bacteria in the mouth are the *streptococcus mutans* and *lactobacillus*. These bacteria may have a beneficial role in that they help to keep out other bacteria.

NUTRIENTS IN DENTAL HEALTH

Healthy gums and teeth are part of a healthy body. Thus, all the nutrients needed for health in blood, membranes, and bone tissues are also needed for healthy teeth and gums. Teeth and gums are not fully developed until some time during the teen years, so malnutrition at any point before this—from the womb—may affect the growth and development of the jaw, the developing teeth, the gingival or periodontal tissue, or the protective substances in saliva.

Throughout life, some of these nutrients do seem to be more important than others in dental health. Calcium is one of the substances in the enamel. An adequate calcium: phosphorus balance in the diet is important to help form the jaw and "mineralize" the teeth. It is a matrix of minerals, including calcium and fluoride, that forms strong enamel. Women with iron and zinc deficiencies during pregnancy seem to have children who are more likely to develop cavities.[4] Fluoride is the mineral that helps strengthen the tooth enamel so it is better able to resist attack from bacterial acid. Vitamin C is extremely important in the healthy development of the gum tissue. In fact, bleeding gums is one of the earliest signs of scurvy or vitamin C deficiency.[5] (Note: a person who meets his Recommended Dietary Allowance for vitamin C—60 mg for adults per day—and notices bleeding gums probably does not have scurvy but should see a dentist to help identify what is wrong.)

Other necessary nutrients include protein for healthy tissue growth, vitamin A for the epithelial cells, folate for healthy blood, and phosphorus for a proper calcium: phosphorus ratio. When all of these together work properly with the inherited structure and tendencies, the result for the individual is the best possible teeth and gums, ready to withstand the environmental damage that constantly threatens in the form of cavities and periodontal disease.

DEVELOPMENT OF CAVITIES AND PERIODONTAL DISEASE

Disease in dentistry may involve the tooth or the gum. It usually results from the environment: the saliva, bacteria, and food.

Dental Caries

Cavities are also called *caries*. Cariogenicity is the tendency to form cavities or caries. Many environmental circumstances, including foods, seem to be cariogenic factors.

Figure 41-2 illustrates just how caries develop. First, teeth must be susceptible. They must be weak enough for bacterial acid to break through the hard enamel surface. Some persons seem totally resistant to caries, probably because of some genetic factor.[3] On the other hand, some persons have highly susceptible teeth and may develop many cavities. Other risk factors that make a tooth more susceptible than necessary include the following:

1. Not enough saliva. Saliva production normally drops during sleep but it may also be cut back as a side-effect of disease, drugs, or head-neck radiation treatments. Teeth that are not exposed to enough saliva develop cavities very quickly.

2. Not enough fluoride. Fluoride is an essential micronutrient, naturally present in some water supplies. Studies have shown that water that is fluoridated at a level of 1 part per million (ppm) or ½ milligram of fluoride in 1 quart of water, has a significant effect on decreasing the incidence of cavities.[3] Fluoride is a trace mineral and it helps to rebuild the minerals on the enamel. The fluoridated tooth is stronger than the nonfluoridated

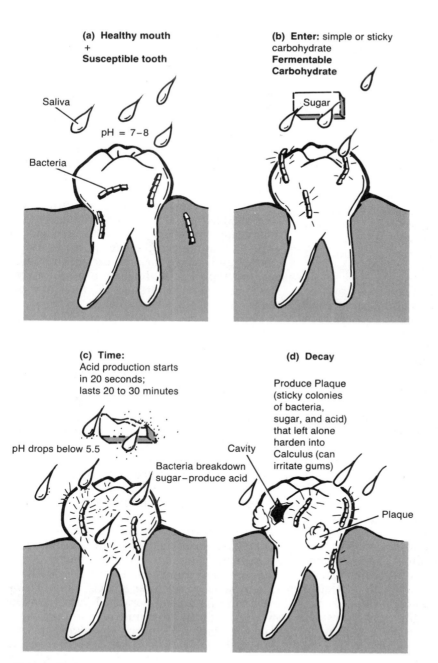

**(a) Healthy mouth
+
Susceptible tooth**

Saliva

pH = 7–8

Bacteria

(b) Enter: simple or sticky carbohydrate
**Fermentable
Carbohydrate**

Sugar

(c) Time:
Acid production starts
in 20 seconds;
lasts 20 to 30 minutes

pH drops below 5.5

Bacteria breakdown
sugar–produce acid

(d) Decay

Produce Plaque
(sticky colonies
of bacteria,
sugar, and acid)
that left alone
harden into
Calculus (can
irritate gums)

Cavity

Plaque

Figure 41-2
The development of caries.

tooth. Since the RDA recommends 1.5 to 2.5 mg of fluoride per day for the average adult, there is no danger of fluoride toxicity in the person who drinks even several quarts of fluoridated water each day.

3. Gum disease that wears away part of the gum and exposes part of the root. Gum disease will be discussed below. The exposed root does not have the protective benefit of enamel. Its covering is the softer, more easily damaged cementum.

4. Excessive acid exposure. This is the cornerstone in the development of caries. Acid on the teeth "burns" or eats away the enamel and creates holes that weaken, pain, and damage the tooth. Acid makes cavities. But what makes acid?

Steps (b), (c), and (d) in Figure 41-2 outline the production of acid. Two agents are needed to make acid: bacteria and food that can be broken down or fermented into acid.

The most highly fermentable foods are the carbohydrates, especially simple sugars or sticky carbohydrate foods. These foods enter the mouth and are broken down by the enzymes in the saliva by the process of chewing.

The bacteria then use these carbohydrates to make acid. As more acid is produced, the pH of the mouth lowers. Normally the pH of the saliva is a little above neutral, or around 7 to 8.[6] Acid production quickly causes it to drop. A pH of 5 to 5.5 may be sufficiently acidic to initiate decay.

The next agent in tooth decay is time (see Fig. 41-2). Bacteria begins to produce acid within 20 seconds of the first contact with food. The production lasts for 20 to 30 minutes after this contact. During this time the tooth is being bathed in a substance that may eat away at its protective surface. If cariogenic foods are introduced once again, the whole process begins anew. Constant snacking on these foods puts teeth at a much higher risk than cariogenic foods spaced several hours apart or taken with meals.

Unless preventive interventions are employed, the natural result of this process is tooth decay. Interventions that may help prevent or slow the process are discussed below.

Preventing Caries

Many persons believe tooth decay can be prevented by simply eliminating table sugar from the diet. As Figure 41-2 illustrates, any sugar, including sucrose, can worsen the problem. Persons who snack frequently on sugary foods might lower their risk by changing their snack patterns and not necessarily their snacks. Children with a diet free of refined sugar may not develop as many cavities as peers who consume high sugar snacks.[7] But there is more to it than this.

Effective prevention involves effective intervention. That is (referring back to Figure 41-2 once again) to prevent cavities it is necessary to protect or strengthen the susceptible tooth; to control and protect against cariogenic foods, and to keep acid production to a minimum. Nutrition is very important in all three of these steps.

Protect or Strengthen the Susceptible Tooth. Protection begins with adequate prenatal nutrition. Genetics cannot be changed but other risks can be minimized. A child then needs to obtain fluoride to help the developing teeth strengthen during the developmental years, from about 3 years to about 18 years. Obtaining fluoride during this "critical" period may decrease the chance of developing caries by up to 60%.[2] Natural fluoride is in some foods (especially seafoods and tea[8]) but the best sources are fluoridated water, fluoridated toothpaste, fluoride treatments, and fluoride rinses. Fluoride treatments are usually recommended for children during the crucial years but may also be used for adults who have periodontal disease if their soft roots have been exposed; the fluoride will strengthen cementum as well as enamel.

It is almost impossible to overdose on fluoride by wise use of these sources alone. However, some naturally fluoridated waters contain high levels of the trace mineral and may cause *fluorosis,* brown or black discoloration. Although these high levels of fluoride darken the teeth, and may discolor them unevenly, they do not seem to pose any health risks.[8] Extremely high levels of fluoride, however, can be toxic, so if water is naturally fluoridated, additional fluoride is not necessary and should not be used.

The professional who is best qualified to advise a person about fluoride is the dentist.

The tooth also needs to be protected by saliva. If some health condition has caused a very dry mouth, the liquid needs to be replaced — but not with sugary fluids! Plain water, sipped frequently, may help. Some tart foods — lemons, limes, artificially sweetened hard candies — help stimulate the glands to make more saliva. Special circumstances may dictate the use of artificial saliva.

A tooth is less suceptible to caries when it is *clean.* Frequent consistent brushing, flossing, and professional cleaning help keep teeth clean.

Control and Protect Against Cariogenic Foods. The sugars — sucrose, glucose, fructose and, to a lesser extent, lactose — seem to cause the most problems. In addition, the longer food is in the mouth, the more acid it will produce and the more damage it can do. Consequently, the foods that seem to be most likely to cause cavities are simple carbohydrate foods that stick to the teeth or are held in the mouth a long time. Some of these are listed opposite.

Just as some foods seem to be especially cariogenic, some foods seem to be protective. If they are included in a meal, together with a cariogenic food, there may be less risk of caries.

Protein is one of these foods. Protein foods may help stimulate saliva production and keep the *p*H of the saliva near or above neutral.[3,4] Fat is another food that may also affect *p*H, although its full role is not clear. Chocolate, although high in fat, does not seem to be as cariogenic as sugars without chocolate that are exposed for an equally long period of time to the teeth. High in both fat and protein, cheeses eaten after a meal or after a sugary snack seem to protect the tooth significantly against caries.[3,4,6]

Other foods, called "detergent foods," are often recommended because their naturally abrasive texture may help to "clean" the teeth. Celery and apples are two of these foods. They are certainly less cariogenic snacks than candy. However, they are not an adequate replacement for dental floss and a tooth brush. They cannot clean out tiny, hard-to-reach cracks and may leave food debris of their own.

Some sweeteners are also safe for the teeth,

FOODS ESPECIALLY LIKELY TO CAUSE CAVITIES, WITH SUGGESTED ALTERNATIVES

I. May Lead Rapidly to Cavities

A. Foods that stick

Candy apples
Caramel popcorn
Cookies
Dry fruit (including raisins)
Honey
"Natural" fruit rolls
Pie, cake, and sweet rolls
Potato chips
Toffee

B. Foods that may be constantly sucked or chewed

Chewy candy
Gum
Hard candy
Juice or milk in baby bottle
Regular carbonated beverages
Any caloric beverage frequently sipped

C. Highly acidic foods that may be sucked or chewed

Chewable vitamin C tablets
"Sour lemon"-type hard candies

II. Suggested Alternative Snack Foods

Cheese
Crackers with peanut butter
Fresh fruit
Milk
Peanuts
Pickles
Popcorn
Pretzels
Raw vegetables
Sugarless gum
Tomato and vegetable juices
Yogurt

since they have only a slight tendency to cause cavities. Non-nutritive sweeteners (aspartame, saccharin) do not contain much or any fermentable carbohydrate. Sugar alcohols (sorbitol, used in sugarless gums, xylitol, and mannitol) may be broken down in the mouth but they do not seem to promote acid production.[2,4]

Keep Acid Production to a Minimum. To minimize acid production, it is essential to control the *time* that cariogenic foods are exposed to bacteria. This can be done in several ways:

a. By brushing/flossing immediately after every meal or snack (which also minimizes "bad breath")

b. By eating snacks at well-spaced intervals and within planned time limits

c. By eating cariogenic foods only at mealtimes, when other foods may help protect the teeth.

All three of these decrease the time in which bacteria can create acid.

Nursing Bottle Syndrome

Nursing bottle syndrome is the name of a common cause of severe tooth decay in infants and young children. Infants often "break" their first tooth between 4 months and 6 months, but may not begin brushing until age two or later. Since cavities can form as soon as teeth are exposed to acid, these months may put baby teeth — and the permanent teeth growing beneath them — at a very high risk. The greatest risk is from the bottle.

The bottle may come in contact with the tooth more often and stay in the mouth much longer than foods. Anything in the bottle that contains calories from carbohydrate can cause cavities. Milk, juice, sugar water, or other sweet beverages all contain fermentable carbohydrates. When these beverages are exposed frequently to the teeth (or for a long, steady period when there is not much saliva, *e.g.,* when the child is sleeping) then teeth decay. They often decay badly. The front teeth, which suck on the nipple, are damaged the worst. This rampant caries in infants and children still on bottles is called "nursing bottle caries" or "nursing bottle mouth." Decayed baby teeth give children an unattractive appearance, make eating difficult and painful (at a time when food is especially critical for growth), and may affect the shape of the jaw or the space and positions of the underlying adult teeth. This syndrome is the product of neglect and can be prevented by limiting a child's exposure to sugars in the bottle, and weaning to a cup as early as possible. Outlined below are some basic guidelines for preventing nursing bottle syndrome.

PREVENTING NURSING BOTTLE SYNDROME

1. Begin keeping infant's teeth clean as soon as they erupt through the gum. Clean with plain wet washcloth or gauze

2. Limit bottle feedings
a. Give plain water or pacifier (or nothing) during nap and nighttimes
b. Never let child lie down for extended time to suck on bottle containing any caloric beverage such as milk, juice, fruit drinks, or sweetened water

3. If child carries bottle everywhere, like a "security blanket," fill it with plain water only

4. Wean from bottle to cup as soon as possible (12 months to 18 months)

5. Encourage child to imitate adults and use toothbrush (with or without toothpaste) as soon as possible (18 months to 24 months)

Periodontal Disease

Periodontal disease is defined as a "painless, slowly progressing disease characterized by microbial colonization of plaque on adjacent tooth surfaces extending into deeper periodontal tissue."[5] Figure 41-1 illustrates some aspects of gum or periodontal disease: gingivitis or an inflamed gingiva (the surface tissue in direct contact with the tooth), and periodontitis, the inflamed periodontal membranes.

Periodontal disease is the primary reason persons over age 35 lose their teeth.[9] Because it is painless periodontal disease is often undetected until it is too late. Many people lose otherwise healthy teeth prematurely, simply because the gums have become so weak, worn away, and diseased that they can no longer hold the teeth securely.

Most important, periodontal disease is as preventable as caries. The causal factors can be minimized and the gums protected.

Cause

Periodontal disease begins with an irritant. The most common irritant is *plaque,* illustrated in diagram (d) of Figure 41-2. Plaque is a sticky substance that bacteria can create and in which it can grow. Bacteria make plaque with the acid by-products of fermentable carbohydrate. Plaque then sticks to the teeth and may build up in areas that are not thoroughly cleaned, for example, the cracks and crevices where the tooth and the gingiva come together. Plaque that is not removed can harden to form mineral deposits called *calculus.*

Calculus is an irritant to gums. Calculus and bacteria on new plaque can work together to inflame the gingiva. This inflammation, gingivitis, is the earliest type of periodontal disease. Inflamed gingiva can then inflame the periodontal membranes under the surface, causing periodontitis. Periodontitis can wear away at the alveolar bone. As bone is destroyed, the tooth is held less securely in the gum. It may loosen and need to be removed.

Periodontal disease may also develop from gums weakened by malnutrition. Malnutrition does not cause periodontal disease, but it may increase the risk by weakening the tissue's ability to resist infection or abrasion.[1,4] Bleeding gums may be a sign of malnutrition, of periodontal disease, or of some other underlying disorder or imbalance.

Gum disease may lead not only to the loss of teeth; gums may also be irritated by the presence of false teeth. Dentures rarely fit as well as natural teeth. They have less sensation and are more awkward to use. If they slip or fit poorly, the gum may be irritated and become diseased.

Prevention

Preventing periodontal disease is far less traumatic than treating it once it occurs. Prevention involves developing habits that, when continued for life, may keep teeth and gums healthy far into old age. Dental problems and tooth loss are not inevitable results of aging; they are predictable results of, for the most part, preventable diseases. Periodontal disease may be prevented and the progress of existing disease may be slowed or stopped by treatment.

A cornerstone of treatment is that of regular checkups and cleaning by a qualified dentist. Floss helps keep teeth and gums clean but only regular dental visits can remove the build-up of calculus, since this hardened plaque sticks like glue and ultimately may appear to be a normal part of the tooth.

A diet that meets the RDA for all nutrients gives the body its best protection against infection. Prevention also involves control of the acid and irritants that begin the process of wearing away the gum. The same dietary changes that help minimize acid production also help keep gums healthy. When less acid is produced, less plaque is likely to form. Dental flossing is usually the most effective means of keeping gums healthy. Floss reaches crevices a toothbrush cannot reach and removes debris. Saliva does not have the same protective effect on the gums that it does on the teeth.

It is interesting to note that among the skeletons found under the ruins of the Mt. Vesuvius eruption on Pompeii and Herculaneum in AD 79, there were few problems with dental caries (probably a result of diet) but there were some signs of periodontal disease in very young adults. "That's why you floss every day," remarked the physical anthropologist involved in this discovery.[10]

SPECIAL PROBLEMS

From the sixth month of life into old age individuals depend on their teeth to chew—and enjoy—nutritious foods. As a result certain dental diseases and chronic states that involve oral damage can form special risks. For example:

1. The elderly often do not have their own teeth, and depend on dentures that can create problems of their own. Many elderly need to modify the texture of their diet in order to adapt to the limitations in chewing or sensing foods. Diets that modify texture were described in Chapter 35.

2. The poor or socially handicapped often eat poorly and do not care properly for their teeth and gums. Malnutrition may weaken their resistance to dental disease. At highest risk in this group are older men who live alone (and who are also at risk for scurvy),[5] mentally or physically handicapped adults, alcoholics, and the undereducated poor whose diet and dental habits are often inadequate and who may be unaware of their risk. These individuals may lose their teeth and develop mechanical feeding problems early in life. By the time they appear at the doctor or the dentist, the damage is done. Treatment should then involve teaching them to compensate, and to begin caring for whatever functions are left.

3. Individuals with certain diseases that affect nutrition or blood flow. There is some de-

Table 41-1

Tips for At-Home Care of Xerostomia

What to Use	Why	Comments
Daily: gently brush gums, tongue, and mouth tissue with (soft!) toothbrush	Stimulates production of saliva; keeps blood flowing to these areas; important for health	Check with health care provider if gums bleed easily
Plain tap or spring water—sip throughout the day	Water is a natural lubricant; provides no calories and no sugar; may contain essential fluoride	There is no need to be concerned about too much water. Water helps prevent constipation. At least 2 quarts of fluids each day are recommended for everyone for general health.
"Dietetic" or "sugar-free" candy, gum, and/or mints	Contain "sorbitol," a natural sugar alcohol that has as many calories as sugar but does not "feed" oral bacteria and cause cavities	A high intake of sorbitol may lead to gas or diarrhea
Beverages—hot or cold—sweetened with artificial sweeteners (*e.g.,* saccharin or aspartame)	Very few calories. Artificial sweeteners do not promote tooth decay	Saccharin has been found to cause cancer in laboratory rats; aspartame has not been found to cause cancer; if in doubt about artificial sweeteners, learn to drink coffee or tea plain
Fruit juices	Contain sugar that does promote cavities but sugar is not "retentive" or sticky so less likely to cause decay. Does provide calories; may also provide vitamins	Limit intake of juices to short-term, occasional, daily use; constant "sipping" on fruit juice may be as cariogenic as other sugar sources.

bate about whether diabetics have a higher-than-normal risk of dental disease resulting from peripheral vascular disease, but this may be true.[3] The teeth and gums may not acquire the blood necessary to keep tissue healthy. Persons with malabsorption syndromes such as celiac sprue or Crohn's ileitis may develop deficiencies in the vitamins and minerals needed for good oral health. Prolonged malnutrition can seriously weaken both teeth and gums.

4. Radiation treatment for oral cancer often destroys or damages salivary glands. Dry mouth and taste changes are common. This syndrome is called *xerostomia.* These cancer patients have an extremely high risk of severe caries unless they somehow replace or restore saliva. Nutritionists and other medical personnel often work intensively with these clients to help find the best alternative for their individual situations. Some tips are listed in Table 41-1.

STUDY QUESTIONS

1. Define the following terms and briefly state the cause:
   - Fluorosis
   - Periodontitis
   - Xerostomia
   - Calculus
   - Nursing bottle syndrome

2. Why is saliva important?

3. What does fluoride do? What are some common sources of fluoride? How long is fluoride necessary in the development of teeth?

4. List and describe at least three separate factors that cause cavities.

5. What types of foods promote cavities? What types of food protect against cavities?

6. "Dental diseases are caused by habits, not foods." How would you respond to this statement?

7. Why do people often lose otherwise healthy teeth as they grow older?

8. List and describe briefly at least two social circumstances or behaviors that may put certain people at special risk for dental disease. Explain the risk.

REFERENCES

1. Jacobs HH: Nutrition and the development of oral tissues. J Am Diet Assoc 83(1): 50–53, July 1983
2. DePaola DP, Alfano MC: Diet and oral health. Nutrition Today, pp 6ff, May–June 1977
3. American Academy of Pedodontics: Changing Perspectives in Nutrition and Caries Research. New York, Medcom, 1979
4. Alfano MC, Diet and nutrition in the etiology and prevention of oral disease. J Dent Res (59)DII: 2194–2202, December 1980
5. Touyz LZG: Vitamin C, oral scurvy and periodontal disease. South African Med J 65: 838–842, May 26, 1984
6. Jenkins N: Diet and dental caries. National Livestock and Meat Board Food and Nutrition News 56(5): 29–32, November–December 1984
7. Silverstein SJ, Knapp JF, Kircos L et al: Dental caries prevalence in children with a diet free of refined sugar. Am J Public Health 73(10): 1196–1199, 1983
8. Shaw JH, Sweeney EA: Nutrition in relation to dental medicine. In Goodhart RE, Shils ME (eds): Modern Nutrition in Health and Disease, 6th ed, pp 852–891. Philadelphia, Lea & Febiger, 1980
9. Fujii DG, Palmer CA: Nutrition in Dentistry for the Nutritionist. Boston, Tufts University School of Dental Medicine/Frances Stern Nutrition Center, 1978
10. Gore R: The dead do tell tales at Vesuvius. National Geographic 165(5): 557–613, 1984

APPENDICES

APPENDIX 1

The Recommended Dietary Allowances

Food and Nutrition Board, National Academy of Sciences —
National Research Council

**Recommended Daily Allowances,[a] Revised 1980 Designed for the Maintenance
of Good Nutrition of Practically all Healthy People in the USA**

	Age	Weight		Height		Energy	Protein	Fat-Soluble Vitamins					
								Vitamin A Activity		Vitamin D		Vitamin E Activity[d]	
	(years)	(kg)	(lbs)	(cm)	(in)	(kcal)	(g)	(re)[b]	(iu)	(iu)	(μg)[c]	(mgα t.e.)	
Infants	0.0–0.5	6	13	60	24	kg × 115	kg × 2.2	420	1,400	400	10	3	
	0.5–1.0	9	20	71	28	kg × 105	kg × 2.0	400	2,000	400	10	4	
Children	1–3	13	29	90	35	1,300	23	400	2,000	400	10	5	
	4–6	20	44	112	44	1,700	30	500	2,500	400	10	6	
	7–10	28	62	132	52	2,400	34	700	3,300	400	10	7	
Males	11–14	45	99	157	62	2,700	45	1,000	5,000	400	10	8	
	15–18	66	145	176	69	2,800	56	1,000	5,000	400	10	10	
	19–22	70	154	177	70	2,900	56	1,000	5,000	300	7.5	10	
	23–50	70	154	178	70	2,700	56	1,000	5,000	200	5.0	10	
	51+	70	154	178	70	2,400[i]	56	1,000	5,000	200	5.0	10	
Females	11–14	46	101	157	62	2,200	46	800	4,000	400	10	8	
	15–18	55	120	163	64	2,100	46	800	4,000	400	10	8	
	19–22	55	120	163	64	2,100	44	800	4,000	300	7.5	8	
	23–50	55	120	163	64	2,000	44	800	4,000	200	5.0	8	
	51+	55	120	163	64	1,800[i]	44	800	4,000	200	5.0	8	
Pregnant						+300	+30	+200	+1,000	+200	+5	+2	
Lactating						+500	+20	+400	+2,000	+200	+5	+3	

[a] The allowances are intended to provide for individual variations among most normal persons as they live in the United States under usual environmental stresses. Diets should be based on a variety of common foods in order to provide other nutrients for which human requirements have been less well defined.

[b] Retinol equivalents. 1 Retinol equivalent = 1 μg retinol or 6 μg Beta carotene.

[c] As cholecalciferol. 10 μg cholecalciferol = 400 I.U. vitamin D.

[d] Alpha tocopherol equivalents. 1 mg d-Alpha-tocopherol = 1 Alpha T.E.

[e] 1 NE (niacin equivalent) is equal to 1 mg of niacin or 60 mg of dietary tryptophan.

Water-Soluble Vitamins							Minerals					
Vita-min C (mg)	Fola-cin^f (μg)	Nia-cin^e (mg n.e.)	Ribo-flavin (mg)	Thia-min (mg)	Vita-min B_6 (mg)	Vita-min B_{12} (μg)	Cal-cium (mg)	Phos-phorus (mg)	Iodine (μg)	Iron (mg)	Magne-sium (mg)	Zinc (mg)
35	30	6	0.4	0.3	0.3	0.5^g	360	240	40	10	50	3
35	45	8	0.6	0.5	0.6	1.5	540	360	50	15	70	5
45	100	9	0.8	0.7	0.9	2.0	800	800	70	15	150	10
45	200	11	1.0	0.9	1.3	2.5	800	800	90	10	200	10
45	300	16	1.4	1.2	1.6	3.0	800	800	120	10	250	10
50	400	18	1.6	1.4	1.8	3.0	1,200	1,200	150	18	350	15
60	400	18	1.7	1.4	2.0	3.0	1,200	1,200	150	18	400	15
60	400	19	1.7	1.5	2.2	3.0	800	800	150	10	350	15
60	400	18	1.6	1.4	2.2	3.0	800	800	150	10	350	15
60	400	16	1.4	1.2	2.2	3.0	800	800	150	10	350	15
50	400	15	1.3	1.1	1.8	3.0	1,200	1,200	150	18	300	15
60	400	14	1.3	1.1	2.0	3.0	1,200	1,200	150	18	300	15
60	400	14	1.3	1.1	2.0	3.0	800	800	150	18	300	15
60	400	13	1.2	1.0	2.0	3.0	800	800	150	18	300	15
60	400	13	1.2	1.0	2.0	3.0	800	800	150	10	300	15
+20	+400	+2	+0.3	+0.4	+0.6	+1.0	+400	+400	+25	h	+150	+5
+40	+100	+5	+0.5	+0.5	+0.5	+1.0	+400	+400	+50	h	+150	+10

^f The folacin allowances refer to dietary sources as determined by *Lactobacillus casei* assay after treatment with enzymes ("conjugases") to make polyglutamyl forms of the vitamin available to the test organism.

^g The RDA for vitamin B_{12} in infants is based on average concentration of the vitamin in human milk. The allowances after weaning are based on energy intake (as recommended by the American Academy of Pediatrics) and consideration of other factors such as intestinal absorption.

^h The increased requirements during pregnancy cannot be met by the iron content of habitual American diets nor by the existing iron stores of many women; therefore the use of 30–60 mg of supplemental iron is recommended. Iron needs during lactation are not substantially different from those of nonpregnant women, but continued supplementation of the mother for 2–3 months after parturition is advisable in order to replenish stores depleted by pregnancy.

^i This is the recommended energy intake for individuals aged 51–75. While nutrient needs for older individuals have not been established, the US RDA recommends energy intake for men over 75 is 2050 kcals, and for women, 1600 kcals.

US Recommended Dietary Allowances (US RDA), used in product labels

	Protein (g)	Vitamin A (iu)	Vitamin D (iu)	Vitamin E (iu)	Vitamin C (mg)	Folic Acid (mg)	Thiamin (mg)	Ribo-flavin (mg)
Infants[1]	18[2] 25	1,500	400	5	35	0.1	0.5	0.6
Children under 4 Years	20[3] 28	2,500	400	10	40	0.2	0.7	0.8
Adults & Children 4 or More Years of Age	45[4] 65	5,000	400	30	60	0.4	1.5	1.7
Pregnant or Lactating Women	[5]	8,000	400	30	60	0.8	1.7	2.0

[1] Infant less than 1 year
[2] 18 g if quality equal to or greater than casein
   25 g if quality less than casein
[3] 20 g if quality equal to or greater than casein
   28 g if quality less than casein
[4] 45 g if quality equal to or greater than casein
   65 g if quality less than casein
[5] No protein stipulation provided for pregnant or lactating women
   (NAS/NRC RDA suggests + 30 g for pregnant and + 20 g for lactating women).

Niacin (mg)	Vitamin B_6 (mg)	Vitamin B_{12} (μg)	Biotin (mg)	Panto-thenic Acid (mg)	Calcium (g)	Phos-phorus (g)	Iodine (μg)	Iron (mg)	Mag-nesium (mg)	Copper (mg)	Zinc (mg)
8	0.4	2	0.15	3	0.6	0.5	45	15	70	0.6	5
9	0.7	3	0.15	5	0.8	0.8	70	10	200	1.0	8
20	2.0	6	0.30	10	1.0	1.0	150	18	400	2.0	15
20	2.5	8	0.30	10	1.3	1.3	150	18	450	2.0	15

APPENDIX 2

Exchange Lists for Meal Planning

LIST 1: MILK LIST
(Includes **Non-Fat,** Low-Fat, and Whole Milk)

One Exchange of Milk contains 12 grams of carbohydrate and 8 grams of protein.

Milk is a basic food for your Meal Plan for very good reasons. Milk is the leading source of calcium. It is a good source of phosphorus, protein, some of the B-complex vitamins, including folacin and vitamin B_{12}, and vitamins A and D. Magnesium is also found in milk.

Since it is a basic ingredient in many recipes you will not find it difficult to include milk in your Meal Plan. Milk can be used not only to drink but can be added to cereal, coffee, tea and other foods.

This List shows the kinds and amounts of milk or milk products to use for one Milk Exchange. Those which appear in **bold type** are **non-fat.** Low-Fat and Whole Milk contain saturated fat.

Non-Fat Fortified Milk

Skim or non-fat milk	1 cup
Powdered (non-fat dry, before adding liquid)	1/3 cup
Canned, evaporated — skim milk	1/2 cup
Buttermilk made from skim milk	1 cup

(Source: Exchange Lists for Meal Planning prepared by American Diabetes Association/American Dietetic Association. Adapted from © 1976, © 1986 editions. Reprinted with permission.)

Yogurt made from skim milk (plain, unflavored)	1 cup
Low-Fat Fortified Milk	
1% fat fortified milk	1 cup
2% fat fortified milk	1 cup
Yogurt made from 2% fortified milk (plain, unflavored)	1 cup
Whole Milk	
Whole milk	1 cup
Canned, evaporated whole milk	1/2 cup
Buttermilk made from whole milk	1 cup
Yogurt made from whole milk (plain, unflavored)	1 cup

Fat content and calories respectively for skim, 2% lowfat and whole milk are: trace fat, 90 calories; 5 grams fat and 120 calories; 8 grams fat and 150 calories.

LIST 2: VEGETABLE LIST

One Exchange of Vegetables contains about 5 grams of carbohydrate, 2 grams of protein and 25 calories.

The generous use of many vegetables, served either alone or in other foods such as casseroles, soups or salads, contributes to sound health and vitality.

Dark green and deep yellow vegetables are among the leading sources of vitamin A. Many of the vegetables in this group are notable sources of vitamin C—asparagus, broccoli, brussels sprouts, cabbage, cauliflower, collards, kale, dandelion, mustard and turnip greens, spinach, rutabagas, tomatoes and turnips. A number, including broccoli, brussels sprouts, beet greens, chard and tomato juice, are particularly good sources of potassium. High folacin values are found in asparagus, beets, broccoli, brussels sprouts, cauliflower, collards, kale and lettuce. Moderate amounts of vitamin B_6 are supplied by broccoli, brussels sprouts, cauliflower, collards, spinach, sauerkraut and tomatoes and tomato juice. Fiber is present in all vegetables.

Whether you serve them cooked or raw, wash all vegetables even though they look clean. If fat is added in the preparation, omit the equivalent number of Fat Exchanges. The average amount of fat contained in a Vegetable Exchange that is cooked with fat meat or other fats is one Fat Exchange.

This List shows the kinds of **vegetables** to use for one Vegetable Exchange. One Exchange is ½ cup.

Asparagus	**Greens:**
Bean Sprouts	**Mustard**
Beets	**Spinach**
Broccoli	**Turnip**
Brussels Sprouts	**Mushrooms**
Cabbage	**Okra**
Carrots	**Onions**
Cauliflower	**Rhubarb**
Celery	**Rutabaga**
Eggplant	**Sauerkraut**
Green Pepper	**String Beans, green or**
Greens:	**yellow**
Beet	**Summer Squash**
Chards	**Tomatoes**
Collards	**Tomato Juice**
Dandelion	**Turnips**
Kale	**Vegetable Juice Cocktail**
	Zucchini

The following **raw vegetables** may be used as desired:

Chicory	**Lettuce**
Chinese Cabbage	**Parsley**
Endive	**Radishes**
Escarole	**Watercress**

Starchy Vegetables are found in the Bread Exchange List.

LIST 3: FRUIT LIST

One Exchange of Fruit contains 15 grams of carbohydrate and 60 calories.

Everyone likes to buy fresh fruits when they are in the height of their season. But you can also buy fresh fruits and can or freeze them for off-season use. For variety serve fruits as a salad or in combination with other foods for dessert.

Fruits are valuable for vitamins, minerals and fiber. Vitamin C is abundant in citrus fruits and fruit juices and is found in raspberries, strawberries, mangoes, cantaloupes, honeydews and papayas. The better sources of vitamin A among these fruits include fresh or dried apricots, mangoes, cantaloupes, nectarines, yellow peaches and persimmons. Oranges, orange juice and cantaloupe provide more folacin than most of the other fruits in this listing. Many fruits are a valuable source of potassium, especially apricots, bananas, several of the berries, grapefruit, grapefruit juice, mangoes, cantaloupes, honeydews, nectarines, oranges, orange juice and peaches.

Fruit may be used fresh, dried, canned or frozen, cooked or raw, as long as no sugar is added.

This List shows the kinds and amounts of **fruits** to use for one Fruit Exchange.

Apple	1 small
Apple Juice	1/2 cup
Applesauce (unsweetened)	1/2 cup
Apricots, fresh	4 medium
Apricots, dried	7 halves
Banana (9 in. long)	1/2
Berries	
Blackberries	3/4 cup
Blueberries	3/4 cup
Raspberries	1 cup
Strawberries	1-1/4 cup
Cherries	12 large
Cider	1/2 cup
Dates	2-1/2
Figs, fresh	2
Figs, dried	1-1/2
Grapefruit	1/2
Grapefruit Juice	1/2 cup
Grapes	15
Grape Juice	1/3 cup
Mango	1/2 small

Melon

Cantaloupe	1/3 small
Honeydew	1/8 medium
Watermelon	1-1/4 cup
Nectarine	1 small
Orange	1 small
Orange Juice	1/2 cup
Papaya	1 cup
Peach	1 medium
Pear	1 small
Persimmon, native	2 medium
Pineapple	3/4 cup
Pineapple Juice	1/2 cup
Plums	2 medium
Prunes	3 medium
Prune Juice	1/3 cup
Raisins	2 tablespoons
Tangerine	2 medium

Cranberries may be used as desired if no sugar is added.

LIST 4: STARCH/BREAD LIST
(Includes **Bread, Cereal** and **Starchy Vegetables**)

One Exchange of Bread contains 15 grams of carbohydrate, 3 grams of protein and 80 calories.

In this List, whole-grain and enriched breads and cereals, germ and bran products and dried beans and peas are good sources of iron and among the better sources of thiamin. The whole-grain, bran and germ products have more fiber than products made from refined flours. Dried beans and peas are also good sources of fiber. Wheat germ, bran, dried beans, potatoes, lima beans, parsnips, pumpkin and winter squash are particularly good sources of potassium. The better sources of folacin in this listing include whole-wheat bread, wheat germ, dried beans, corn, lima beans, parsnips, green peas, pumpkin and sweet potato.

Starchy vegetables are included in this List, because they contain the same amount of carbohydrate and protein as one slice of bread.

Bread

White (including French and Italian)	1 slice
Whole Wheat	1 slice
Rye or Pumpernickel	1 slice
Raisin	1 slice
Bagel, small	1/2
English Muffin, small	1/2
Plain Roll, bread	1
Frankfurter Roll	1/2
Hamburger Bun	1/2
Dried Bread Crumbs	3 Tbs.
Tortilla, 6″	1

This List shows the kinds and amounts of **Beans, Cereals, Starchy Vegetables** and Prepared Foods to use for one Bread Exchange. Those which appear in **bold type** are **low-fat.**

Cereal

Bran Flakes	1/2 cup
Other ready-to-eat unsweetened Cereal	3/4 cup
Puffed Cereal (unfrosted)	1-1/2 cups
Cereal (cooked)	1/2 cup
Grits (cooked)	1/2 cup
Rice or Barley (cooked)	1/3 cup
Pasta (cooked), Spaghetti, Noodles, Macaroni	1/2 cup
Popcorn (popped, no fat added)	3 cups
Cornmeal (dry)	2-1/2 Tbs.
Flour	2-1/2 Tbs.
Wheat Germ	3 Tbs.

Crackers

Animal Crackers	8
Graham, 2-1/2″ sq.	3
Matzoth	3/4 oz.
Oyster	24
Pretzels	3/4 oz.
Rye Wafers, 2″ × 3-1/2″	4
Saltines	6
Whole Wheat Crackers	3/4 oz.

Dried Beans, Peas and Lentils

Beans, Peas, Lentils (dried and cooked)	1/3 cup
Baked Beans, no pork (canned)	1/4 cup

Starchy Vegetables

Corn	1/2 cup
Corn on Cob (6 in. long)	1
Lima Beans	1/2 cup
Peas, Green (canned or frozen)	1/2 cup
Plantain	1/2 cup
Potato, White	1 small
Potato (mashed)	1/2 cup

Pumpkin	3/4 cup
Winter Squash, Acorn or Butternut	3/4 cup
Yam or Sweet Potato	1/3 cup

Starch Foods Prepared with Fat
 Count as one starch/bread
 serving plus one fat serving:

Biscuit 2-1/2 ″ dia.	1
Chow Mein Noodles	1/2 cup
Corn Bread, 2″ cube	1
Crackers, round butter type	6
French Fried Potatoes, 2″ – 3-1/2″ long	10 (1-1/2 oz.)
Muffin, plain, small	1
Pancake, 4″ across	2
Stuffing Bread (prepared)	1/4 cup
Taco Shell, 6″ dia.	2
Waffle, 4-1/2″ square	1
Whole Wheat Crackers, fat added (e.g., Triscuit®)	4 – 6 (1 oz.)

LIST 5: MEAT LIST
Lean and Medium Fat Choices

One Exchange of Meat (1 oz.) contains 7 grams of protein. One lean choice has 3 grams fat and 55 calories; one medium fat choice has 5 grams fat and 75 calories.

All of the foods in the Meat Exchange Lists are good sources of protein and many are also good sources of iron, zinc, vitamin B_{12} (present only in foods of animal origin) and other vitamins of the vitamin B-complex.

Cholesterol is of animal origin. Foods of plant origin have no cholesterol.

Oysters are outstanding for their high content of zinc. Crab, liver, trimmed lean meats, the dark muscle meat of turkey, dried beans and peas and peanut butter all have much less zinc than oysters but are still good sources.

Dried beans, peas and peanut butter are particularly good sources of magnesium; also potassium.

Your choice of meat groups through the week will depend on your blood lipid values. Consult with your diet counselor and your physician regarding your selection.

You may use the meat, fish or other Meat choices that are prepared for the family when no fat or flour have been added. If meat is fried, use the fat included in the Meal Plan. Meat juices with the fat removed may be used with your meat or vegetables for added flavor. Be certain to trim off all visible fat and measure meat after it has been cooked. A three-ounce serving of cooked meat is about equal to four ounces of raw meat.

To plan a diet low in saturated fat and cholesterol, choose only those Exchanges in **bold type.**

Beef:	**USDA Good or Choice grades of lean beef such as Round, Sirloin Flank, Tenderloin, Chipped Beef;** Ground Beef, Roast, Steaks and Meatloaf	1 oz.
Lamb:	Most Lamb (e.g., chops, legs, roast) is medium-fat	1 oz.
Pork:	**Ham, Canadian Bacon, Tenderloin,** Boston Butt, Chops, Loin Roast	1 oz.
Veal:	**Leg, Loin, Rib, Shank, Shoulder,** Cutlets	1 oz.
Poultry:	**Meat without skin of Chicken, Turkey, Cornish Hen,** Duck, Goose, Ground Turkey	1 oz.
Fish:	**Any fresh or frozen Mackerel, Crab and Lobster,** Tuna, Salmon (in oil)	1oz. 1/4 cup
	Clams, Oysters, Scallops, Shrimp,	5 or 1 oz.
	Sardines, drained	3
Diet Cheese (less than 80 cals/oz.)		1 oz.
Grated Parmesan		2 Tbs.
Cottage Cheese, Dry and 2% butterfat or part-skim ricotta		1/4 cup
Egg substitutes		1/4 cup
Eggs (high cholesterol; limit to 3 per week)		1
Tofu (2-1/2″ × 2-3/4″ × 1″)		4 oz.
Liver, Heart, Kidney, Sweet Breads		1 oz.

High Fat Meats and Substitutes

These are high in saturated fat, cholesterol and calories and should be used only 3 times per week. One exchange contains 7 grams protein, 8 grams fat and 100 calories.

Beef:	USDA Prime cuts, as Ribs, Corned Beef	1 oz.
Lamb:	Ground Patties	1 oz.
Pork:	Spare Ribs, Ground Pork, Pork Sausage	1 oz.
Fish:	Any fried fish product	1 oz.
Cheese:	All regular cheeses, as American, Blue, Cheddar, Monterey, Swiss	1 oz.
Other:	Luncheon Meat, Sausage,	1 oz.
	Knockwurst, Bratwurst	1 frank
	Chicken or Turkey	(1/10
	Frankfurter	lb.)
	Peanut Butter (unsaturated fat)	1 Tbs.

Beef or pork frankfurters count as 1 high fat meat plus one fat choice.

LIST 6: FAT EXCHANGES

One Exchange of Fat contains 5 grams of fat and 45 calories.

Fats are of both animal and vegetable origin and range from liquid oils to hard fats.

Oils are fats that remain liquid at room temperature and are usually of vegetable origin. Common fats obtained from vegetables are corn oil, olive oil and peanut oil. Some of the common animal fats are butter and bacon fat.

Since all fats are concentrated sources of calories, foods on this List should be measured carefully to control weight. Margarine, butter, cream and cream cheese contain vitamin A. Use the fats on this List in the amounts on the Meal Plan.

This List shows the kinds and amounts of Fat-Containing Foods to use for one Fat Exchange. To plan a diet low in Saturated Fat select only those Exchanges which appear in **bold type.** They are **Polyunsaturated.**

Margarine, soft, tub or stick*	1 teaspoon
Avocado (4″ in diameter)**	1/8
Oil, Corn, Cottonseed, Safflower, Soy, Sunflower	1 teaspoon
Oil, Olive**	1 teaspoon
Oil, Peanut**	1 teaspoon
Olives**	10 small or 5 large
Almonds**	6 whole
Pecans**	2 large whole
Peanuts**	
Spanish	20 whole
Virginia	10 whole
Walnuts	2 whole
Nuts, other**	1 tablespoon
Seeds; Pinenuts, Sunflower (without shells)	1 tablespoon
Pumpkin Seeds	2 teaspoons
Margarine, regular stick	1 teaspoon
Butter	1 teaspoon
Bacon fat	1 teaspoon
Bacon, crisp	1 strip
Cream, light	2 tablespoons
Cream, sour	2 tablespoons
Cream, heavy	1 tablespoon
Cream Cheese	1 tablespoon
French dressing***	1 tablespoon
Italian dressing***	1 tablespoon
Lard	1 teaspoon
Mayonnaise***	1 teaspoon
Salad dressing, mayonnaise type ***	2 teaspoons
Salad dressing, reduced calorie	2 tablespoons
Salt pork	1/4 oz.

---

* Made with corn, cottonseed, safflower, soy or sunflower oil only

** Fat content is primarily monounsaturated

*** If made with corn, cottonseed, safflower, soy or sunflower oil can be used on fat modified diet

For more information or an updated copy of the Exchange List booklet for use with patients, write to:

The American Diabetes Association
1660 Duke St.
Alexandria, VA 22314
OR
The American Dietetic Association
430 North Michigan Ave.
Chicago, IL 60611

GLOSSARY

Note: Number (in parentheses) at the end of each listing indicates the chapter in which the word first appears.

Absorption Passage of digested food and nutrients through the walls of the cell, blood vessels, or into some other segment of the digestive tract. (1)

Achiote Ground annato seeds, a common coloring and seasoning in Hispanic foods. (18)

Acid Substance with a pH between 0 and 6.9 on a scale of 14. Opposite: basic or alkaline. (1)

Acidosis Life-threatening state in which the pH of the body fluids drops below 7.3. May be caused by disorders of respiration (breathing) or metabolism. (28)

Aerobic Using oxygen. (17)

Aflotoxin A poisonous mold that may grow on peanuts. (40)

Alcohol A chemical substance produced by distillation or fermentation of carbohydrate foods (ethyl alcohol) or wood (methyl alcohol, which is toxic). Ethyl alcohol provides 7 kilocalories per gram of alcohol. (11)

Alkalosis Life-threatening state in which the pH of body fluids rises above 7.4. May be caused by disorders of respiration (breathing) or metabolism. (28)

Alimentary Pertaining to feeding. (1)

Alimentary Canal See *Digestive tract.* (1)

Alimentary Tract See *Digestive tract.* (1)

Alimentation Feeding. (1)

Alkaline The quality of having a pH between 7.1 and 14 on a scale of 14. Also called *basic.* Opposite: acidic. (1)

Allergen An antigen whose presence in the blood causes an allergic reaction. Most allergenic substances are normal plants or foods to which an individual has developed a sensitivity. (40)

Allergy An extreme sensitivity to one or more substances. The immune system reacts to the presence of these substances (in the air or in food) as if they were germs or a virus. See also *Food sensitivity.* (40)

Amino Acid The "building blocks" that make proteins. There are 22 amino acids present in food. Only 8 (9 in infants) are "essential" parts of the diet. The body can form the "nonessential" amino acids in the body from the essential amino acids. Different types of proteins contain different groups of the amino acids in varying proportions. (3)

Amygdalin See *Laetrile.* (30)

Amylopectin Starch made of branching or networklike structures of glucose. (4)

Amylose Starch made of long polysaccharide chains of glucose. (4)

Anorexia Loss of appetite. (29)

Anorexia Nervosa A rare self-starving syndrome chiefly of women. Usually begins before age 25 and, untreated, may persist for years. Women (or men) fear food, the loss of control, deny their extreme thinness, may exercise vigorously to prevent weight gain, and usually require intense, long-term medical care, including psychiatric counseling, before recovery can begin. (29)

Anthropometrics Physical measurements of parts of the human body. May include height, weight, triceps skinfold thickness (TSF), mid-arm muscle circumference (MAMC), and other measures. (12)

Antibody Protein substance formed by the body to help destroy or rid the body of foreign agents (called antigens), such as germs, viruses, or allergenic substances. (3)

Antigen Foreign substance (i.e., not part of the body) such as a germ, virus, or allergen that enters the body and causes the immune system to produce antibodies. (40)

Antioxidant A substance that helps protect cells from the destruction and changes that may occur after exposure to oxygen. Lemon juice acts as a antioxidant on apples and prevents the cut fruit from turning brown from oxygen exposure. (30)

Arachidonic Acid An essential fatty acid that can be produced by the body. (5)

Ascites The presence of excess fluid in the extracellular space of the peritoneal cavity (the tissuelike sack in the abdomen that encloses the major organs). Often results from fluid seeping from the cells as the result of osmolar or nutrient imbalances. (28)

Ascorbic Acid Vitamin C. (7)

Aspiration Inhaling into the lungs (38)

Atherosclerosis Also called arteriosclerosis; a common form of heart disease characterized by layers of fat, cholesterol, and other plaque deposits that build up on the inner wall of the blood vessels and may lead to blockage and heart attacks. (5)

ATP Adenosine triphosphate. The form of energy used by the body for life and growth. (2)

Avidin A protein in raw egg white that may combine with the vitamin, biotin, and prevent biotin from being absorbed. (7)

Basal Metabolic Rate The amount of energy needed for a person to maintain life when the body is at rest. (2)

Basic Four General division of all foods grouped by necessary nutrients (other than energy and fat). Four groups include dairy, meat and meat substitutes, fruits and vegetables, and grains and cereals. An inexact but helpful guideline for planning and preparing nutritionally balanced meals. (12)

Benign Harmless (30)

Beriberi Thiamin deficiency disease. (7)

Bile Liquid that helps digest fats or lipids. Made in the gallbladder and released into the duodenal area of the small intestine via the "common bile duct." (1)

Blood Sugar Blood concentration of the monosaccharide glucose. (4)

BMR See *Basal metabolic rate.* (2)

Bolus Feeding Feeding of a large amount of nutrients at one time. (38)

Botulism Food poisoning caused by spores of the organism, *clostridium botulinum.* May contaminate unopened foods that have not been prepared properly. Reactions may be very serious and sometimes lead to death. Must be treated immediately. (15)

Bran The outer hull of a grain. Also called the chaff. Is not completely digestible and is therefore considered fiber. (10)

Buffers Systems and substances that help keep normal body acid-base balance. Buffers help protect against extreme change. (28)

Bulimarexia The disorder of anorexia nervosa that also involves the practice of bulimia. (37)

Bulimia The regular practice of eating very large quantities of food at one sitting. May be followed by intentional purging through vomiting or laxative abuse in order to prevent weight gain. (37)

Cachexia Extreme emaciation, malnutrition, and weakness following some disease, trauma, or starvation syndrome. Common in some cancers. A cachectic person is hypermetabolic, has low immunity, and may easily die from minor illnesses. (30)

CAD Coronary artery (or heart) disease. (25)

Calculus Mineral deposits on the tooth formed from hardened plaque that has not been removed. (41)

Calorie The amount of heat (i.e., energy) needed to raise one gram of water from 15 to 16 degrees Celsius. Food energy is commonly measured in kilocalories (1 kilocalorie or Kcal equals 1000 calories). Calorie is also the common, lay term used to describe kilocalories. (2)

CAPD Continuous ambulatory peritoneal dialysis. See *Peritoneal dialysis.* (23)

Cancer The abnormal, uncontrolled growth of some lump or mass ("tumor") of abnormal cells in the body. (30)

Carbohydrate A group of substances, including sugar, glycogen, starch, dextrins, and fiber, that are made of carbon, oxygen, and hydrogen. May be abbreviated CHO. One gram of CHO is used by the body to produce about 4 kilocalories of food energy. (2)

Carcinogens Substances that may induce or lead to the development of some type of cancer. Many additives (now off the market), natural food substances, and environmental chemicals are known carcinogens. (17)

Caries Tooth cavities; holes eaten into tooth enamel by bacteria. May cause pain and/or become channels for bacteria to cause deeper tooth or gum infections. (41)

Cariogenicity The ability of a substance to create or induce caries. In general, carbohydrates are more cariogenic than proteins or fats. (41)

Carotene A substance in plants that can be converted (in the body) to vitamin A. Carotene gives carrots their orange color. High levels of carotene may discolor the skin but do not seem to be harmful. (6)

Celiac Sprue A genetic defect that results in lifelong hypersensitivity to gliadin, a part of gluten, a protein in grains. Treatment requires a lifelong, gluten-free diet. Also called nontropical sprue or gluten-sensitive enteropathy. (24)

Cellulose A form of insoluble fiber naturally present in fruits, vegetables, and legumes. (10)

Cementum A thin, protective covering between the soft dentin and the hard enamel surface of the tooth. (41)

Central TPN Total parenteral nutrition (TPN) given through a large intravenous "line" or needle into a large, subclavian vein. (38)

Cheilosis Cracking and sores at the corners of the mouth. May be one symptom of certain vitamin deficiency diseases. (7)

Chemically Defined Formulas Also called *isotonic.* Liquid formulas with protein, carbohydrate, and fat sources predigested into smaller molecules. Some digestion (to the "elemental" forms) must still occur within the intestines. (38)

Chemotherapy A cancer treatment using carefully controlled high levels of toxic chemicals in an attempt to destroy specific cancer cells. (30)

Chinese Restaurant Syndrome A sensitivity or allergic reaction to monosodium glutamate. (40)

Chitterlings Called "chitlins," these are pig intestines. They are thoroughly cleaned, chopped fine, and boiled with spices and seasonings. (18)

Cholecalciferol Another name for vitamin D, one of the fat-soluble vitamins. (6)

Cholecystitis Inflammation of the gallbladder. (25)

Cholesterol A complex lipid produced naturally by animals and man. Contained in animal products, especially organ meats, egg yolk, and shrimp. Plant products contain no cholesterol, though they may contain fat. (5)

Chromosome Microscopic bodies in each cell of the body carrying the genes that determine what hereditary characteristics will be present in an individual. (34)

Chylomicrons The most lightweight of the lipoproteins, made primarily of triglycerides, the form into which food fat is first digested. (5)

Chyme Partially digested mass of foods in the stomach. (1)

Cilantro Coriander leaves, a commonly used seasoning in Hispanic foods. (18)

Compliance Cooperation. (31)

Congee A watery mixture of cooked rice and water. Used in Chinese culture for infants and as a broth believed to be "healthful" during illness. (18)

Cobalamin Vitamin B_{12}. (7)

Coded Dating Stamped numbers and/or letters on food products that indicate where, when, and in what batch a food was made. Not easily interpreted by consumers. (19)

Colitis See *Ulcerative colitis.* (33)

Colon The section of the digestive tract along the last five feet of the tract; a large, smooth muscle-lined tissue that is involved in fluid balance but not in nutrient absorption. (1)

Colostrum Fluid from the breasts that nourishes breast-fed infants during the first few days of life. Contains high levels of essential minerals and antibacterial substances produced by the mother. (14)

Common Bile Duct The channel that connects the small intestines, the pancreas, and the gallbladder; carries the fluids produced by the latter two into the small intestine. (1)

Common Metabolic Pathway The set of chemical reactions that carbohydrate, protein, and fat must experience in the cell in order to be used and to produce ATP for energy; also called the Krebs or citric acid cycle. (2)

Complementary Proteins Protein foods that are eaten together at the same meal to allow for the maximal use of the protein by combining amino acids in a proportion that will be used most effectively. Proteins are combined to compensate for "limiting amino acids" in vegetarian sources of protein. (3)

Complete Proteins Food (or food combinations) containing each of the essential amino acids in proportions that allow for maximal use of the protein by the body. Animal proteins are all "complete proteins." Vegetarian sources are usually deficient in one or more essential amino acids and must be combined with a "complementary" protein source to form a complete protein. (3)

Compliance Cooperation. (31)

Congee A watery mixture of cooked rice and water. Used in Chinese culture for infants and as a broth believed to be "healthful" during illness. (18)

Continuous Feeding Constant feeding of very small quantities of nutrients, usually through a feeding tube and regulated by a feeding pump. (38)

Crohn's Ileitis Also called ileitis or Crohn's disease; an inflammatory bowel disease that may affect the entire length of the digestive tract from mouth to anus. (33)

Crude Fiber Portion of indigestible fiber in a food that is left over after artificial "digestion" of the food with acid. Used to measure food fiber before more exact testing methods were available. Not a measure of total fiber content. (10)

Curreri's Equation An equation used to estimate the energy needs of a burn patient. Kcals needed equals $(25 \times wt\ (kg)) + (40 \times \%$ total body surface burned). (39)

Cutin An insoluble fiber present in the skin of fruit, vegetables, and legumes. (10)

Cyclamate An artificial sweetener discovered in 1937 and used widely until it was banned in 1970 when it was proved to be a carcinogen. As a sweetener, cyclamate did not leave the bitter aftertaste that characterized saccharin. (17)

Dehydration Inadequate body water. (28)

Dentin The soft substance surrounding the pulp of the tooth (41)

Dextrin Partially digested starch. (4)

Diabetes, Adult-Onset Also called type II or non-insulin dependent diabetes (NIDDM). Usually begins after age 35. The body continues to produce insulin but is not able to use it properly. Insulin injections or oral hypoglycemic agents are sometimes used in treatment but weight loss is almost always the most effective treatment. (31)

Diabetes, Gestational Diabetes that develops during the physical stress of pregnancy. Women with gestational diabetes have a 50% chance of becoming permanently diabetic later. Controlled by diet and, sometimes, insulin injections. (31)

Diabetes, Juvenile-Onset Also called type I or insulin-dependent diabetes mellitus (IDDM). Usually begins in childhood, adolescence, or early adulthood. The natural production of insulin stops and daily injections of the hormone become necessary. (31)

Diabetes Mellitus Usually called simply diabetes, a disorder of insulin-blood sugar balance. May be type I, type II, or gestational (above). The body is unable automatically to control blood sugar levels. Treatments may include insulin injections, oral hypoglycemic agents (pills), and diet to help normalize blood sugar and prevent as many complications of the disorder as possible. (31)

Dialysis Filtering waste products (or other substances) out of the blood. (28)

Diet Order The recommendation by a physician for a particular type of diet for a hospitalized or institutionalized person. Menus are prepared according to a particular diet order, which controls for any particular nutrient needs or restrictions. (21)

Diet Therapy See *Therapeutic nutrition.* (21)

Dietary Fiber Amount of total digestible and indigestible fiber in a food. Crude plus soluble fibers. (10)

Digestive Tract The channel in the body beginning at the mouth and ending at the anus, along which food, beverages, medications, and liquids are broken down, digested and/or absorbed. Also called alimentary tract, alimentary canal, gut, or intestinal tract. (1)

Diglyceride Lipid containing two fatty acids. (5)

Disaccharide Sugar that contains two monosaccharides per molecule. The three major disaccharides are sucrose (table sugar), lactose (milk sugar), and maltose. (4)

Diverticulitis Inflammation of the diverticuli present in diverticulosis. (24)

Diverticulosis The presence of forced pouchlike spaces (diverticuli) in the walls of the intestine. May be aggravated by a chronic low-fiber diet that exerts constant, high pressure on these walls. (24)

Dolomite Over-the-counter substance used as a calcium supplement but that may also contain traces of toxic minerals such as lead. (8)

Dopamine Tyraminelike substance. See *Tyramine.* (36)

Dumping Syndrome Diarrhea and nutrient malabsorption that may result from hyperosmolarity or a surgically shortened or damaged intestinal tract. (9)

Duodenum The first of the three sections of the small intestine. Extends from stomach to jejunum. (1)

Dysgeusia An altered sense of taste, usually resulting from some physical disorder. (30)

Dysphagia A swallowing disorder. (35)

Edema Swelling caused by too much water in the spaces between the cells. (2)

Electrolytes Elemental particles with an electrical force or charge. The most plentiful electrolytes in human metabolism are sodium (Na+), potassium (K+) and Chloride (Cl−). Minerals also function as electrolytes. (1)

Elemental Formula Liquid formula containing nutrients in their most chemically simple, "elemental" form. (38)

Elimination Diet A diet that is used to identify food allergies or sensitivities by eliminating suspected foods from the diet. Elimination diets are sometimes very strict and may be inadequate in certain nutrients. (40)

-emia Relating to the blood. (27)

Endosperm The central, largest portion of grain. White flour is made from the endosperm of the wheat kernel and does not include the germ or bran. (10)

Enteral Nutrition Food given via the digestive tract, orally, or through a tube. (38)

Enteric Coated Referring to substances treated with a coating that protects them from being digested by stomach acid. Many medications are enteric coated to enable them to pass whole through the stomach and break down in an area further on in the digestive tract where they will be effectively absorbed. (1)

Enzyme A protein substance with a specific action that allows a specific reaction (in digestion or cell metabolism) to occur. Most enzymes work best only in a certain part of the body or cell; many different enzymes are essential for proper metabolism. Enzymes may easily be destroyed by changes in environment, especially temperature or acidity. (1)

Esophageal Sphincter A muscular "door" between the esophagus and the stomach that, with the help of the diaphragm, is normally kept closed, except during swallowing; may be forced open in vomiting and hiatal hernia, allowing stomach acid to damage the esophageal walls. (1)

Esophagitis Sensitive, irritated, and painful esophagus damaged by acid, usually from the stomach. (33)

Esophagus 25 centimeters of digestive tract between the pharynx and the stomach. Carries food but has no role in digestion. Its sensitive tissue walls can easily be damaged by stomach acid. (1)

Essential Amino Acids The amino acids that cannot be synthesized by the body and so must be provided via the diet; includes isoleucine, leucine, lysine, methionine, phenylalanine, threonine, tryptophan, valine, and (in infants) histidine. (3)

Essential Fatty Acids EFAs, long-chain fats essential for the proper working of the body; includes linoleic, linolenic, and arachidonic acid. (5)

Exchanges Units that can be interchanged equally with other, similar units. (22)

Extracellular Outside the cell. (9)

Failure-to-Thrive A syndrome of inadequate growth in infants and young children; results from some unknown medical (organic) or a social, or family (inorganic) disorder. (29)

Fasting Abstaining from all foods or beverages that contain energy or any other nutrient except water. (20)

Fat See *Lipid.* (2)

Fat-Soluble Vitamins Vitamins that are most effectively digested and absorbed in fat or lipid substances; includes vitamins A, D, E, and K. Excessive doses of fat-soluble vitamins are stored in the fat cells of the body and, at a certain point, may produce toxic effects. (6)

Fatty Acid Part of a lipid molecule, made of a string of carbon atoms. (5)

FDA Food and Drug Administration, a US government agency that regulates and monitors food and drug production and sales, laws, and safety standards. (19)

Feingold Diet A diet that omits all food and drugs containing salicylates, artificial colors, flavors, and preservatives. Claimed to help control 50% of childhood hyperactivity, a claim that has not been effectively proven by controlled studies. The diet may be inadequate in vitamin C. (40)

FEP Free erythrocyte protoporphyrin; high FEP may be a sign of iron deficiency. (27)

Fetus Latin for "young one;" refers to an infant during the rapid growth period between conception and birth. (13)

Fiber The indigestible carbohydrate portion of a food. May include cellulose, hemicellulose, lignins, pectins, cutins, and gums. (4)

Fistula An abnormal opening between two parts of the body that are not normally connected, or an opening to the outside of the body. (41)

Fluoridated Water Water that has had the essential mineral fluoride added to a level of 1 part fluoride (Fl−) to 1 million parts water (i.e., 1 part per million or ppm); water may also be naturally fluoridated and levels of the mineral may vary widely. (8)

Fluorosis Brown or black discoloring of the teeth caused by high levels of fluoride in the water or diet. Although it is unattractive, it does not seem to be dangerous. (41)

Food Jag Usually refers to a young child's persistent desire for only one or a few foods; a normal but unpredictable part of childhood development that may last several days to a week. (16)

Food Sensitivity An abnormal reaction (e.g., swelling, rash, difficulty breathing, itching) to one or more particular foods. Unlike an allergy, a food sensitivity may not involve the immune system. (40)

Free Erythrocyte Protoporphyrin See *FEP.* (27)

Fructose A monosaccharide common in fruits and vegetables; the sweetest of the sugars. (4)

Galactose A monosaccharide (sugar) in dairy products; galactose is part of the lactose (milk sugar) molecule, together with glucose. (4)

Galactosemia Disorder caused by a genetic defect in the ability of galactose to be converted to glucose for energy; usually treated with a galactose-free diet throughout infancy. (34)

Gastric Reflux The "backup" of gastric juice or acid from the stomach into the esophagus, causing heartburn, pain, and discomfort. (33)

Gastroenteritis Inflammation and irritation of the stomach and small intestine; usually results in diarrhea and sometimes vomiting. (28)

Gestational Diabetes See *Diabetes, gestational.* (31)

Germ The central, most concentrated fat- and protein-containing portion of a grain, such as wheat germ. (10)

Gingiva The surface tissue of the gums. (41)

Glomerular Filtration The process of blood filtering through the glomeruli, part of the nephrons of the kidney, to help filter out waste products into the urine. (9)

Glucose The monosaccharide (sugar) most used in the body for energy; carbohydrate, fat, and protein may all be broken down into glucose to produce energy. (4)

Glucose Tolerance Test GTT, a 3–5-hour test measuring blood glucose after an initial dose of a sweetened, glucose-containing drink. Used by physicians to identify reactive hypoglycemia; for most accurate results, individuals are often required to include at least 150 grams of carbohydrate in their diet each day for three days before the test. (24)

Gluten A carbohydrate substance common in many grains including wheat, rye, oats, barley, and many grain products and processed foods. Gluten is what makes bread dough "elastic" during kneading. (24)

Glycemic Index The relative measure of how fast certain carbohydrate foods elevate blood sugar (glucose) levels. (24)

Glycirrhizic Acid A drug in natural licorice that may be dangerous for individuals on diuretic or hypertension medications (36)

Glycogen A polysaccharide most common as the storage form of energy in the liver and muscle tissue. (4)

Glycogen Storage Disease A disease caused by an inborn error of metabolism of glycogen; at least nine different disorders may relate to this type of error; survival and growth may be possible in certain types of GSD's with early detection and careful diet control. (34)

Goiter Ringlike mass of flesh around the neck caused by iodine imbalance; usually a result of long-term iodine deficiency; some foods are also believed to induce goiters in certain sensitive persons. (8)

Goiter Belt Geographical area where the soil is deficient in iodine and consequently the development of goiters has been common. (27)

Goitrin A substance in some vegetables that slows thyroid production in experimental animals. Sensitive persons who eat large amounts of goitrin-containing foods may develop goiter even without an iodine deficiency. (27)

Goitrogens Foods that contain goitrins. (27)

GRAS List List of additives "generally recognized as safe" by the FDA. (40)

Growth Spurt A period of time characterized by especially rapid growth. This may occur in adolescence just prior to sexual maturation; nutrient needs are higher during a growth spurt than at other times. (17)

Gum A soluble fiber naturally present in oats, legumes, and certain vegetables, trees and sea plants. (10)

Gut See *Digestive tract.* (1)

Harris-Benedict Equation Set of two equations (one for men and one for women) that can be used to help determine the resting energy needs of adults, based on age, height, and weight. (12)

Health Care Team Team of medical and support persons who work together with patients in health care to help treat diseases. May be formal or informal; usually directed or guided by physician(s). (21)

Health Food A vague term referring to foods for which some special nutrition or health claim (often unfounded or false) is made. (20)

Hematocrit Percent of total blood volume made up of red blood cells. (27)

Heme The organic, protein-bound form of iron. The iron found in animal products is in the form of heme iron; more readily absorbed than the iron in plant (nonheme) sources. (27)

Hemicellulose A soluble fiber naturally present in grain hulls and bran. (10)

Hemochromatosis Too much iron in the blood. (27)

Hemoglobin The portion of the red blood cell that carries iron and is responsible for transport, storage, and proper use of oxygen throughout the body. (27)

Hepatic Referring to the liver, where many drugs and nutrients undergo chemical changes required for proper metabolism. (23)

Hepatic Encephalopathy A syndrome of severe confusion and delirium that may occur in alcoholics whose damaged liver is unable to handle properly the protein in the diet. (23)

Hiatus Hernia Protrusion of part of the stomach up through the muscle of the diaphragm; a hiatus (or hiatal) hernia forces an opening between the esophagus and the stomach and results in painful gastric reflux. (33)

Homocystinuria Disorder caused by a genetic defect in the metabolism of the essential amino acid methionine. Normal growth and survival may be possible only on a methionine-controlled diet. (34)

Homogenized Milk Milk forced through a process that evenly distributes the fat particles throughout the milk and prevents separation or rising of cream to the top. (19)

Hormones Protein substances made by various glands or other parts of the body in very small quantities that are then carried through the blood and play a vital role in triggering important chemical actions within the body. (3)

Hospice An organization of volunteer and professional personnel that works to provide support and encouragement to the terminally ill. (30)

Hydrogenated A term used to describe unsaturated fats that have been saturated (fully or partially) by the addition of hydrogen. (5)

Hyper- Greater than normal. (27)

Hyperalimentation A technically incorrect term that refers to tube or intravenous feeding. Methods may be combined with oral feeding or with each other. (23)

Hyperglycemia Blood sugar levels above the normal range. Normal ranges depend on whether blood is taken during fasting or after a meal. Uncontrolled, long-term hyperglycemia may be a sign of disease and may damage the blood vessels. (4)

Hyperinsulinism The overproduction of insulin from the pancreas in response to increased blood sugar. Leads to hypoglycemia. (24)

Hyperlipidemia See *Hyperlipoproteinemia*. (25)

Hyperlipoproteinemia A group of at least five different disorders characterized by elevated levels of lipoproteins in the blood. Also called hyperlipidemia. (25)

Hypermetabolism Metabolism that is more rapid than normal, often as a result of disease, stress, or trauma. (23)

Hypo- Lower than normal. (27)

Hypoglycemia Blood sugar levels below the normal range. Persistent, uncontrolled hypoglycemia may be a sign of disease and may be harmful. (4)

IBD Inflammatory bowel disease; a group of diseases whose cause and cure is unknown and that may flare up sporadically causing severe intestinal pain, diarrhea, sometimes leading to bleeding and hospitalization. Most common IBDs are Crohn's ileitis and ulcerative colitis. (33)

Ileum End and longest segment of the small intestine; responsible for digestion and absorption of many nutrients. (1)

Ileus A blockage in the intestines due to trauma, bacterial growth, or disease. (39)

Inborn Errors of Metabolism Mutations (inherited or induced) in a gene that result in some abnormality of metabolism, usually a missing enzyme; inborn errors are present at birth and may cause early death, severe mental retardation, or malnutrition if they cannot be detected or treated effectively. (34)

Inflammatory Bowel Disease See *IBD*. (33)

Insulin A hormone that the pancreas produces and releases into the blood; helps "carry" blood glucose into the cells. (24)

Intermittent Feeding Feeding a small amount of nutrients at frequent or intermittent intervals. (38)

Intracellular Within the cell. (9)

Intravenous Line Passage made by a needle inserted into a major blood vessel; used to give medications or parenteral nutrition. (9)

Intrinsic Factor A protein substance in the liquid of the small intestines that facilitates B_{12} absorption into the blood. (7)

Inverted Nipples Nipples that contract or "back up" into the breast when the nipple area is squeezed, as in breast-feeding. Infants cannot grasp an inverted nipple well enough to get the available milk. Inversion can usually be corrected. (14)

Iodized Salt Salt supplemented with the essential mineral iodine to provide 76 micrograms of iodine per gram of salt. Iodized salt may be the major source of iodine for people living in "goiter belt" areas. (8)

Jejunum Second of the three segments of the small intestine; involved in digestion of many nutrients. (1)

Joule An international unit of energy measured electrically: a joule is "the work done in one second by a current of one ampere against a resistance of one ohm." One calorie equals approximately 4.2 joules. (2)

Junk Food Foods that contain energy from sugar and/or fat but little or no other nutrients. (16)

Ketones Byproducts of fat breakdown. (24)

Kilocalorie 1000 calories; a kilocalorie is the common term used to describe food energy and is usually called a calorie. Also called Kcals. (2)

Kosher Refers to strict orthodox diet followed by some Jewish groups and individuals. Foods forbidden by the Mosaic Law are forbidden and all dairy products must be kept, prepared, and consumed separately from all meat products. (18)

Krebs Cycle See *Common metabolic pathway*. (2)

Kwashiorkor Literally "red or golden boy;" a form of malnutrition that occurs when the diet contains enough energy but not enough protein. Common in children in underdeveloped countries who have been weaned from the breast but not then given a diet containing adequate protein; disorder was named by Africans whose children's hair changed pigment as a result of the malnutrition; children or adults with kwashiorkor often appear bloated and puffy as a result of fluid imbalance. (2)

Lactase The enzyme in the small intestine that digests lactose (milk sugar) into galactose and glucose. (24)

Lactation Breast-feeding. (14)

Lactobacillus A bacteria common in the mouth; ferments carbohydrate into lactic acid, which is what "sours" milk. (41)

Lacto-Ovo Vegetarian A vegetarian who will eat dairy products and eggs. (18)

Lactose "Milk sugar," a disaccharide made of glucose and galactose; the least sweet sugar. (4)

Lactose Intolerance An inability to adequately digest lactose in milk products as a result of inadequate production of lactase enzyme in the small intestines. Many persons have mild intolerance and can consume small portions of foods with lactose; symptoms of intolerance include gas, cramps, diarrhea; may be inherited or induced by disease or antibiotics. (24)

Laetrile A toxic substance derived from powdered apricot pits; illegal in the US. Claims that laetrile "cure" cancer have no valid scientific base; also called amygdalin or vitamin B_{17}. (30)

Let-Down Reflex Hormonally-controlled reaction that causes breast milk to be released from the glands and into the nipple for lactation. (14)

Lignin An insoluble fiber naturally present in plant and grain stems, hulls, straw, and in tannin. (10)

Limiting Amino Acid The essential amino acid that is low or deficient in a protein food. The body requires the eight (or nine in infants) essential amino acids in a particular ratio and the ability to use a protein (PER or protein efficiency ratio) depends on the quantity of the least available amino acid, the "limiting amino acid." (3)

Linoleic Acid An essential fatty acid that must be present in the diet for health since it cannot be produced by the body. (5)

Linolenic Acid An essential fatty acid that may also be produced naturally in the body. (5)

Lipase An enzyme that breaks down lipid. (25)

Lipid A substance that is chemically composed of triglyceride and fatty acids; also called *fat*. Lipids cannot dissolve in water unless they are attached to a water-soluble complex (e.g., lipoprotein molecule). One gram of fat is used by the body to produce about 9 kilocalories of energy. (2)

Lipoproteins Complex molecules (of varying weight and density) made up of protein combined with a lipid (may be cholesterol, triglycerides, or phospholipids); the forms in which fat is carried through the blood. (5)

Long-Chain Triglyceride Triglyceride molecule with fatty acids ranging in length from 14 to 24 carbons. The most common natural form of lipids. (5)

Macrobiotic Diet A strict vegan diet that has evolved from certain Eastern religious philosophies; of the many "levels" of the diet, the strictest are deficient in certain major nutrients and could lead to serious deficiencies. (30)

Macrocytic Anemia Anemia resulting from red blood cells that are large, immature, and unable to carry the normal amount of iron-containing hemoglobin. (7)

Malignant Quickly growing; potentially harmful or life-threatening; cancerous. (30)

Malta A sweet, nonalcoholic beverage common in the Hispanic culture. Made from malt extract, sugar, and caramel, with little or no vitamins or minerals. (18)

Maltose Malt sugar, a disaccharide most common in grains and partly digested starch. (4)

Mannitol A *sugar alcohol.* (4)

Maple Syrup Urine Disease Also called MSUD or branched-chain ketoaciduria, an inborn error of metabolism that requires a special diet for survival to tightly control three essential amino acids. (34)

Marasmus Severe protein-calorie malnutrition that puts a child (or adult) at high risk for infections and serious illness or death from minor diseases. (2)

Marginal Barely sufficient or slightly inadequate. (27)

Masa Harina Cornmeal that has been treated with lime. Common in Mexican and some South American diets. (26)

MCT Medium-chain triglyceride; a triglyceride molecule with 3 fatty acids that are each 8 to 12 carbon atoms in length. MCTs are useful in the diet control of some diseases but are not naturally present in food. (5)

MCV Mean corpuscular volume; the average volume of the red blood cells. (27)

Mean Corpuscular Volume See *MCV.* (27)

Mechanical Soft Diet A diet restricting foods to those that may be chewed easily and swallowed. Used when some physical impairment makes chewing difficult. (24)

Medium-Chain Fatty Acids A fatty acid containing 8 to 12 carbon atoms; see also *MCT.* (5)

Megaloblastic Anemia Anemia that is caused either by vitamin B_{12} or folacin deficiency; under a microscope the red blood cells appear much larger than normal. (26)

Megavitamin A vitamin supplement that contains far more of the vitamin than is needed or recommended by the RDA. Certain vitamins in high doses may have toxic or druglike effects on the body. (30)

Metabisulfite See *Sulfites.* (40)

Metabolism Conversion of nutrients into energy for use by the body. (1)

Metastases Cancerous tumors that begin to grow in areas of the body far from the location of the original tumor. Metastases are a sign that the original cancer has spread. (30)

Mineral Inorganic natural elements that contain charges, causing them to combine with other elements and substances; 12 minerals are known to be essential in minute quantities for normal human nutrition. (8)

Monosaccharides The simplest unit of sugar; glucose, fructose, and galactose are all monosaccharides. (4)

Monosodium Glutamate See *MSG.* (40)

Monounsaturated Fat A lipid with one point on each molecule that is not totally saturated with hydrogen; olive oil is a monounsaturated fat. (5)

Motility Movement, often referring to the self-propelling movement of substances along the digestive tract. (1)

MSG Monosodium glutamate; an additive that contains sodium and that, especially in Asian cooking, is used to enhance the flavor of food. (40)

Nasogastric From the nose to the stomach; also called NG. (38)

Nasogastric Tube A feeding tube that enters the nose and descends into the gastric area (the stomach). Used for feeding when oral feeding is not possible or is not adequate. (23)

Negative Nitrogen Balance A net loss of nitrogen; the body is in negative nitrogen balance when it excretes more nitrogen than is being replaced by dietary protein. (3)

Neonatal The first 30 days of human life after birth. (13)

Nephrons Networking channels in the kidney that help filter wastes and excess substances out of the blood and into the urine. Normally all the blood in the body is filtered through the kidneys in this way. (9)

Nephrotic Syndrome Medical symptoms accompanying progressive kidney failure; often includes anorexia. (23)

Net Weight Weight of solids in canned foods minus the weight of the surrounding liquids, broth, or other packing material. (19)

Neuropathy Nerve damage, a common complication of diabetes mellitus; may involve extremities, leading to loss of feeling in toes, fingers, or other parts of the body. (31)

Night Blindness The inability to readjust the eyes to night lights, sometimes as a result of vitamin A deficiency. (6)

Nitrogen Balance The state in which the body's intake of nitrogen equals output (or excretion). (3)

NPO A diet order that literally means "nil per os," or nothing by mouth; common before and immediately after surgery or certain test procedures. (21)

Nursing Bottle Syndrome Rampant tooth decay in infants and young children usually caused by overuse of the bottle and constant sucking on energy-containing liquids. (15)

Obesity Weight that is 20% or more above ideal body weight as a result of excess fat stores. (32)

Open Dating Easily understood dates marked on food products that usually indicate how long a food will remain fresh. (19)

Oral Cavity The mouth and throat. (1)

Oral Hypoglycemic Agent OHA, pills used in type II diabetes, that stimulate the pancreas to produce insulin. (31)

Oral Rehydration Therapy An inexpensive and easily mixed solution developed by the World Health Organization (WHO) to help correct fluid and electrolyte imbalances that often cause death quickly in poor, undernourished children with diarrhea. (28)

Organic Food An incorrect term used to refer to foods grown in soil treated with "organic" or "natural" fertilizers; in reality, every food is organic since it comes from a living organism; many foods grown with "organic" fertilizers still contain residues of chemical pesticides. (20)

Osmolarity Pressure that results from the concentration of particles in a certain volume of fluid. Fluids with high osmolarity tend to attract water from nearby low osmolarity fluids; also called osmolality; measured in milliosmoles; (m/Osm); normal osmotic pressure in the blood is 280–290 m/Osm per kilogram of plasma. (9)

Osteomalacia Bone disease that occurs in adults and is usually caused by imbalance in vitamin D metabolism. (6)

Osteopenia Not enough bone. (27)

Osteoporosis Progressive loss of bone that is not related to any known disease; can become a major handicap; may be preventable through lifelong diet, exercise, and close medical attention. (27)

Oxalate An indigestible substance naturally present in certain foods that may combine with minerals and prevent them from being absorbed. (8)

Pancreatic Amylase The enzyme produced by the pancreas that breaks down starch. (4)

Parenteral Nutrition Nutrients given directly into the blood via an intravenous needle. (38)

Pareve A term referring to kosher food practices; foods that are "pareve" are "neutral" and may be prepared and served with either "meat" or "milk" meals. (18)

Pasteurized Milk Milk that has been heat treated to kill certain dangerous bacteria. (19)

PCM See *Protein-calorie malnutrition.* (23)

Peak Height Velocity Time when growth (in height and weight) is occurring most quickly. (17)

Pectin A soluble fiber naturally present in fruit pulp, legumes, and certain plants. (10)

Pellagra Niacin deficiency disease. (7)

PEM See *Protein-calorie malnutrition.* (23)

Periodontal Disease Gum disease caused by long-term irritation of food particles and calculus; occurs slowly, painlessly, over many years, and may be slowed or prevented by regular dental care. (41)

Peripheral TPN Total parenteral nutrition given through a needle into a "peripheral" blood vessel, usually on the arm or hand. (38)

Peristalsis The involuntary muscle contractions of the walls of the digestive tract that propel digesting substances. (1)

Peritoneal Dialysis Artificial filtering out of waste products from the body, used when the kidneys fail. Involves forcing a hyperosmolar solution into the peritoneal cavity and later discarding and replacing it. May be done in a hospital or by a frequently replaced bag of fluid worn around the waist; this process is called continuous ambulatory peritoneal dialysis (CAPD). (23)

Pernicious Anemia Anemia resulting from a B_{12} deficiency that cannot be corrected by diet; usually treated with periodic B_{12} injections. (7)

Pharynx Section of the digestive tract extending from the nose to the esophagus; used for breathing and carrying food. (1)

Phenylalanine An amino acid needed for normal protein metabolism that may build up dangerously in the blood in certain diseases (e.g., PKU) and cause brain damage. (23)

Phenylethylamine A tyraminelike substance; see *Tyramine*. (36)

Phenylketonuria See *PKU*.

Phospholipid Lipid made of two fatty acids and some type of nitrogen-phosphate complex. (5)

Phytates Naturally occurring substances in certain foods that are indigestible and may combine with certain nutrients to result in poor absorption of those nutrients. (8)

Pica The practice of eating nonfood substances, such as clay, dirt, laundry starch, ice, or other nonfoods. (13)

PKU Phenylketonuria; a genetic error of metabolism that is detected within the first week of life. Children with PKU will become permanently and severely mentally retarded unless they are treated with a strict, phenylalanine-controlled diet. They may be able to live an otherwise normal life of normal intelligence on this diet and with ongoing medical care. (23)

Placebo A substance used in medicine, especially in research, that closely resembles another drug or substance but does not act in the body in the same way and may have no medicinal value. Placebos are used in research to help prevent bias that might occur if researcher or subject knew which substance was being given. (40)

Placenta The organ that grows in the womb with the fetus and that provides nourishment for the fetus. Nutrients and drugs pass from the mother's blood through the placenta into the infant's blood. Also called the afterbirth. (13)

Plaque A sticky mixture of fermented carbohydrate, bacteria, and other substances that is formed on the teeth within 20 minutes after meals containing carbohydrates. May act as "breeding ground" for more bacteria if it is not promptly and completely removed. (41) Plaque may also refer to deposits of cholesterol in blood vessels. (25)

Polenta Cornmeal. (18)

Polysaccharide Starches, long-connecting carbohydrate molecules of mono- or disaccharides, usually glucose. (4)

Polyunsaturated Fat A lipid with several places on each molecule that are not completely saturated with hydrogen and may attract other substances. Polyunsaturated fatty acids are abbreviated PUFA. Most PUFAs are vegetable oils; fish oil is also high in PUFA. (5)

Portal Vein A blood vessel that directly connects the intestinal bloodstream with the liver. Some nutrients, such as MCTs, can be absorbed directly into the blood through this vein and thus bypass the digestive process of the small intestines. (4)

Protein A group of substances that contain compounds of nitrogen and that are naturally present in animals and plants; one gram of protein is used by the body to produce about 4 Kcals of energy. The nitrogen in protein is essential to maintain body protein, including muscles, enzymes, hormones, and immune factors. (2)

Protein-Calorie Malnutrition Sometimes called PEM or protein-energy malnutrition; starvation resulting from a diet inadequate in protein and energy. Most common in children in underdeveloped nations and in adults with certain diseases. (2)

Protein-Sparing Modified Fast Abbreviated PSMF; a special diet used by some physicians to treat life-threatening (morbid) obesity. It involves fasting that is modified by including a small amount of daily protein. Should never be used without close medical supervision since electrolyte imbalances may develop. (23)

P:S Ratio A quality of a fat indicating the ratio of polyunsaturated to saturated fat. (5)

Pulmonary Relating to the lungs. (28)

Pulp The center of the tooth, filled with blood vessels that keep the teeth healthy, and nerves that sense pain and pressure. (41)

Pyloric Sphincter The valvelike muscle between the stomach and the small intestine that controls the release of chyme from the stomach. (1)

Pyridoxal Vitmin B_6; also called pyridoxine or pyridoxamine. (7)

Pyridoxamine Vitamin B_6. (7)

Pyridoxine Vitamin B_6. (7)

Radiation Therapy A cancer treatment using high doses of radiation, carefully directed only to the cancerous areas of the body. Radiation exposure kills cells, including normal cells, so its use is limited to several days or weeks of treatment. Also called therapeutic radiology (TR), X-ray or cobalt therapy. (30)

Recommended Dietary Allowances National guidelines based on extensive, recent research that list all nutrients known to be essential for health and the recommended daily intake that will meet the needs of 99% of the population; also called the *RDA;* useful in assessing diets and planning menus for groups but may overestimate needs of some persons. (3)

Renal Referring to the kidneys, where waste products are filtered out of the blood and urine is formed. (23)

Residue Leftover; see *Fiber.* (24)

Rickets Deficiency disease in children caused by inadequate vitamin D and poor calcium metabolism; usully results in soft bowed legs and skeletal abnormalities. (6)

Ringer's Lactate Solution Also called *lactated ringer's solution,* a mixture of sterile water and electrolytes used to restore fluids lost, as in severe burns. (39)

Roughage A common term for fiber; see *Fiber.* (10)

Saccharin The first artificial sweetener, discovered in 1879 and currently used in many "dietetic" products; has been proven to cause cancer in laboratory animals but its safety in humans is still controversial. (17)

Salicylates Natural substances present in many foods and added to drugs, flavorings, and beverages. (40)

Satiety The feeling of fullness, as from a large meal. (30)

Saturated Fats Fatty acids that contain as much carbon and hydrogen as possible and that are therefore usually stiff and hard even at room temperature. A diet high in saturated fats may play a role in heart disease. Includes most animal fats as well as palm and coconut oil. (5)

Scurvy Disease caused by long-term vitamin C deficiency. (7)

Sepsis Serious infection in the blood that causes fever and threatens health. (39)

Shock A syndrome, usually a result of trauma, in which the body systems suddenly slow down, depriving the cells of oxygen and the heart of adequate blood; may lead to coma and death if not treated rapidly. (39)

Short-Chain Fatty Acids A fatty acid containing 2 to 6 carbons in each chain. (5)

Sickle Cell Anemia An inherited disease most common in blacks of African descent. Red blood cells are shaped like a "sickle" rather than like the normal disk; this may cause blockage in blood vessels, intense pain, disability, and sometimes organ failure; no known cure. (27)

Sippy Diet A diet no longer in use that was part of ulcer treatment in the past; included frequent intake ("sips") of milk or cream and a very bland diet. (33)

Small Intestine Segment of the digestive tract, lined with hairy folds of tissues called *villi,* and bathed with digestive liquids; involved in digestion and absorption of almost all major nutrients. (1)

Sodium Bisulfite See *Sulfites.* (40)

Sofrito A prepared sauce used in Hispanic meals to season cooked dry beans; usually made at home but also commercially produced; high in sodium and fat. (18)

Sorbitol A sugar alcohol commonly used to sweeten sugarless gum; overconsumption sometimes leads to diarrhea, gas, and cramping. (4)

Starch Carbohydrates made of many long, connected units of mono- and disaccharides; also called polysaccharides. (4)

Stasis Lack of movement, as when peristalsis slows down. (38)

Streptococcus Mutans A variety of bacteria most common in the mouth. (41)

Stress State in which nutrient needs change as a result of physical trauma, infection, disease, or starvation. (39)

Stunting Low height (usually under the 3rd percentile) for age, resulting from long-term borderline or acute malnutrition during normal periods of growth. (2)

Substrate Substance involved in an enzymatic or other chemical reaction in which changes occur. (1)

Sucrase The enzyme in the small intestine that digests sucrose into glucose and fructose. (24)

Sucrose Table sugar; a disaccharide found in cane or beet sugar; it is composed of glucose and fructose, and is the second sweetest sugar. (4)

Sugar Alcohol A natural product similar to the monosaccharides that is digested more slowly than other sugars; contains the same concentration of energy as disaccharides, i.e., 4 Kcals per gram of carbohydrate. Includes sorbitol, mannitol, and xylitol. (4)

Sulfites Preservatives added to many fresh, cut, or processed foods. Certain persons may have severe allergic reactions to these substances; also called sodium metabisulfite, sodium bisulfite, sodium sulfite, potassium bisulfite, potassium metabisulfite or sulfur dioxide. (40)

Sulfur Dioxide See *Sulfites*. (40)

Tartrazine FD & C yellow food dye #5. (40)

Test Diet A short-term diet modifying or controlling one or more nutrients in order to test for some disease, malabsorption, or intolerance. (39)

Thalassemia Genetic disorder causing defects in hemoglobin; no known cure. Complications depend on the severity of the disorder; most common in people of Mediterranean or African descent. (27)

Therapeutic Nutrition The application of nutritional science to the supportive use of nutrition in disease. (21)

Thyrotoxicosis Disease caused by too much iodine. (6)

TIBC Total iron binding capacity (of the blood). (27)

Tocopherol Vitamin E. (6)

Tofu Soybean curd; a soft white, crumbly substance resembling ricotta or farmer's cheese that is made from coagulated, mashed soybeans; high in protein and may be high in calcium; little flavor but absorbs seasonings well in cooking. (18)

Total Iron Binding Capacity See *TIBC*. (27)

Total Parenteral Nutrition See *TPN*. (38)

Toxicity Poisoning. (7)

TPN Total parenteral nutrition, feeding by an intravenous needle into the blood; also called *intravenous hyperalimentation* (*IVH*). (38)

Transferrin The form of iron present in blood serum. (27)

Transit Time The time needed for food to pass through the entire length of the digestive tract and to be excreted. (10)

Trauma A physical wound or injury, including surgery and burns. (39)

Triceps Skinfold Thickness The thickness of the flesh that can be "pinched" away from the triceps muscle in the upper arm; used to assess body fat and muscle stores; usually measured by special calipers; results may differ widely depending on how the measurement is taken. (12)

Triglyceride Lipid containing three fatty acids. (5)

Tube Feeding Feeding of nutrients in liquid form through a tube extending from the nose or mouth to some point in the small intestine; may be combined with oral or parenteral feeding. (38)

Tubular Resorption The return of essential substances through the filtering tubes of the kidney into the blood, conserving them from being excreted and allowing them to be recycled in the metabolic process. (9)

Tumor An abnormal growth or mass of cells in some part of the body; may be harmless or cancerous. (30)

Tyramine Protein substances that are naturally present in many aged or fermented foods; may cause severe reactions in persons on certain medications. (36)

Ulcer An area of the intestinal or stomach wall that has been worn away by acid, forming a crater and causing great pain, discomfort, and sometimes bleeding; most common ulcers are in the duodenum or the stomach. (33)

Ulcerative Colitis An inflammatory bowel disease that affects the colon only. (33)

Underweight Ten percent or more below established weight standards for height; usually a sign of very few fat stores. May also put a person at risk for infection and prolonged illness due to lowered immunity and inadequate nutrient stores. (22)

Unit Pricing Labels placed in most grocery stores to indicate the price-per-pound of each individual brand item. Unit pricing is designed to help shoppers compare foods and food costs. (19)

Unsaturated Fats Lipids that are not completely saturated by hydrogen and, therefore, that are often soft or liquid at room temperature; fish oils are naturally unsaturated. (5)

USRDA US Recommended Dietary Allowances, broad categories of nutrient standards used primarily for food labelling; not to be confused with the RDA, which list recommendations by more specific age and sex groups (see Appendices). (12)

Vegans Persons whose diets contain no animal products of any kind; the vegan diet may be deficient in several nutrients. (7)

Vegetarian One who eats no meat or flesh of any living animal; may eat eggs and dairy products (lacto-ovo) or only dairy products (lacto-) in addition to plants and grains. (18)

Vianda Starchy root vegetables commonly included in Hispanic meals; may be boiled or fried; includes varieties such as plantains, batata, namé, yautio, malanga, and apio. (18)

Villi Hairy or tentaclelike projections lining the folds of tissues along the walls of the small intestine; healthy villi are essential for normal digestion and absorption of nutrients. (1)

Vitamins A group of complex organic (carbon-containing) substances that are necessary in very small quantities for normal body functions; provide no energy and must be included in the diet because the body cannot produce them in sufficient quantities. (6)

Vitamin B$_{17}$ See *Laetrile*. (30).

Water-Soluble Vitamins Vitamins that can be digested and absorbed in water. Excesses are usually excreted readily, although a very high intake from supplements may cause retention and lead to potential toxicity problems. (6)

Xerophthalmia Night blindness, a sign of vitamin A deficiency; the eyes cannot adjust quickly to darkness after sudden, bright light. (26)

Xerostomia Dry mouth caused by damage to the salivary glands; common after cancer treatments to the head and neck area; may lead to serious dental problems if teeth and gums are not kept moist and clean. (41)

Xylitol The sweetest of the sugar alcohols; not in common use because of questions about its safety in food. (4)

INDEX

Numbers followed by an *f* indicate a figure; *t* following a page number indicates tabular material.

hepatic encephalopathy, in protein-controlled diets, 197
herbal medicine, 327–329. *See also* drug(s)
hiatal hernia, 307–308
Hispanic-Americans, food patterns of, 144–146
homocystinuria, 317f
hormones
 nitrogen and, 17
 vitamin D as, 37
hospice care, in terminal illness, 271–272
hospitalization, in eating disorders, 342
Hot-cold theory, in Chinese-American diet, 143–144
hydrogenated oil, 29–30
hyperalimentation. *See* enteral nutrition; parenteral nutrition
hyperglycemia, 24
 in diabetes mellitus, 277
 symptoms of, 282f
hyperinsulinism, carbohydrate-controlled diet in, 203
hyperkalemia, fluid-controlled diet in, 245
hyperlipidemias, 213, 215, 216t
hyperlipoproteinemia. *See* hyperlipidemia
hypermetabolism, in protein-controlled diet, 197
hypersensitivity. *See* allergy
hypertension
 calcium deficiency in, 229
 fluid-controlled diet in, 249–251
 sodium restriction in, 249–251
hypertonic dehydration, 242
hypochromic anemia, copper therapy in, 237
hypoglycemia, 24
 carbohydrate-controlled diet in, 203–204
 in diabetes mellitus, 277
 sample menu for, 204
 symptoms of, 282f
hypothyroidism, 237

ileitis, 311
ileum, 7
infancy. *See* infant(s)
infant(s)
 allergy to milk in, 372
 death rates in, by method of feeding, 111f
 energy needs in, 113
 feeding guide for, 116t
 feeding practices in, 119–120
 Chinese-American, 143
 Italian-American, 146–147
 kosher, 147–148
 Mexican-American, 145

Puerto Rican, 146
 Southeast Asian, 149
 Southern (USA), 150
 vegetarian, 151
 fluoride, recommended for, 114
 formula, 115
 introduction of solid foods to, 115–120, 116t
 iron needs in, 114
 mortality rates in, 90f
 nutrition in, 113–120
 protein needs in, 113–114
 vitamin D needs in, 114
infection
 in enteral feeding, 353–354
 in parenteral feeding, 353–354
 stress in, 362
inflammatory bowel diseases, 311
ingredients on food labels, 155
inherited inborn errors of metabolism. *See* metabolic defects
injury
 energy needs in, 362–363
 protein-controlled diet in, 200
 as trauma, 362–363
insulin, 202
 in blood sugar control, 276f, 282
 in diabetes control, 282–283
 preparations, 284f
 pumps, 288–289
 reaction, 287
 in trauma, 365
intestines, food sensitivity symptoms in, 370
intracellular fluid, 54
intravenous hyperalimentation, 348. *See also* parenteral nutrition
intravenous line, 57
intrinsic factor, vitamin B_{12} and, 43, 223
iodide. *See* iodine
iodine, 51
 goiter and, 51
 Recommended Dietary Allowances of, 49t, 85t
 therapy, in disease, 236–237
 thyrotoxicosis and, 51
iodized salt, 51
iron, 50
 absorption of, 231, 234f
 effect of ascorbic acid on, 235f
 effect of protein on, 235f
 deficiency syndromes, 232–234
 dietary, 234f
 excretion of, 233
 food sources of, 50, 236
 metabolism, 232
 needs in infancy, 114
 needs in pregnancy, 93–94, 94f